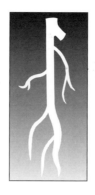

Review of
Vascular
Surgery

Companion to
Vascular Surgery, 6th Edition

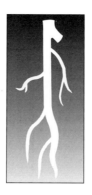

Review of
Vascular
Surgery

Companion to *Vascular Surgery, 6th Edition*

SECOND EDITION

Robert B. Rutherford, MD, FACS, FRCS Hon. (Glasg)

Emeritus Professor of Surgery
University of Colorado School of Medicine
Denver, Colorado

with the collaboration of Jack L. Cronenwett, MD; Peter Gloviczki, MD; K. Wayne Johnston, MD; William C. Krupski, MD; Kenneth Ouriel, MD; Anton N. Sidawy, MD; Hugh G. Beebe, MD; Kimberly J. Hansen, MD; Gregory L. Moneta, MD; Mark R. Nehler, MD; William A. Pearce, MD; Bruce A. Perler, MD; John J. Ricotta, MD; Russell H. Samson, MD; James M. Seeger, MD; R. James Valentine, MD; Thomas W. Wakefield, MD; Fred A. Weaver, MD

ELSEVIER
SAUNDERS

1600 John F. Kennedy Boulevard
Suite 1800
Philadelphia, PA 19103-2899

Review of Vascular Surgery:
Companion to *Vascular Surgery, 6th Edition*
Second Edition

ISBN: 1-4160-2515-4

NOTICE

Knowledge and best practice in this field are constantly changing. As new research and experience broaden our knowledge, changes in practice, treatment, and drug therapy may become necessary or appropriate. Readers are advised to check the most current information provided (i) on procedures featured or (ii) by the manufacturer of each product to be administered, to verify the recommended dose or formula, the method and duration of administration, and contraindications. It is the responsibility of the practitioner, relying on his or her own experience and knowledge of the patient, to make diagnoses, to determine dosages and the best treatment for each individual patient, and to take all appropriate safety precautions. To the fullest extent of the law, neither the Publisher nor the Editors assume any liability for any injury and/or damage to persons or property arising out or related to any use of the material contained in this book.

Previous edition copyrighted 1995.

International Standard Book Number 1-4160-2515-4

Publishing Director: Anne Lenehan
Publisher: Natasha Andjelkovic
Developmental Editor: Donna L. Morrissey
Project Manager: Cecelia Bayruns
Marketing Manager: Ethel Cathers

Printed in the United States of America.

Last digit is the print number: 9   8   7   6   5   4   3   2   1

Dedication

To William Krupski, who always gave his very best to his patients, students, and colleagues.

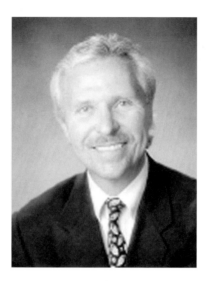

William C. Krupski, MD
1947–2004

Editors

Editor-in-Chief

ROBERT B. RUTHERFORD, MD, FACS, FRCS Hon. (Glasg)
Emeritus Professor of Surgery, University of Colorado School of Medicine, Denver, Colorado.

Associate Editors

JACK L. CRONENWETT, MD, FACS
Professor of Surgery, Dartmouth Medical School, Hanover, New Hampshire.
Chief, Section of Vascular Surgery, Dartmouth-Hitchcock Medical Center, Lebanon, New Hampshire.

PETER GLOVICZKI, MD, FACS
Professor of Surgery, Mayo Clinic College of Medicine.
Chair, Division of Vascular Surgery and Director, Gonda Vascular Center, Mayo Clinic, Rochester, Minnesota.

K. WAYNE JOHNSTON, MD, FACS, FRCSC
Professor and R. Fraser Elliott Chair in Vascular Surgery, Department of Surgery, University of Toronto Faculty of Medicine.
Vascular Surgeon, Toronto General Hospital, Toronto, Ontario, Canada.

WILLIAM C. KRUPSKI, MD, FACS*
Formerly Clinical Professor of Surgery, University of California, San Francisco, School of Medicine.
Attending Vascular Surgeon, The Kaiser Permanente Medical Group, San Francisco, California.

KENNETH OURIEL, MD, FACS, FACC
Professor of Surgery, Cleveland Clinic Lerner College of Medicine of Case Western Reserve University.
Chairman, Division of Surgery, Cleveland Clinic Foundation, Cleveland, Ohio.

ANTON N. SIDAWY, MD, FACS
Professor of Surgery, George Washington University School of Medicine.
Chief of Surgery, VA Medical Center, Washington, D.C.

---

* Deceased

Assistant Editors

HUGH G. BEEBE, MD, FACS
Director Emeritus, Jobst Vascular Center, The Toledo Hospital, Toledo, Ohio.

KIMBERLEY J. HANSEN, MD, FACS
Professor of Surgery and Head, Section on Vascular Surgery, Division of Surgical Sciences, Wake Forest University School of Medicine, Winston-Salem, North Carolina.

GREGORY L. MONETA, MD, FACS
Professor of Surgery, Oregon Health and Sciences University School of Medicine.
Chief, Division of Vascular Surgery, Portland, Oregon.

MARK R. NEHLER, MD, FACS
Associate Professor of Surgery, University of Colorado Health Sciences Center School of Medicine.
Program Director, Surgical Residency Program, University of Colorado Health Sciences Center, Denver, Colorado.

WILLIAM H. PEARCE, MD, FACS
Violet R. and Charles A. Baldwin Professor of Vascular Surgery, Northwestern University Feinberg School of Medicine.
Chief, Vascular Surgery Division, Northwestern Memorial Hospital, Chicago, Illinois.

BRUCE A. PERLER, MD, MBA, FACS
Julius H. Jacobson II Professor of Surgery, Johns Hopkins University School of Medicine.
Chief, Division of Vascular Surgery, Johns Hopkins Hospital, Baltimore, Maryland.

JOHN J. RICOTTA, MD, FACS, FACS
Professor and Chair, Department of Surgery, State University of New York at Stony Brook School of Medicine.
Surgeon in Chief, University Hospital at Stony Brook, Stony Brook, New York.

RUSSELL H. SAMSON, MD, FACS, RVT
Former Associate Professor of Surgery, Albert Einstein College of Medicine of Yeshiva University, New York, New York.
Staff, Sarasota Memorial Hospital.
President, Mote Vascular Foundation, Inc., Sarasota, Florida.

JAMES M. SEEGER, MD, FACS
Professor of Surgery, University of Florida College of Medicine.
Chief, Division of Vascular Surgery and Endoscopic Therapy, Shands at University of Florida, Gainesville, Florida.

R. JAMES VALENTINE, MD, FACS
Frank H. Kidd, Jr., Distinguished Professor and Vice-Chairman, Department of Surgery, University of Texas Southwestern Medical Center, Dallas, Texas.

THOMAS W. WAKEFIELD, MD, FACS
S. Martin Lindenauer Collegiate Professor of Surgery, University of Michigan Medical School.
Staff Surgeon, Section of Vascular Surgery, Department of Surgery, University of Michigan Hospital and Ann Arbor Veterans Administration Medical Center, Ann Arbor, Michigan.

FRED A. WEAVER, MD, FACS
Professor of Surgery, University of Southern California Keck School of Medicine.
Chief of Vascular Surgery, University of Southern California Hospital.
Attending Surgeon, Vascular Surgery, Los Angeles County–University of Southern California Medical Center, Los Angeles, California.

Contributors

AHMED M. ABOU-ZAMZAM, JR., MD
Associate Professor, Division of Vascular Surgery, Loma Linda University School of Medicine, Loma Linda, California.
Lower Extremity Amputation: Indications, Patient Evaluation, and Level Determination

ALI F. ABURAHMA, MD
Professor, Department of Surgery, West Virginia University School of Medicine; Chief, Vascular Section, Robert C. Byrd Health Sciences Center; Co-Director, Vascular Center of Excellence, Charleston Area Medical Center, Charleston, West Virginia.
Causalgia and Post-traumatic Pain Syndromes; Lumbar Sympathectomy: Indications and Technique

ERIC D. ADAMS, MD
Adjunct Assistant Professor of Surgery, Uniformed Services University of the Health Sciences, Bethesda, Maryland; Fellow, Vascular Surgery, Washington Hospital Center and Georgetown University, Washington, D.C.
Nonthrombotic Complications of Arteriovenous Access for Hemodialysis

SAMUEL S. AHN, MD
Professor of Surgery, David Geffen School of Medicine at UCLA; Attending Surgeon, UCLA Center for the Health Sciences, Los Angeles, California.
Upper Extremity Sympathectomy

JAMES C. ANDREWS, MD
Gonda Vascular Center, Mayo Clinic, Rochester, Minnesota.
Surgical Treatment of Superior Vena Cava Syndrome

ENRICO ASCHER, MD
Professor of Surgery, Division of Vascular Surgery, Maimonides Medical Center, Brooklyn, New York.
Secondary Arterial Reconstructions in the Lower Extremity

ZAKARIA I. ASSI, MD
Diagnostic Radiologist, Department of Interventional Radiology, The Toledo Hospital; Director, Interventional Radiology, Flower Hospital, Toledo, Ohio.
Catheter-Based Interventions for Acute Deep Venous Thrombosis

JUAN AYERDI, MD
Assistant Professor of Surgery, Department of General Surgery, Division of Surgical Sciences, Wake Forest University School of Medicine, Winston-Salem, North Carolina.
Principles of Arteriography; Fundamental Techniques in Endovascular Surgery; Open Surgical Repair of Renovascular Disease

MARTIN R. BACK, MD, FACS
Associate Professor of Surgery, University of South Florida College of Medicine, Tampa, Florida.
Infection in Prosthetic Vascular Grafts

J. DENNIS BAKER, MD
Professor of Surgery, David Geffen School of Medicine at UCLA; Chief, Vascular Surgery Section, West Los Angeles VA Medical Center, Los Angeles, California.
The Vascular Laboratory

WILLIAM H. BAKER, MD, FACS
Emeritus Professor of Surgery, Loyola University–Chicago Stritch School of Medicine, Maywood, Illinois.
Arteriovenous Fistulae of the Aorta and Its Major Branches

JEFFREY L. BALLARD, MD
Clinical Professor of Surgery, University of California, Irvine, School of Medicine; Staff Vascular Surgeon, St. Joseph Hospital of Orange, Orange, California.
Carotid and Vertebral Artery Injuries

DENNIS F. BANDYK, MD, FACS
Professor of Surgery, University of South Florida College of Medicine, Tampa, Florida.
Infection in Prosthetic Vascular Grafts

JOHN BARTHOLOMEW, MD
Head, Section of Vascular Medicine, Department of Cardiovascular Medicine, Cleveland Clinic, Cleveland, Ohio.
Atheromatous Embolization

MICHEL A. BARTOLI, MD
Fellow, Department of Vascular Surgery, Hospital La Timone, Marseille, France.
Neurogenic Thoracic Outlet Syndrome

HISHAM S. BASSIOUNY, MD
Professor of Surgery, The University of Chicago Pritzker School of Medicine; Attending Surgeon, The University of Chicago Hospitals and Clinics and Louis A. Weiss Memorial Hospital, Chicago, Illinois.
Diagnosis and Treatment of Nonocclusive Mesenteric Ischemia

B. TIMOTHY BAXTER, MD
Professor of Surgery, Cell Biology, and Anatomy, University of Nebraska College of Medicine, Omaha, Nebraska.
Arterial Aneurysms: Etiologic Considerations

HUGH G. BEEBE, MD
Director Emeritus, Jobst Vascular Center, The Toledo Hospital, Toledo, Ohio.
3D Image Processing

MARSHALL E. BENJAMIN, MD
Medical Director, Vascular Laboratory, Maryland Vascular Center, University of Maryland Medical Center, Baltimore, Maryland.
Endovascular Treatment of Renovascular Disease

JOHN J. BERGAN, MD, FACS, FRCS Hon. (Eng.)
Professor of Surgery, UCSD School of Medicine, San Diego; Attending Surgeon, Scripps Memorial Hospital, La Jolla, California.
Varicose Veins: Treatment by Intervention Including Sclerotherapy

RAMON BERGUER, MD, PhD
Frankel Professor of Vascular Surgery and Professor of Engineering, School of Medicine and Cullen College of Engineering, University of Michigan, Ann Arbor, Michigan; Vascular Surgeon, University of Michigan Health System.
Brachiocephalic Vessel Reconstruction; Vertebrobasilar Ischemia: Indications, Techniques, and Results of Surgical Repair

JOSHUA W. BERNHEIM, MD
Vascular Surgery Fellow, New York Presbyterian Hospital, New York.
Renal Artery Imaging and Physiologic Testing

KERSTIN BETTERMANN, MD, PhD
Assistant Professor, Department of Neurology, Wake Forest University School of Medicine; Neurologist, North Carolina Baptist Hospital of Wake Forest University, Winston-Salem, North Carolina.
Diagnostic Evaluation and Medical Management of Patients with Ischemic Cerebrovascular Disease

RODGER L. BICK, MD, PhD, FACP
Clinical Professor of Pathology, University of Texas Southwestern Medical Center; Director, Dallas Thrombosis Hemostasis and Difficult Hematology Clinical Center, Dallas, Texas.
Normal and Abnormal Coagulation

JAMES H. BLACK III, MD
Assistant Professor of Surgery, Johns Hopkins University School of Medicine; Vascular Surgeon, Division of Vascular and Endovascular Surgery, Johns Hopkins Hospital, Baltimore, Maryland.
Aortic Dissection: Perspectives for the Vascular/ Endovascular Surgeon

W. TODD BOHANNON, MD
Assistant Professor of Surgery, Texas A & M University Health Science Center; Scott & White Memorial Hospital and Clinic, Temple, Texas.
Venous Transpositions in the Creation of Arteriovenous Access

THOMAS C. BOWER, MD
Professor of Surgery, Mayo Clinic College of Medicine; Consultant, Division of Vascular Surgery, Mayo Clinic, Rochester, Minnesota.
Evaluation and Management of Malignant Tumors of the Inferior Vena Cava

JOHN G. BRAWLEY, MD
Fellow, Vascular Surgery, University of Texas Southwestern Medical Center, Dallas, Texas.
Traumatic Arteriovenous Fistulae

DAVID C. BREWSTER, MD
Clinical Professor of Surgery, Harvard Medical School; Vascular Surgeon, Division of Vascular Surgery, Massachusetts General Hospital, Boston, Massachusetts.
Direct Reconstruction for Aortoiliac Occlusive Disease

PATRICIA E. BURROWS, MD
Professor of Radiology, Harvard Medical School; Staff Radiologist, Children's Hospital, Boston, Massachusetts.
Endovascular Treatment of Vascular Anomalies

RUTH L. BUSH, MD
Assistant Professor, Division of Vascular Surgery and Endovascular Therapy, Michael E. DeBakey Department of Surgery, Baylor College of Medicine, Houston, Texas.
Complications of Endovascular Procedures; Management of Thrombosed Dialysis Access

JACOB BUTH, MD, PhD
Consultant Vascular Surgeon, Department of Surgery, Catharina Hospital, Eindhoven, The Netherlands.
Endovascular Treatment of Aortic Aneurysms

KEITH D. CALLIGARO, MD
Chief, Section of Vascular Surgery, Department of
Surgery, Pennsylvania Hospital, Philadelphia,
Pennsylvania.
Renal Artery Aneurysms and Arteriovenous Fistulae

RICHARD P. CAMBRIA, MD
Professor of Surgery, Harvard Medical School; Chief,
Division of Vascular and Endovascular Surgery, and Co-
Director, Thoracic Aortic Center, Massachusetts General
Hospital, Boston, Massachusetts.
*Aortic Dissection: Perspectives for the Vascular/
Endovascular Surgeon*

TERESA L. CARMAN, MD
Attending, Vascular Medicine, Jobst Vascular Center, The
Toledo Hospital, Toledo, Ohio.
Thrombolytic Agents and Their Actions

JEFFREY P. CARPENTER, MD
Professor, Department of Surgery; Director, Vascular
Laboratory, Hospital of the University of Pennsylvania,
Philadelphia, Pennsylvania.
Magnetic Resonance Imaging and Angiography

PATRICK J. CASEY, MD
Vascular Surgery Fellow, Division of Vascular and
Endovascular Surgery, Massachusetts General Hospital,
Boston, Massachusetts.
Anastomotic Aneurysms

JOAQUIN J. CERVEIRA, MD
Assistant Professor of Surgery and Chief, Endovascular
Surgery, Kaiser Permanente Medical Center, Panorama
City, California.
The Pathophysiology of Chronic Venous Disorders

JAE-SUNG CHO, MD
Assistant Professor, Department of Surgery, University of
Pittsburgh Medical Center, Pittsburgh, Pennsylvania.
*Surgical Treatment of Chronic Occlusions of the
Iliac Veins and the Inferior Vena Cava*

G. PATRICK CLAGETT, MD
Professor, Division of Vascular Surgery, University of
Texas Southwestern Medical Center, Dallas, Texas.
Upper Extremity Aneurysms

HARRY CLOFT, MD, PhD
Associate Professor, Radiology, Mayo Medical School;
Senior Associate Consultant, Department of Radiology,
Mayo Clinic, Rochester, Minnesota.
Carotid Angioplasty and Stenting

RAUL COIMBRA, MD, PhD
Associate Professor, Department of Surgery, Division of
Trauma Medicine, University of California, San Diego,
School of Medicine; Associate Director of Trauma,
Department of Surgery, Division of Trauma, UCSD
Medical Center, San Diego, California.
*Epidemiology and Natural History of Vascular
Trauma*

ANTHONY J. COMEROTA, MD, FACS
Clinical Professor of Surgery, University of Michigan
Medical School; Director, Jobst Vascular Center, The
Toledo Hospital, Toledo, Ohio.
*Thrombolytic Agents and Their Actions; Catheter
Directed Thrombolytic Therapy; Catheter Based
Interventions for Acute Deep Venous Thrombosis*

JOHN P. CONNORS III, MD
Resident, Department of Plastic and Reconstructive
Surgery, Brigham and Women's Hospital, Boston,
Massachusetts.
Vascular Tumors and Malformations in Childhood

MICHAEL S. CONTE, MD
Associate Professor of Surgery, Harvard Medical School;
Associate Surgeon (Vascular), Brigham and Women's
Hospital, Boston, Massachusetts.
*Molecular Biology and Gene Therapy in Vascular
Disease*

JUDITH W. COOK, MD
Fellow, Division of Vascular Surgery, Department of
Surgery, University of Washington School of Medicine,
Seattle, Washington.
*Clinical and Diagnostic Evaluation of the Patient
with Deep Venous Thrombosis*

MICHAEL J. COSTANZA, MD
Clinical Associate Professor, Division of Vascular
Surgery, Department of Surgery, SUNY Upstate Medical
Center, Syracuse, New York.
Endovascular Treatment of Renovascular Disease

JACK L. CRONENWETT, MD
Professor of Surgery, Dartmouth Medical School,
Hanover; Chief, Section of Vascular Surgery, Dartmouth-
Hitchcock Medical Center, Lebanon, New Hampshire.
*Overview [Arterial Aneurysms]; Abdominal Aortic
and Iliac Aneurysms*

JOHN A. CURCI, MD
Assistant Professor of Surgery, Washington University
School of Medicine, St. Louis, Missouri.
Arterial Aneurysms: Etiologic Considerations

JACOB CYNAMON, MD
Professor of Clinical Radiology, Albert Einstein College of Medicine of Yeshiva University; Director, Vascular and Interventional Radiology, Montefiore Medical Center, Bronx, New York.
Techniques for Thromboembolectomy of Native Arteries and Bypass Grafts

MICHAEL D. DAKE, MD
Professor of Radiology, Medicine, and Surgery, University of Virginia; Professor and Chairman, Department of Radiology, University of Virginia Health System, Charlottesville, Virginia.
Endovascular Treatment of Vena Caval Occlusions

MICHAEL DALSING, MD
Professor of Surgery, Indiana University School of Medicine; Director of Vascular Surgery, Clarian Health, Indianapolis, Indiana.
The Surgical Treatment of Deep Venous Valvular Incompetence

R. CLEMENT DARLING III, MD
Professor of Surgery, Albany Medical College; Chief, Division of Vascular Surgery, Albany Medical Center Hospital, Albany, New York.
Arterial Thromboembolism

MARK G. DAVIES, MD, PhD
Associate Professor, Department of Vascular and Endovascular Surgery, University of Rochester School of Medicine and Dentistry; Medical Director, Vascular Diagnostic Laboratory, Vascular Biology and Therapeutics Program and Endovascular Therapy Program; Division of Vascular Surgery, Strong Heart and Vascular Center; Attending Physician, Strong Memorial Hospital, Rochester, New York.
Intimal Hyperplasia: Basic Response to Vascular Injury and Reconstruction

RAJEEV DAYAL, MD
Clinical Instructor in Surgery, Weill Medical College of Cornell University; Fellow, Vascular Surgery, New York–Presbyterian Hospital, New York, New York.
Standardized Reporting Practices

RICHARD H. DEAN, MD
Professor of Surgery, Wake Forest University School of Medicine; President and CEO, Wake Forest University Health Sciences, Winston-Salem, North Carolina.
Atherosclerotic Renovascular Disease and Ischemic Nephropathy

DEMETRIOS DEMETRIADES, MD, PhD, FACS
Professor of Surgery, University of Southern California School of Medicine; Director, Division of Trauma and SICU, Los Angeles County–University of Southern California Medical Center, Los Angeles, California.
Abdominal Vascular Injuries

RALPH G. DE PALMA, MD, FACS
National Director of Surgery, Department of Veterans Affairs, Medical-Surgical Group; Professor of Surgery, Uniformed Services University of the Health Sciences F. Edward Hébert School of Medicine; Staff Surgeon, Veterans Affairs Medical Center, Washington, D.C.
Atherosclerosis: Plaque Characteristics and Concepts of Evolution; Postoperative Sexual Dysfunction After Aortoiliac Interventions; Vasculogenic Erectile Dysfunction; Superficial Thrombophlebitis: Diagnosis and Management

TINA R. DESAI, MD
Assistant Professor of Surgery, The University of Chicago Pritzker School of Medicine; Attending Surgeon, The University of Chicago Hospitals and Clinics, Chicago, Illinois.
Diagnosis and Treatment of Nonocclusive Mesenteric Ischemia; Acute Renovascular Occlusive Events

LARRY-STUART DEUTSCH, MD, CM, FRCPC, FACR
Chief-of-Service, Vascular and Interventional Radiology Section, Good Samaritan Regional Medical Center and St. Joseph's Hospital and Medical Center; Chair, Department of Medical Imaging, Clinical Diagnostic Radiology Inc., Phoenix, Arizona.
Anatomy and Angiographic Diagnosis of Extracranial and Intracranial Vascular Disease

MATTHEW J. DOUGHERTY, MD
Attending Surgeon, Department of Surgery, Pennsylvania Hospital, Philadelphia, Pennsylvania.
Renal Artery Aneurysms and Arteriovenous Fistulae

WALTER N. DURAN, PhD
Professor of Physiology and Surgery, UMDNJ–New Jersey Medical School, Newark, New Jersey.
The Pathophysiology of Chronic Venous Disorders

MATTHEW J. EAGLETON, MD
Assistant Professor of Surgery, Section of Vascular Surgery, University of Michigan Medical School, Ann Arbor, Michigan.
Perioperative Considerations: Coagulopathy and Hemorrhage

JAMES M. EDWARDS, MD
Associate Professor, Division of Vascular Surgery, Department of Surgery, Oregon Health and Science University School of Medicine; Chief of Surgery, Portland Veterans Affairs Medical Center, Portland, Oregon.
Upper Extremity Revascularization

MATTHEW S. EDWARDS, MD
Assistant Professor of Surgery, Section on Vascular Surgery, Wake Forest University School of Medicine, Winston-Salem, North Carolina.
Endovascular Treatment of Renovascular Disease; Open Surgical Repair of Renovascular Disease

BO EKLOF, MD, PhD
Emeritus Professor of Surgery, University of Hawaii John A. Burns School of Medicine, Honolulu, Hawaii.
Surgical Thrombectomy for Acute Deep Venous Thrombosis

ERIC D. ENDEAN, MD, FACS
Gordon L. Hyde Professor of Surgery, Department of Surgery, University of Kentucky College of Medicine; Chief, Division of General and Vascular Surgery, University of Kentucky Chandler Medical Center; Attending Surgeon, Lexington Veterans Affairs Medical Center, Lexington, Kentucky.
Treatment of Acute Intestinal Ischemia Caused by Arterial Occlusions

MARK S. ESKANDARI, MD
Assistant Professor of Surgery, Division of Vascular Surgery, Northwestern University Feinberg School of Medicine; Attending Surgeon, Division of Vascular Surgery, Northwestern Memorial Hospital, Chicago, Illinois.
Occupational Vascular Problems

ANTHONY L. ESTRERA, MD
Assistant Professor, Department of Cardiothoracic and Vascular Surgery, University of Texas at Houston Medical School; Attending, Hermann Memorial City Hospital, Houston, Texas.
Thoracoabdominal Aortic Aneurysms

JAWED FAREED, PhD
Professor, Department of Pathology and Pharmacology; Director, Special Coagulation Laboratory and the Hemostasis and Thrombosis Research Program, Loyola University Medical Center, Maywood, Illinois.
Normal and Abnormal Coagulation

SCOTT R. FECTEAU, MD
Fellow in Training (Vascular Surgery), Albany Medical Center Hospital, Albany, New York.
Arterial Thromboembolism

MARK F. FILLINGER, MD
Associate Professor of Surgery, Dartmouth Medical School, Hanover; Faculty (Section of Vascular Surgery), Dartmouth-Hitchcock Medical Center, Lebanon, New Hampshire.
Computed Tomography in Vascular Disease; 3D Image Processing

MICHELLE FLORIAN-KUJAWSKI, BS
Department of Pharmacology, Loyola University Medical Center, Maywood, Illinois.
Normal and Abnormal Coagulation

VIVIAN GAHTAN, MD
Chief, Section of Vascular Surgery, Department of Surgery, SUNY Upstate Medical University College of Medicine; Vascular Surgeon, Surgery Service, Syracuse Veterans Affairs Medical Center, Syracuse, New York.
Molecular Biology and Gene Therapy in Vascular Disease

GAIL L. GAMBLE, MD
Assistant Professor of Physical Medicine and Rehabilitation, Mayo Clinic College of Medicine, Rochester, Minnesota.
Nonoperative Management of Chronic Lymphedema

NICHOLAS J. GARGIULO, MD
Assistant Professor of Surgery, Albert Einstein College of Medicine of Yeshiva University; Attending Surgeon, Weiler Hospital, Bronx, New York.
Techniques for Thromboembolectomy of Native Arteries and Bypass Grafts; Secondary Arterial Reconstructions in the Lower Extremity

BRUCE L. GEWERTZ, MD, FACS
Dallas B. Phemister Professor and Chairman, Department of Surgery, The University of Chicago Pritzker School of Medicine; Attending Surgeon, The University of Chicago Hospitals and Clinics, Chicago, Illinois.
Acute Renovascular Occlusive Events

JOSEPH GIORDANO, MD
Professor and Chairman, Department of Surgery, George Washington University School of Medicine; Chief of Surgery, George Washington University Hospital, Washington, D.C.
Embryology of the Vascular System

MARY E. GISWOLD, MD
Resident, Department of Surgery, Oregon Health and Sciences University School of Medicine, Portland, Oregon.
Nonoperative Treatment of Chronic Venous Insufficiency

SEYMOUR GLAGOV, MD
Professor Emeritus, Department of Pathology, The University of Chicago Pritzker School of Medicine; Pathologist, University of Chicago Hospitals and Clinics, Chicago, Illinois.
Artery Wall Pathology in Atherosclerosis

PETER GLOVICZKI, MD
Professor of Surgery, Mayo Clinic College of Medicine; Chair, Division of Vascular Surgery and Director, Gonda Vascular Center, Mayo Clinic, Rochester, Minnesota.
Principles of Venography; Lymphatic Complications of Vascular Surgery; Introduction and General Considerations [The Management of Venous Disorders]; Management of Perforator Vein Incompetence; Surgical Treatment of Chronic Occlusions of the Iliac Veins and the Inferior Vena Cava; Surgical Treatment of Superior Vena Cava Syndrome; Lymphedema: An Overview; Clinical Diagnosis and Evaluation of Lymphedema; Nonoperative Management of Chronic Lymphedema; Surgical Treatment of Chronic Lymphedema and Primary Chylous Disorders

JERRY GOLDSTONE, MD, FACS, FRCS
Professor of Surgery, Case School of Medicine, Case Western Reserve University; Chief, Division of Vascular Surgery, University Hospitals of Cleveland, Cleveland, Ohio.
Aneurysms of the Extracranial Carotid Artery

MICHAEL J. V. GORDON, MD
Director, The Hand Center, Division of Plastic Surgery; Assistant Professor, Department of Surgery, University of Colorado Health Sciences Center, Denver, Colorado.
Upper Extremity Amputation

RICHARD M. GREEN, MD
Chairman, Department of Surgery, Lenox Hill Hospital, New York, New York.
Training in Endovascular Surgery; Subclavian-Axillary Vein Thrombosis

LAZAR J. GREENFIELD, MD
Professor of Surgery and Chair Emeritus, Department of Surgery, University of Michigan, Ann Arbor, Michigan.
Vena Caval Interruption Procedures

HOWARD P. GREISLER, MD
Professor of Surgery and Professor of Cell Biology, Neurobiology, and Anatomy, Loyola University Chicago Stritch School of Medicine, Maywood; Attending Surgeon, Loyola University Medical Center, Maywood; Staff Surgeon, Edward Hines Jr. VA Hospital, Hines, Illinois.
Prosthetic Grafts

NAVYASH GUPTA, MD, FACS
Assistant Professor, Department of Surgery, University of Pittsburgh School of Medicine; Attending Surgeon, University of Pittsburgh Hospitals and Clinics, Pittsburgh, Pennsylvania.
Acute Renovascular Occlusive Events

ALLEN D. HAMDAN, MD
Assistant Professor of Surgery, Harvard Medical School; Attending Vascular Surgeon and Director of Clinical Research, Department of Vascular Surgery, Beth Israel Deaconess Medical Center, Boston, Massachusetts.
Management of Foot Ulcers in Diabetes Mellitus

JAAP F. HAMMING, MD, PhD
Department of Surgery, Leiden University Medical Center, Leiden, The Netherlands.
Lower Extremity Aneurysms

KIMBERLEY J. HANSEN, MD, FACS
Professor of Surgery and Head, Section on Vascular Surgery, Division of Surgical Sciences, Wake Forest University School of Medicine, Winston-Salem, North Carolina.
Renal Complications; Renovascular Disease: An Overview; Atherosclerotic Renovascular Disease and Ischemic Nephropathy; Open Surgical Repair of Renovascular Disease

LINDA M. HARRIS, MD
Assistant Professor of Surgery, University of Buffalo School of Medicine and Biomedical Sciences; Program Director, Vascular Surgery Residency, and Interim Division Chief, Vascular Surgery, Millard Fillmore Hospital, Buffalo, New York.
The Modified Biograft; Endovascular Treatment of Aortic Aneurysms

PETER L. HARRIS, MD, FRCS
Director, Vascular and Transplant Services, Regional Vascular Unit, Royal Liverpool University Hospital, England, United Kingdom.
Endovascular Treatment of Aortic Aneurysms

PETER K. HENKE, MD
Assistant Professor, Section of Vascular Surgery, Department of Surgery, University of Michigan Medical School; Chief, Vascular Surgery, Ann Arbor Veterans Affairs Hospital, Ann Arbor, Michigan.
Vascular Thrombosis Due to Hypercoagulable States; Vena Caval Interruption Procedures

WILLIAM R. HIATT, MD
Professor of Medicine, Division of Vascular Medicine, University of Colorado Health Sciences Center School of Medicine, Denver, Colorado.
Atherogenesis and the Medical Management of Atherosclerosis

KIM J. HODGSON, MD
Professor and Chairman, Division of Vascular Surgery, Department of Surgery, Southern Illinois University School of Medicine, Springfield, Illinois.
Principles of Arteriography; Fundamental Techniques in Endovascular Surgery

DEBRA A. HOPPENSTEADT, PhD
Assistant Professor, Department of Pathology; Technical Director, Hemostasis and Thrombosis Research Program, Loyola University Medical Center, Maywood, Illinois.
Normal and Abnormal Coagulation

DAVID B. HOYT, MD, FACS
Professor, Department of Surgery, Division of Trauma, Burns, and Critical Care, University of California, San Diego, School of Medicine; Attending Surgeon, Trauma Center, UCSD Medical Center–Hillcrest, San Diego, California.
Epidemiology and Natural History of Vascular Trauma

THOMAS S. HUBER, MD, PhD
Associate Professor of Surgery, University of Florida College of Medicine, Gainesville, Florida.
Chronic Mesenteric Ischemia

JOSEPH HUH, MD
Assistant Professor, Department of Cardiothoracic Surgery, Baylor College of Medicine; Attending Surgeon, Veterans Affairs Medical Center Houston, Houston, Texas.
Thoracic Vascular Trauma

RUSSELL D. HULL, MBBS, MSc
Professor of Medicine, University of Calgary Faculty of Medicine; Director, Thrombosis Research Unit, Foothills Hospital, Calgary, Alberta, Canada.
Prevention and Medical Treatment of Acute Deep Venous Thrombosis

TAM T. HUYNH, MD
Assistant Professor, Department of Cardiothoracic and Vascular Surgery, University of Texas at Houston Medical School; Attending, Hermann Memorial City Hospital, Houston, Texas.
Thoracoabdominal Aortic Aneurysms

ERIK K. INSKO, MD, PhD
Adjunct Assistant Professor of Radiology, University of Pennsylvania School of Medicine; Attending, Hospital of the University of Pennsylvania, Philadelphia, Pennsylvania; Director of Cardiovascular Imaging, Mecklenburg Radiology Associates, Presbyterian Hospital, Charlotte, North Carolina.
Magnetic Resonance Imaging and Angiography

OMER IQBAL, MD
Assistant Professor, Department of Pathology, Hemostasis and Thrombosis Research Program, Loyola University Medical Center, Maywood, Illinois.
Normal and Abnormal Coagulation

GLENN R. JACOBOWITZ, MD
Associate Professor of Surgery, New York University School of Medicine; Attending Physician, New York University Medical Center, Bellevue Hospital, and New York Harbor VA Medical Center, New York, New York.
Surgical Management of Congenital Vascular Malformations

WALTER P. JESKE, PhD
Associate Professor, Departments of Pathology and Thoracic and Cardiovascular Surgery, Hemostasis and Thrombosis Research Laboratories, Loyola University Medical Center, Maywood, Illinois.
Normal and Abnormal Coagulation

KAJ JOHANSEN, MD, PhD
Clinical Professor of Surgery, University of Washington School of Medicine; Director of Surgical Education, Swedish Medical Center, Providence Campus, Seattle, Washington.
Vascular Pain; Compartment Syndrome: Pathophysiology, Recognition, and Management; Portal Hypertension: Surgical Management of Its Complications

K. WAYNE JOHNSTON, MD, FRCSC
Professor and R. Fraser Elliott Chair in Vascular Surgery, Department of Surgery, University of Toronto Faculty of Medicine; Vascular Surgeon, Toronto General Hospital, Toronto, Ontario, Canada.
Ischemic Neuropathy; The Chronically Ischemic Leg: An Overview

PETER G. KALMAN, MD, FRCSC, FACS
Professor, Departments of Surgery and Radiology, Loyola University Chicago Stritch School of Medicine; Chief, Division of Vascular Surgery, Loyola University Medical Center, Maywood, Illinois.
Profundaplasty: Primary and Secondary Applications

MANJU KALRA, MBBS
Assistant Professor of Surgery, Mayo Clinic College of Medicine; Consultant, Division of Vascular Surgery, Mayo Clinic, Rochester, Minnesota.
Management of Perforator Vein Incompetence; Surgical Treatment of Superior Vena Cava Syndrome

VIKRAM S. KASHYAP, MD
Associate Professor of Surgery, Cleveland Clinic Lerner College of Medicine of Case Western Reserve University; Staff, Department of Vascular Surgery, Cleveland Clinic Foundation, Cleveland, Ohio.
Aortoenteric Fistulae

KARTHIKESHWAR KASIRAJAN, MD, FACS
Assistant Professor of Surgery, Emory University School of Medicine; Attending Surgeon, Emory University Hospital, Atlanta, Georgia.
Acute Limb Ischemia

K. CRAIG KENT, MD
Professor and Vice Chairman, Department of Surgery, Weill Medical College of Cornell University; Professor of Surgery, Columbia University College of Physicians and Surgeons; Director, Vascular Center, and Chief, Combined Columbia and Cornell Division of Vascular Surgery, New York–Presbyterian Hospital, New York, New York.
Standardized Reporting Practices; Renal Artery Imaging and Physiologic Testing

GEORGE E. KOPCHOK, BS (Biomed.Eng.)
Research Associate, Harbor-UCLA Medical Center, Torrance, California.
Intravascular Ultrasound

TIMOTHY F. KRESOWIK, MD
Professor of Surgery, University of Iowa Carver College of Medicine; Attending Surgeon, University of Iowa Hospitals and Clinics, Iowa City, Iowa.
Complications Following Carotid Endarterectomy and Perioperative Management

WILLIAM C. KRUPSKI, MD*
Formerly Clinical Professor of Surgery, University of California, San Francisco, School of Medicine; Attending Vascular Surgeon, The Kaiser Permanente Medical Group, San Francisco, California.
Endarterectomy; Cardiac Complications: Screening and Prevention; Indications, Surgical Technique, and Results for Repair of Extracranial Occlusive Lesions; Uncommon Disorders Affecting the Carotid Arteries

BRAJESH K. LAL, MD
Assistant Professor of Surgery; Assistant Professor of Vascular Surgery; Assistant Professor of Pharmacology/Physiology, UMDNJ–New Jersey Medical School, Newark, New Jersey.
The Pathophysiology of Chronic Venous Disorders

GLENN M. LaMURAGLIA, MD
Associate Professor of Surgery, Harvard Medical School; Attending Surgeon, Division of Vascular and Endovascular Surgery, Massachusetts General Hospital, Boston, Massachusetts.
Anastomotic Aneurysms

W. ANTHONY LEE, MD
Assistant Professor of Surgery, University of Florida College of Medicine, Gainesville, Florida.
Chronic Mesenteric Ischemia

LEWIS J. LEVIEN, MBBCh, PhD, FCSSA
Consultant Vascular Surgeon, Department of Surgery, Milpark Hospital, Johannesburg, South Africa.
Nonatheromatous Causes of Popliteal Artery Disease

PETER H. LIN, MD
Associate Professor, Division of Vascular Surgery and Endovascular Therapy, Michael E. DeBakey Department of Surgery, Baylor College of Medicine, Houston, Texas.
Complications of Endovascular Procedures; Management of Thrombosed Dialysis Access

THOMAS F. LINDSAY, MD, MDCM, FRCS, FACS
Associate Professor, Division of Vascular Surgery, University of Toronto Faculty of Medicine; Staff Surgeon, Division of Vascular Surgery, Toronto General Hospital, University Health Network, Toronto, Ontario, Canada.
Ruptured Abdominal Aortic Aneurysms

PAMELA A. LIPSETT, MD, FACS, FCCM
Professor of Surgery, ACCM, and Nursing; Surgical Critical Care Fellowship Director, Johns Hopkins University School of Medicine, Baltimore, Maryland.
Respiratory Complications in Vascular Surgery

EVAN C. LIPSITZ, MD
Assistant Professor of Surgery, Albert Einstein College of Medicine of Yeshiva University; Attending Surgeon, Montefiore Medical Center, Bronx, New York.
Techniques for Thromboembolectomy of Native Arteries and Bypass Grafts; Secondary Arterial Reconstructions in the Lower Extremity

JAYME E. LOCKE, MD
Department of Surgery, Johns Hopkins University School of Medicine, Baltimore, Maryland.
Respiratory Complications in Vascular Surgery

FRANK W. LoGERFO, MD
William V. McDermott Professor of Surgery, Harvard Medical School; Chief, Division of Vascular Surgery, Beth Israel Deaconess Medical Center, Boston, Massachusetts.
The Autogenous Vein; Management of Foot Ulcers in Diabetes Mellitus

G. MATTHEW LONGO, MD
Instructor, Department of Surgery, Northwestern University Feinberg School of Medicine; Vascular Surgery Fellow, Northwestern Memorial Hospital, Chicago, Illinois.
Evaluation of Upper Extremity Ischemia

*Deceased.

ROBERT C. LOWELL, MD, FACS, RVT
Horizon Vascular Surgery, PC, Gainseville, Georgia.
Lymphatic Complications of Vascular Surgery

ALAN B. LUMSDEN, MD, FACS
Professor and Chief, Division of Vascular Surgery and
Endovascular Therapy, Michael E. DeBakey Department
of Surgery, Baylor College of Medicine, Houston, Texas.
*Complications of Endovascular Procedures;
Management of Thrombosed Dialysis Access*

M. ASHRAF MANSOUR, MD, FACS
Associate Professor of Surgery, Michigan State University
College of Human Medicine, East Lansing; Vascular
Surgery Program Director, Grand Rapids Medical
Education and Research Center, Grand Rapids, Michigan.
*Arteriovenous Fistulae of the Aorta and Its Major
Branches*

WILLIAM A. MARSTON, MD
Associate Professor, Division of Vascular Surgery,
University of North Carolina at Chapel Hill School of
Medicine, Chapel Hill, North Carolina.
Physiologic Assessment of the Venous System

JON S. MATSUMURA, MD
Associate Professor of Surgery, Division of Vascular
Surgery, Northwestern University Feinberg School of
Medicine; Staff Physician, Division of Vascular Surgery,
Northwestern Memorial Hospital, Chicago, Illinois.
*Arterial Complications of Thoracic Outlet
Compression*

KENNETH L. MATTOX, MD
Professor and Vice Chair, Department of Surgery, Baylor
College of Medicine; Chief of Staff and Chief of Surgery,
Ben Taub General Hospital, Houston, Texas.
Thoracic Vascular Trauma

JAMES MAY, MD, MS, FRACS, FACS
Bosch Professor of Surgery, University of Sydney Faculty
of Medicine; Vascular Surgeon, Royal Prince Alfred
Hospital, Sydney, New South Wales, Australia.
Basic Techniques of Endovascular Aneurysm Repair

MICHAEL A. McKUSICK, MD
Assistant Professor of Radiology, Mayo Clinic College of
Medicine, Rochester, Minnesota.
Principles of Venography

ROBERT B. McLAFFERTY, MD
Associate Professor of Surgery, Division of Vascular
Surgery, Southern Illinois University School of Medicine;
Memorial Medical Center; St. John's Hospital,
Springfield, Illinois.
Revascularization Versus Amputation

MARK H. MEISSNER, MD
Associate Professor, Division of Vascular Surgery,
University of Washington School of Medicine, Seattle,
Washington.
*Venous Duplex Scanning; Antithrombotic Therapy;
Pathophysiology and Natural History of Acute Deep
Venous Thrombosis; Clinical and Diagnostic
Evaluation of the Patient with Deep Venous
Thrombosis*

ROBERT R. MENDES, MD
Division of Vascular Surgery, University of North
Carolina at Chapel Hill School of Medicine, Chapel Hill,
North Carolina.
Physiologic Assessment of the Venous System

LOUIS M. MESSINA, MD
Professor of Surgery, and Chief, Division of Vascular
Surgery, University of California San Francisco; Director,
UCSF Heart and Vascular Center, UCSF Medical Center,
San Francisco, California.
*Endarterectomy; Renal Artery Fibrodysplasia and
Renovascular Hypertension*

CHARLES C. MILLER III, PhD
Associate Professor, Department of Cardiothoracic and
Vascular Surgery, University of Texas at Houston
Medical School, Houston, Texas.
Thoracoabdominal Aortic Aneurysms

JOSEPH L. MILLS, SR., MD
Professor of Surgery, University of Arizona College of
Medicine; Chief, Division of Vascular and Endovascular
Surgery, University Medical Center, Tucson, Arizona.
Infrainguinal Bypass

MARC E. MITCHELL, MD
Assistant Professor of Surgery, University of Pennsylvania
School of Medicine; Chief of Surgery, Philadelphia VA
Medical Center, Philadelphia, Pennsylvania.
*Basic Considerations of the Arterial Wall in Health
and Disease*

J. GREGORY MODRALL, MD
Associate Professor, Department of Surgery, University of
Texas Southwestern Medical Center at Dallas
Southwestern Medical School; Chief, Section of Vascular
Surgery, Dallas Veterans Affairs Medical Center, Dallas,
Texas.
Traumatic Arteriovenous Fistulae

GREGORY L. MONETA, MD
Professor of Surgery, Oregon Health and Sciences
University School of Medicine; Chief, Division of
Vascular Surgery, OHSU Hospitals and Clinics, Portland,
Oregon.
*Nonoperative Treatment of Chronic Venous
Insufficiency*

SAMUEL R. MONEY, MD, MBA, FACS
Clinical Associate Professor of Surgery, Tulane University
School of Medicine; Chief, Vascular Surgery, Ochsner
Clinic Foundation, New Orleans, Louisiana.
Medical Treatment of Intermittent Claudication

ERIN MARC MOORE, MD
Clinical Instructor in Surgery, University of Kentucky
College of Medicine; Staff, Department of Surgery,
Section of Vascular Surgery, University of Kentucky
Chandler Medical Center and Veterans Affairs Hospital
Lexington, Lexington, Kentucky.
*Treatment of Acute Intestinal Ischemia Caused by
Arterial Occlusions*

WESLEY S. MOORE, MD
Professor of Surgery, Division of Vascular Surgery, David
Geffen School of Medicine at UCLA; Vascular Surgeon,
Division of Vascular Surgery, UCLA Medical Center, Los
Angeles, California.
*Fundamental Considerations in Cerebrovascular
Disease; Indications and Surgical Technique for
Repair of Extracranial Occlusive Lesions*

MARK D. MORASCH, MD
Assistant Professor of Surgery, Division of Vascular
Surgery, Northwestern University Feinberg School of
Medicine; Attending Surgeon, Division of Vascular
Surgery, Northwestern Memorial Hospital, Chicago,
Illinois.
*Brachiocephalic Vessel Reconstruction; Intestinal
Ischemia Caused by Venous Thrombosis;
Vertebrobasilar Ischemia: Indications, Techniques,
and Results of Surgical Repair*

JOHN B. MULLIKEN, MD
Professor of Surgery, Division of Plastic Surgery, Harvard
Medical School; Director, Craniofacial Centre, and Co-
Director, Vascular Anomalies Center, Children's Hospital
Boston, Boston, Massachusetts.
Vascular Tumors and Malformations in Childhood

PETER NEGLÉN, MD, PhD
Vascular Surgeon, River Oaks Hospital, Jackson,
Mississippi.
*Endovascular Treatment of Chronic Occlusions of
the Iliac Veins and the Inferior Vena Cava*

MARK R. NEHLER, MD
Associate Professor of Surgery, University of Colorado
Health Sciences Center School of Medicine; Program
Director, Surgical Residency Program, University of
Colorado Health Sciences Center, Denver, Colorado.
*Selection of Patients for Vascular Interventions;
Natural History and Nonoperative Treatment of
Chronic Lower Extremity Ischemia; Amputation: An
Overview; Revascularization versus Amputation*

AUDRA NOEL, MD
Assistant Professor of Surgery, Mayo Clinic College of
Medicine; Consultant, Division of Vascular Surgery,
Mayo Clinic, Rochester, Minnesota.
*Surgical Treatment of Chronic Lymphedema and
Primary Chylous Disorders*

PATRICK J. O'HARA, MD
Professor of Surgery, Cleveland Clinic Lerner College of
Medicine; Staff, Department of Vascular Surgery,
Cleveland Clinic Foundation, Cleveland, Ohio.
Aortoenteric Fistulae

W. ANDREW OLDENBURG, MD, FACS
Associate Professor of Surgery, Mayo Medical School,
Rochester, Minnesota; Head, Section of Vascular Surgery,
Mayo Clinic, Jacksonville, Florida.
*Primary Tumors of Major Blood Vessels: Diagnosis
and Management*

JEFFREY W. OLIN, DO
Professor of Medicine, Mount Sinai School of Medicine;
Director, Vascular Medicine, Zena and Michael A.Wiener
Cardiovascular Institute, Mount Sinai Medical Center,
New York, New York.
*Thromboangiitis Obliterans (Buerger's Disease);
Atheromatous Embolization*

KENNETH OURIEL, MD, FACS, FACC
Professor of Surgery, Cleveland Clinic Lerner College of
Medicine of Case Western Reserve University; Chairman,
Division of Surgery, Cleveland Clinic Foundation,
Cleveland, Ohio.
*Perioperative Considerations: Coagulopathy and
Hemorrhage; Training in Endovascular Surgery;
Acute Limb Ischemia*

FRANK T. PADBERG, JR., MD, FACS
Professor of Surgery, Division of Vascular Surgery,
UMDNJ–New Jersey Medical School, Newark; Chief,
Section of Vascular Surgery, VA New Jersey Health Care
System, East Orange, New Jersey.
*Classification and Clinical and Diagnostic
Evaluation of Patients with Chronic Venous
Disorders*

PETER J. PAPPAS, MD
Professor of Surgery, UMDNJ–New Jersey Medical
School; Director, Division of Vascular Surgery; Director,
General Surgery Residency Program; Director, Vascular
Surgery Residency Program, UMDNJ–Newark, New
Jersey.
The Pathophysiology of Chronic Venous Disorders

JEFFREY D. PEARCE, MD
Research Fellow in Vascular Surgery, Department of
General Surgery, Division of Surgical Sciences, Wake
Forest University School of Medicine, Winston-Salem,
North Carolina.
Renal Complications

WILLIAM H. PEARCE, MD
Violet R. and Charles A. Baldwin Professor of Vascular
Surgery, Northwestern University Feinberg School of
Medicine; Chief, Vascular Surgery Division, Northwestern
Memorial Hospital, Chicago, Illinois.
*Overview [Neurovascular Conditions Involving the
Upper Extremity]; Evaluation of Upper Extremity
Ischemia*

DEBORAH PEATE, RVT
Senior Technologist, David B. Pilcher Vascular
Diagnostic Laboratory, Division of Vascular Surgery,
Fletcher Allen Health Care, Burlington, Vermont.
*The Role of Noninvasive Studies in the Diagnosis
and Management of Cerebrovascular Disease*

ERIC K. PEDEN, MD
Assistant Professor, Division of Vascular Surgery and
Endovascular Therapy, Michael E. DeBakey Department
of Surgery, Baylor College of Medicine, Houston, Texas.
*Complications of Endovascular Procedures;
Management of Thrombosed Dialysis Access*

BRUCE A. PERLER, MD, MBA
Julius H. Jacobson II Professor of Surgery, Johns Hopkins
University School of Medicine; Chief, Division of
Vascular Surgery, Johns Hopkins Hospital, Baltimore,
Maryland.
*Overview [Complications of Vascular Surgery and
Ischemia: Prevention and Management]*

DAPHNE M. PIERRE-PAUL, MD
Clinical Assistant Instructor, Department of Surgery,
Section of Vascular Surgery, SUNY Upstate Medical
University College of Medicine, Syracuse, New York.
*Molecular Biology and Gene Therapy in Vascular
Disease*

GRAHAM F. PINEO, MD
Professor of Medicine, University of Calgary Faculty of
Medicine; Director, Thrombosis Research Unit, Foothills
Hospital, Calgary, Alberta, Canada.
*Prevention and Medical Treatment of Acute Deep
Venous Thrombosis*

FRANK B. POMPOSELLI, JR., BS, MD
Associate Professor of Surgery, Harvard Medical School;
Clinical Chief of Vascular Surgery, Beth Israel Deaconess
Medical Center, Boston, Massachusetts.
The Autogenous Vein

MARY C. PROCTOR, MD
Senior Research Associate, Department of Surgery,
University of Michigan School of Medicine, Ann Arbor,
Michigan.
Vena Caval Interruption Procedures

WILLIAM J. QUINONES-BALDRICH, MD
Professor of Surgery, Division of Vascular Surgery,
University of California Los Angeles, Los Angeles,
California.
Takayasu's Disease: Nonspecific Aortoarteritis

JOYESH K. RAJ, MD
Attending Surgeon, Fairview Hospital, Cleveland Clinic
Health System, Westlake, Ohio.
Upper Extremity Amputation

SESHADRI RAJU, MD
Emeritus Professor of Surgery, University of Mississippi
School of Medicine; Honorary Surgeon, University
Hospital, Jackson, Mississippi.
*Endovascular Treatment of Chronic Occlusions of
the Iliac Veins and the Inferior Vena Cava*

JOHN E. RECTENWALD, MD
Clinical Assistant Professor of Surgery and Radiology,
University of Michigan, Department of Surgery,
University of Michigan, Ann Arbor, Michigan.
Vena Caval Interruption Procedures

DANIEL J. REDDY, MD, FACS
D. Emerick and Eve Szilagyi Chair in Vascular Surgery,
Henry Ford Health System, Detroit, Michigan.
Infected Aneurysms

MICHAEL A. RICCI, MD
Roger H. Allbee Professor of Surgery, Division of
Vascular Surgery, University of Vermont College of
Medicine, Burlington, Vermont.
*The Role of Noninvasive Studies in the Diagnosis
and Management of Cerebrovascular Disease*

JOHN J. RICOTTA, MD, FACS
Professor and Chair, Department of Surgery, State
University of New York at Stony Brook School of
Medicine; Surgeon in Chief, University Hospital at Stony
Brook, Stony Brook, New York.
*General Strategies: Choice of Procedure and
Technique [Open Vascular Surgery: Basic
Considerations]; Vascular Conduits: An Overview*

DAVID A. RIGBERG, MD
Assistant Professor of Surgery, Division of Vascular
Surgery, David Geffen School of Medicine at UCLA, Los
Angeles, California.
Takayasu's Disease: Nonspecific Aortoarteritis

THOMAS S. RILES, MD
George David Stewart Professor and Chair, Department of
Surgery, New York University School of Medicine, New
York, New York.
*Surgical Management of Congenital Vascular
Malformations*

KYUNG M. RO, MD
Resident, Department of Radiology, UCDavis Medical
Center, Sacramento, California.
Upper Extremity Sympathectomy

SEAN P. RODDY, MD
Associate Professor of Surgery, Albany Medical College;
Attending Vascular Surgeon, Albany Medical Center
Hospital, Albany, New York.
Arterial Thromboembolism

THOM ROOKE, MD
Krehbiel Professor of Vascular Medicine, Mayo Clinic
College of Medicine; Head, Section of Vascular Medicine,
Mayo Clinic, Rochester, Minnesota.
*Uncommon Arteriopathies; Nonoperative
Management of Chronic Lymphedema*

RANDI ROSE, MD
Clinical Instructor, Department of Surgery, Mount Sinai
School of Medicine; Staff, Zena and Michael A.Wiener
Cardiovascular Institute, Mount Sinai Medical Center,
New York, New York.
Atheromatous Embolization

VINCENT L. ROWE, MD
Assistant Professor of Surgery, University of Southern
California Keck School of Medicine; Attending Surgeon,
LosAngeles County–University of Southern California
Medical Center, Los Angeles, California.
Vascular Injuries of the Extremities

C. VAUGHAN RUCKLEY, MB, ChM, FRCSE
Emeritus Professor of Vascular Surgery, University of
Edinburgh; Former Consultant Surgeon, Royal Infirmary,
Edinburgh, Lothian, Scotland, United Kingdom.
*Lower Extremity Amputation: Technique and
Perioperative Care*

**ROBERT B. RUTHERFORD, MD, FACS, FRCS
Hon. (Glasg.)**
Emeritus Professor of Surgery, University of Colorado
School of Medicine, Denver, Colorado.
*Essentials of Clinical Evaluation; Selection of
Patients for Vascular Interventions; Essential
Considerations in Evaluating the Results of
Treatment; Basic Vascular Surgical Techniques;
Causalgia and Post-traumatic Pain Syndromes;
Lumbar Sympathectomy: Indications and Technique;
Overview [Arteriovenous Fistulas, Congenital
Vascular Malformations, and Vascular Tumors];
Diagnostic Evaluation of Arteriovenous Fistulas and
Vascular Anomalies; Surgical Thombectomy for
Acute Deep Venous Thrombosis*

EVA M. RZUCIDLO, MD
Assistant Professor, Department of Vascular Surgery,
Dartmouth Medical School; Vascular Surgeon, Dartmouth
Hitchcock Medical Center, Lebanon, New Hampshire.
Arterial Duplex Scanning

HAZIM J. SAFI, MD
Professor and Chairman, Department of Cardiothoracic
and Vascular Surgery, University of Texas at Houston
Medical School; Vascular Surgeon, Hermann Memorial
City Hospital, Houston, Texas.
Thoracoabdominal Aortic Aneurysms

RUSSELL H. SAMSON, MD, FACS, RVT
Former Associate Professor of Surgery, Albert Einstein
College of Medicine of Yeshiva University, New York,
New York; Staff, Sarasota Memorial Hospital; President,
Mote Vascular Foundation, Inc., Sarasota, Florida.
*Maintaining a Computerized Vascular Registry;
Overview: Medical Management in a Vascular
Surgery Practice; Hypertension and Patients with
Vascular Disorders*

MARC L. SCHERMERHORN, MD
Assistant Professor of Surgery, Harvard Medical School;
Chief, Section of Interventional and Endovascular
Surgery, Beth Israel Deaconess Medical Center, Boston,
Massachusetts.
Abdominal Aortic and Iliac Aneurysms

ALVIN SCHMAIER, MD
Professor of Internal Medicine and Pathology; Course
Director, M2 Hematology Sequence, University of
Michigan Medical School; Director, Coagulation
Laboratory, University of Michigan Hospitals and Health
Centers, Ann Arbor, Michigan.
*Vascular Thromboses Due to Hypercoagulable
States*

DARREN B. SCHNEIDER, MD
Assistant Professor of Surgery and Radiology, University
of California San Francisco; Attending Surgeon, Division
of Vascular Surgery, UCSF Medical Center, San
Francisco, California.
*Renal Artery Fibrodysplasia and Renovascular
Hypertension*

JOSEPH R. SCHNEIDER, MD, PhD
Professor of Surgery, Division of Vascular Surgery,
Northwestern University Feinberg School of Medicine,
Chicago; Senior Attending, Evanston Northwestern Health
Care, Evanston, Illinois.
Extra-Anatomic Bypass

PETER A. SCHNEIDER, MD
Vascular and Endovascular Surgeon, Division of Vascular
Therapy, Hawaii Permanente Medical Group, Honolulu,
Hawaii.
*Endovascular Surgery in the Management of
Chronic Lower Extremity Ischemia; Endovascular
and Surgical Management of Extracranial Carotid
Fibromuscular Arterial Dysplasia*

JAMES M. SEEGER, MD
Professor of Surgery, University of Florida College of
Medicine; Chief, Division of Vascular Surgery and
Endovascular Therapy, Shands at University of Florida,
Gainesville, Florida.
Chronic Mesenteric Ischemia

TAQDEES SHEIKH, MD
Associate Professor, Department of Anesthesiology,
Loyola University Health System, Maywood, Illinois.
Normal and Abnormal Coagulation

ROGER F. J. SHEPHERD, MB, BCH
Assistant Professor of Medicine, Mayo College of
Medicine; Staff, Gonda Vascular Center, Mayo Clinic,
Rochester, Minnesota.
*Uncommon Arteriopathies; Raynaud's Syndrome:
Vasospastic and Occlusive Arterial Disease
Involving the Distal Upper Extremity*

KEVIN M. SHERIDAN, MD
Resident (General Surgery), Department of Surgery,
Indiana University Hospital; Division of Vascular
Surgery, Clarian Health Hospitals, Indianapolis, Indiana.
*The Surgical Treatment of Deep Venous Valvular
Incompetence*

ANTON N. SIDAWY, MD, MPH
Professor of Surgery, George Washington University
School of Medicine; Chief of Surgery, VA Medical
Center, Washington, D.C.
*Basic Considerations of the Arterial Wall in Health
and Disease; Hyperglycemia, Diabetes, and
Syndrome X; Strategies of Arteriovenous Dialysis
Access; Nonthrombotic Complications of
Arteriovenous Access for Hemodialysis*

MICHAEL B. SILVA, JR., MD
Professor of Surgery, Texas Tech University Health
Sciences Center; Vice-Chairman, Department of Surgery;
Chief, Vascular Surgery and Vascular Interventional
Radiology, University Medical Center, Lubbock, Texas.
*Venous Transpositions in the Creation of
Arteriovenous Access*

JAMES C. STANLEY, MD
Professor and Associate Chair, Department of Surgery,
University of Michigan Medical School; Co-Director,
University of Michigan Cardiovascular Center, and Head,
Section of Vascular Surgery, University Hospital, Ann
Arbor, Michigan.
*Arterial Fibrodysplasia; Splanchnic Artery
Aneurysms; Renal Artery Fibrodysplasia and
Renovascular Hypertension*

W. CHARLES STERNBERGH III, MD
Clinical Assistant Professor of Surgery, Tulane University
School of Medicine; Program Director, Vascular Surgery,
Ochsner Clinic Foundation, New Orleans, Louisiana.
Medical Treatment of Intermittent Claudication

RONALD J. STONEY, MD
Professor Emeritus, Division of Vascular Surgery,
University of California-SanFrancisco School of
Medicine, SanFrancisco, California.
Endarterectomy

EUGENE STRANDNESS, JR., MD*
Formerly Professor of Surgery and Chief, Vascular
Surgery, University of Washington School of Medicine,
Seattle, Washington.
*Pathophysiology and Natural History of Acute Deep
Venous Thrombosis*

RICHARD J. STRILKA, MD, PhD
Division of Vascular Surgery, Department of Surgery,
University of Maryland, Baltimore, Maryland.
Endovascular Treatment of Renovascular Disease

TIMOTHY M. SULLIVAN, MD, FACS
Associate Professor of Surgery, Division of Vascular
Surgery, Mayo Clinic, Rochester, Minnesota.
Carotid Angioplasty and Stenting

DAVID S. SUMNER, MD
Distinguished Professor of Surgery Emeritus, Department
of Surgery, Division of Peripheral Vascular Surgery,
Southern Illinois University School of Medicine,
Springfield, Illinois.
*Vascular Physiology: Essential Hemodynamic
Principles; Physiologic Assessment of Peripheral
Arterial Occlusive Disease; Evaluation of Upper
Extremity Ischemia*

PETER R. TAYLOR, MA, MChir, FRCS
Consultant Vascular and Endovascular Surgeon, Guy's
and St. Thomas' NHS Foundation Trust, London, United
Kingdom.
*Functional Outcome and Natural History of Major
Lower Extremity Amputation*

THEODORE H. TERUYA, MD
Clinical Assistant Professor of Surgery, University of
Hawaii John A. Burns School of Medicine, Honolulu,
Hawaii.
Carotid and Vertebral Artery Injuries

---
* Deceased.

ROBERT W. THOMPSON, MD
Professor of Surgery, Radiology, and Cell Biology and Physiology, Washington University School of Medicine; Attending Surgeon, Barnes–Jewish Hospital, St.Louis, Missouri.
Arterial Aneurysms: Etiologic Considerations; Neurogenic Thoracic Outlet Syndrome

MAHMUT TOBU, MD
Department of Pathology, Loyola University Medical Center, Maywood, Illinois.
Normal and Abnormal Coagulation

JAMES F. TOOLE, MD
The Walter C. Teagle Professor of Neurology and Professor of Public Health Sciences, Wake Forest University School of Medicine; Past President of the International Stroke Society and the World Federation of Neurology, Winston-Salem, North Carolina.
Diagnostic Evaluation and Medical Management of Patients with Ischemic Cerebrovascular Disease

J. JEAN E. TURLEY, MD, FRCPC
Associate Professor, Department of Medicine (Neurology), University of Toronto Faculty of Medicine; Staff, St. Michael's Hospital, Toronto, Ontario, Canada.
Ischemic Neuropathy

GILBERT R. UPCHURCH, JR., MD
Associate Professor of Surgery and Leland Ira Doan Research Professor of Vascular Surgery, University of Michigan Medical School, Ann Arbor, Michigan.
Splanchnic Artery Aneurysms

R. JAMES VALENTINE, MD
Frank H. Kidd Jr. Distinguished Professor and Vice-Chairman, Department of Surgery, University of Texas Southwestern Medical Center, Dallas, Texas.
Anatomy of Commonly Exposed Arteries

J. HAJO VAN BOCKEL, MD, PhD
Professor, Department of Surgery, Leiden University Medical Center, Leiden, The Netherlands.
Lower Extremity Aneurysms

FRANK J. VEITH, MD
Professor and Vice Chairman, Department of Surgery, Albert Einstein College of Medicine of Yeshiva University; William J.von Liebig Chair in Vascular Surgery, Montefiore Medical Center, Bronx, New York.
Techniques for Thromboembolectomy of Native Arteries and Bypass Grafts; Secondary Arterial Reconstructions in the Lower Extremity

HEINZ W. WAHNER, MD
Professor Emeritus of Radiology, Mayo Clinic, Rochester, Minnesota.
Clinical Diagnosis and Evaluation of Lymphedema

THOMAS W. WAKEFIELD, MD
S. Martin Lindenauer Collegiate Professor of Surgery, University of Michigan Medical School; Staff Surgeon, Section of Vascular Surgery, Department of Surgery, University of Michigan Hospital and Ann Arbor Veterans Administration Medical Center, Ann Arbor, Michigan.
Arterial Fibrodysplasia; Vascular Thromboses Due to Hypercoagulable States; Vena Caval Interruption Procedures

MATTHEW J. WALL, JR., MD
Associate Professor, Michael E. DeBakey Department of Surgery, Baylor College of Medicine; Deputy Chief of Surgery and Chief of Cardiothoracic Surgery, Ben Taub General Hospital, Houston, Texas.
Thoracic Vascular Trauma

DANIEL WALSH, MD
Professor of Surgery (Vascular), Dartmouth Medical School, Hanover; Vice-Chair, Department of Surgery, Dartmouth-Hitchcock Medical Center, Lebanon, New Hampshire.
Postoperative Graft Thrombosis: Prevention and Management

MARYANNE WATERS, RN, RVT
Instructor in Surgery, Department of Surgery, Division of Vascular Surgery, University of Vermont College of Medicine, Burlington, Vermont.
The Role of Noninvasive Studies in the Diagnosis and Management of Cerebrovascular Disease

JAMES C. WATSON, MS, MD
Clinical Instructor in Surgery, University of Washington School of Medicine, Seattle, Washington.
Compartment Syndromes: Pathophysiology, Recognition, and Management

FRED A. WEAVER, MD
Professor of Surgery, University of Southern California Keck School of Medicine; Chief of Vascular Surgery, University of Southern California University Hospital; Attending Surgeon, Vascular Surgery, Los Angeles County–University of Southern California Medical Center, Los Angeles, California.
Vascular Injuries of the Extremities

MITCHELL R. WEAVER, MD
Vascular Surgery Fellow, Henry Ford Health System, Detroit, Michigan.
Infected Aneurysms

JONATHAN M. WEISWASSER, MD
Assistant Professor of Surgery, George Washington University School of Medicine; Chief, Vascular Surgery, Washington VA Medical Center, Washington, D.C.
Hyperglycemia, Diabetes, and Syndrome X; Strategies of Arteriovenous Dialysis Access

GEOFFREY H. WHITE, MD, FRACS
Associate Professor of Surgery, University of Sydney
Faculty of Medicine; Head, Department of Vascular
Surgery, Royal Prince Alfred Hospital, Sydney, New
South Wales, Australia.
Basic Techniques of Endovascular Aneurysm Repair

JOHN V. WHITE, MD
Clinical Professor of Surgery, University of Illinois
School of Medicine, Chicago; Chairman, Department of
Surgery, Advocate-Lutheran General Hospital, Park
Ridge, Illinois.
*Proper Outcomes Assessment: Patient-Based and
Economic Vascular Interventions; Evaluation of the
Patient with Chronic Lower Extremity Ischemia*

RODNEY A. WHITE, MD
Professor of Surgery, David Geffen School of Medicine at
UCLA, Los Angeles; Associate Chair, Department of
Surgery, Harbor-UCLA Medical Center, Torrance,
California.
Intravascular Ultrasound

DAVID R. WHITTAKER, MD
Fellow, Section of Vascular Surgery, Dartmouth-
Hitchcock Medical Center, Lebanon, New Hampshire.
*Computed Tomography, CT Angiography, and 3D
Reconstruction for the Evaluation of Vascular
Disease*

DAVID B. WILSON, MD
Vascular Surgery Fellow, Section of Vascular Surgery,
Department of General Surgery, Wake Forest University
School of Medicine, Winston-Salem, North Carolina.
*Atherosclerotic Renovascular Disease and Ischemic
Nephropathy*

GARY G. WIND, MD, FACS
Professor of Surgery, Uniformed Services University of
the Health Sciences F. Edward Hébert School of
Medicine; Staff Surgeon, Bethesda Naval Hospital,
Bethesda, Maryland.
Anatomy of Commonly Exposed Arteries

CHARLES L. WITTE, MD*
Former Professor of Surgery, University of Arizona
College of Medicine; Former Attending Surgeon, General
Surgery/Trauma, University Medical Center, Tucson,
Arizona.
*Lymph Circulatory Dynamics, Lymphangiogenesis,
and Pathophysiology of the Lymphovascular System*

* Deceased.

MARLYS H. WITTE, MD
Professor of Surgery; Director, Student Research
Programs, University of Arizona College of Medicine;
Attending in Surgery (Lymphology), University Medical
Center; Secretary-General, International Society of
Lymphology, Department of Surgery, University of
Arizona, Tucson, Arizona.
*Lymph Circulatory Dynamics, Lymphangiogenesis,
and Pathophysiology of the Lymphovascular System*

HEATHER WOLFORD, MD
Chief Resident, Department of Surgery, University of
Colorado Health Sciences Center, Denver, Colorado.
*Natural History and Nonoperative Treatment of
Chronic Lower Extremity Ischemia; Amputation:
An Overview; Revascularization versus Amputation*

KENNETH R. WOODBURN, MD, FRCSG (Gen.)
Honorary Clinical Lecturer, Peninsula Medical School,
Devon and Cornwall; Consultant Vascular Surgeon, Royal
Cornwall Hospital, Truro, Cornwall, United Kingdom.
*Lower Extremity Amputation: Technique and
Perioperative Care*

MARK C. WYERS, MD
Assistant Professor, Dartmouth Medical School, Hanover;
Assistant Professor of Surgery, Vascular, Dartmouth-
Hitchcock Medical Center, Lebanon, New Hampshire.
*Physiology and Diagnosis of Splanchnic Arterial
Occlusion*

CHENGPEI XU, MD, PhD
Senior Research Scientist, Department of Surgery,
Division of Vascular Surgery, Stanford University School
of Medicine, Stanford, California.
Artery Wall Pathology in Atherosclerosis

LIAN XUE, MD, PhD
Research Assistant Professor, Loyola University Medical
Center, Chicago, Illinois.
Prosthetic Grafts

JAMES S. T. YAO, MD, PhD
Magerstadt Professor of Surgery, Division of Vascular
Surgery, Northwestern University Feinberg School of
Medicine; Attending Surgeon, Division of Vascular
Surgery, Northwestern Memorial Hospital, Chicago,
Illinois.
Occupational Vascular Problems

RICHARD A. YEAGER, MD
Professor of Surgery, Oregon Health and Sciences
University; Vascular Chief, Portland VA Medical Center,
Portland, Oregon.
*Lower Extremity Amputation: Perioperative
Complications*

ALBERT E. YELLIN, MD, FACS
Professor of Surgery, Division of Vascular Surgery, University of Southern California Keck School of Medicine; Associate Chief of Staff and Medical Director, Surgical Services, Los Angeles County–University of Southern California Medical Center, Los Angeles, California.
Vascular Injuries of the Extremities

CHRISTOPHER K. ZARINS, MD
Professor of Surgery, Stanford University School of Medicine; Chief, Division of Vascular Surgery, Stanford University Medical Center, Stanford, California.
Artery Wall Pathology in Atherosclerosis

GERALD B. ZELENOCK, MD
Chair, Department of Surgery, and Chief of Surgical Services, William Beaumont Hospital, Royal Oak, Michigan.
Splanchnic Artery Aneurysms

R. EUGENE ZIERLER, MD
Professor of Surgery, University of Washington School of Medicine; Medical Director, Vascular Diagnostic Service, University of Washington Medical Center, Seattle, Washington.
Vascular Physiology: Essential Hemodynamic Principles; Physiologic Assessment of Peripheral Arterial Occlusive Disease

ROBERT M. ZWOLAK, MD, PhD
Professor of Surgery, Dartmouth Medical School; Attending Surgeon, Section of Vascular Surgery, Dartmouth-Hitchcock Medical Center, Lebanon, New Hampshire; Chief, Section of Vascular Surgery, White River Junction Veterans Affairs Medical Center, White River Junction, Vermont.
Arterial Duplex Scanning; Physiology and Diagnosis of Splanchnic Arterial Occlusion

Preface

This is the second time we have produced a companion review book with *Vascular Surgery*. The first one accompanied the fourth edition and was edited by Dr. William Krupski. Being chairman of the vascular surgery examinations committee of the American Board of Surgery at the time, I perceived a potential conflict of interest in editing it myself, so I asked Dr. Krupski to edit it, and, as those of you who enjoyed the first edition will attest, he did a superb job. The first edition was well received, and, based on belated complaints, it was regrettable that we did not produce one with the fifth edition.

Dr. Krupski and I developed plans for this companion review book at the same time the sixth edition of *Vascular Surgery* was planned, and we had looked forward to editing the book together this time. But, on November 27, 2004, before we could start on it, Bill Krupski tragically lost his life. In addition to contributing over 110 original peer review articles and close to 50 book chapters to our literature, Bill was an enthusiastic teacher, receiving a dozen citations for this during his career. He particularly enjoyed the question-and-answer teaching format and worked for a number of years on the SESAP committee. He was committed to excellence in every aspect of his professional career. Needless to say, this companion review book, and our specialty, is much the worse for his loss.

This book differs from the first edition in that it consists of multiple-choice questions, usually three drawn from each chapter of the textbook, *each with five possible answers, only one of which is correct.* The correct answers, accompanied by a point-by-point discussion, are located separately in each section. Clearly, the intention is for the reader to commit to a particular answer before discovering which is correct and why, because it has been shown that one learns more from getting an answer wrong, once explained, than guessing the right one.

This review book is intended to provide a good test of knowledge of vascular disease and its management. As an indicator of the reader's knowledge and understanding of the many topics represented in the textbook, it should pinpoint chapters deserving further study, since chapter numbers are used to identify the questions. This book is intended to be an educational tool and an adjunct to the textbook, which is, by its scope and depth, not likely to be read from cover, but rather will be read topically, serving as a reference for researching problems arising in clinical practice. Although this self-assessment review book may be helpful in preparing for multiple-choice examinations in vascular surgery and the question format is similar, its contents arc quite different in that they are meant to be more educational than just a test of knowledge. The discussions accompanying the correct answer serve this broader purpose and really reach to the core of each question and are the best part, in my view. In most of the discussions, the parts that pertain to each of the five possible answers are keyed to them by A, B, C, D, and E designations inserted in the text.

In addition to its self-assessment role, this review book will find good use as a vehicle for vascular surgery teaching rounds with students, residents, and fellows. The question-and-answer format is an excellent approach to teaching and learning. Having the questions numerically keyed to chapters in the textbook allows individuals to follow through in depth on specific aspects of the diagnosis and management of vascular disease. A systematic topical review of *Vascular Surgery,* assigning the questions from a particular chapter to individual participants in advance of each session, has proved to be a valuable learning experience in the past.

I would like to express my sincere thanks to all the chapter authors who submitted thoughtful questions, for creating good questions is a challenging task, and also to the section editors for taking up the slack and helping with the editing of this book in Bill Krupski's absence. I also wish to acknowledge the support of dedicated staff at Elsevier—publisher Natasha Andjelkovic, developmental editor Donna Morrissey, project manager Cecelia Bayruns, senior book designer Ellen Zanolle, and senior marketing manager Ethel Cathers.

We hope our efforts have resulted in a useful means for vascular surgeons to assess and advance their knowledge of the diagnosis and management of vascular disease.

Robert B. Rutherford, MD

Contents

Section I

BASIC CONSIDERATION FOR CLINICAL PRACTICE   1
  Robert B. Rutherford

Chapter 1
Essentials of Clinical Evaluation   1

Chapter 2
Selection of Patients for Vascular Treatments   1

Chapter 3
Essential Considerations in Evaluating the Results of Treatment   1

Chapter 4
Maintaining a Computerized Vascular Registry   2

Chapter 5
Proper Outcomes Assessment: Patient-Based and Economic Evaluations of Vascular Interventions   2

Chapter 6
Standardized Reporting Practices   3

Answers for Section I   4

Section II

BASIC VASCULAR SCIENCE   9
  Anton N. Sidawy

Chapter 7
Embryology of the Vascular System   9

Chapter 8
Basic Considerations of the Arterial Wall in Health and Disease   9

Chapter 9
Vascular Physiology: Essential Hemodynamic Principles   9

Chapter 10
Artery Wall Pathology in Atherosclerosis   10

Chapter 11
Intimal Hyperplasia: Basic Response to Arterial and Vein Graft Injury and Reconstruction   10

Chapter 12
Molecular Biology and Gene Therapy in Vascular Disease   10

Answers for Section II   12

Section III

THE VASCULAR DIAGNOSTIC LABORATORY: BASIC TECHNIQUES   17
  Gregory L. Moneta

Chapter 13
The Vascular Laboratory   17

Chapter 14
Physiologic Assessment of Peripheral Arterial Occlusive Disease   17

Chapter 15
Physiologic Assessment of the Venous System   18

Chapter 16
Arterial Duplex Scanning   18

Chapter 17
Venous Duplex Scanning   19

Answers for Section III   20

Section IV

VASCULAR IMAGING: BASIC TECHNIQUES AND APPLICATIONS   23
  Hugh G. Beebe

Chapter 18
Principles of Arteriography   23

Chapter 19
Principles of Venography   23

Chapter 20

3D Image Processing 24

Chapter 21

Computed Tomography, CT Angiography, and 3D Reconstruction for the Evaluation of Vascular Disease 24

Chapter 22

Magnetic Resonance Imaging and Angiography 25

Chapter 23

Intravascular Ultrasound 25

Answers for Section IV 26

Section V

ARTERIAL DISEASES: BASIC CONSIDERATIONS 31
R. James Valentine

Chapter 24

Atherosclerosis: Plaque Characteristics and Concepts of Evolution 31

Chapter 25

Thromboangiitis Obliterans (Buerger's Disease) 31

Chapter 26

Takayasu's Disease: Nonspecific Aortoarteritis 31

Chapter 27

Arterial Fibrodysplasia 32

Chapter 28

Uncommon Arteriopathies 32

Chapter 29

Arterial Aneurysms: Etiologic Considerations 33

Answers for Section V 34

Section VI

BLEEDING AND CLOTTING: FUNDAMENTAL CONSIDERATIONS 39
Thomas W. Wakefield

Chapter 30

Normal and Abnormal Coagulation 39

Chapter 31

Antithrombotic Therapy 39

Chapter 32

Thrombolytic Agents and Their Actions 39

Chapter 33

Perioperative Considerations: Coagulopathy and Hemorrhage 40

Chapter 34

Vascular Thrombosis Due to Hypercoagulable States 40

Answers for Section VI 42

Section VII

NONOPERATIVE MANAGEMENT OF PATIENTS WITH VASCULAR DISEASES 45
Russell H. Samson

Chapter 35

Overview: Medical Management in a Vascular Surgery Practice[*]

Chapter 36

Atherogenesis and the Medical Management of Atherosclerosis 45

Chapter 37

Medical Treatment of Intermittent Claudication 45

Chapter 38

Hyperglycemia, Diabetes, and Syndrome X 46

Chapter 39

Hypertension and Patients with Vascular Disorders 46

Chapter 40

Vascular Pain 46

Answers for Section VII 48

Section VIII

OPEN VASCULAR SURGERY: BASIC CONSIDERATIONS 51
John J. Ricotta

Chapter 41

General Strategies: Choice of Procedure and Technique 51

---

[*] Asterisks denote chapters without questions.

Chapter 42

Anatomy of Commonly Exposed Arteries 51

Chapter 43

Basic Vascular Surgical Techniques 51

Chapter 44

Techniques for Thromboembolectomy of Native Arteries and Bypass Grafts 52

Chapter 45

Endarterectomy 52

Chapter 46

Vascular Conduits: An Overview 52

Chapter 47

The Autogenous Grafts 53

Chapter 48

The Modified Biograft 53

Chapter 49

Prosthetic Grafts 54

Answers for Section VIII 55

Section IX

ENDOVASCULAR SURGERY: BASIC CONSIDERATIONS 61
Kenneth Ouriel

Chapter 50

Training in Endovascular Surgery 61

Chapter 51

Fundamental Techniques in Endovascular Surgery 61

Chapter 52

Basic Techniques of Endovascular Aneurysm Repair 62

Chapter 53

Intra-arterial Catheter-Directed Thrombolysis 62

Chapter 54

Complications of Endovascular Procedures 62

Answers for Section IX 64

Section X

COMPLICATIONS OF VASCULAR SURGERY AND ISCHEMIA: PREVENTION AND MANAGEMENT 67
Bruce Perler

Chapter 55

Overview[*]

Chapter 56

Cardiac Complications: Screening and Prevention 67

Chapter 57

Respiratory Complications in Vascular Surgery 67

Chapter 58

Renal Complications 68

Chapter 59

Infection in Prosthetic Vascular Grafts 68

Chapter 60

Anastomotic Aneurysms 68

Chapter 61

Aortoenteric Fistula 69

Chapter 62

Ischemic Neuropathy 69

Chapter 63

Lymphatic Complications of Vascular Surgery 69

Chapter 64

Postoperative Sexual Dysfunction after Aortoiliac Interventions 69

Chapter 65

Postoperative Graft Thrombosis: Prevention and Management 70

Answers for Section X 71

Section XI

ACUTE LIMB ISCHEMIA 77
Kenneth Ouriel

Chapter 66

Acute Limb Ischemia 77

[*] Asterisks denote chapters without questions.

Chapter 67

Arterial Thromboembolism 77

Chapter 68

Atheromatous Embolization 78

Answers for Section XI 79

Section XII

VASCULAR TRAUMA 83
Fred A. Weaver

Chapter 69

Epidemiology and Natural History of Vascular Trauma 83

Chapter 70

Carotid and Vertebral Artery Injuries 83

Chapter 71

Thoracic Vascular Trauma 84

Chapter 72

Abdominal Vascular Injuries 84

Chapter 73

Vascular Injuries of the Extremities 84

Chapter 74

Compartment Syndromes: Pathophysiology, Recognition, and Management 85

Chapter 75

Causalgia and Post-traumatic Pain Syndromes 86

Answers for Section XII 87

Section XIII

MANAGEMENT OF CHRONIC ISCHEMIA OF THE LOWER EXTREMITIES 93
K. Wayne Johnston

Chapter 76

The Chronically Ischemic Leg: An Overview[*]

Chapter 77

Natural History and Nonoperative Treatment of Chronic Lower Extremity Ischemia 93

_____

[*] Asterisks denote chapters without questions.

Chapter 78

Evaluation of the Patient with Chronic Lower Extremity Ischemia 93

Chapter 79

Direct Reconstruction for Aortoiliac Occlusive Disease 94

Chapter 80

Extra-Anatomic Bypass 94

Chapter 81

Infrainguinal Bypass 94

Chapter 82

Profundaplasty: Isolated and Adjunctive Applications 95

Chapter 83

Secondary Arterial Reconstructions in the Lower Extremity 95

Chapter 84

Endovascular Surgery in the Management of Chronic Lower Extremity Ischemia 96

Chapter 85

Lumbar Sympathectomy: Indications and Technique 96

Chapter 86

Nonatheromatous Causes of Popliteal Artery Disease 96

Chapter 87

Management of Foot Ulcers in Diabetes Mellitus 97

Chapter 88

Vasculogenic Erectile Dysfunction 97

Answers for Section XIII 98

Section XIV

NEUROVASCULAR CONDITIONS INVOLVING THE UPPER EXTREMITY 107
William H. Pearce

Chapter 89

Overview[*]

Chapter 90

Evaluation of Upper Extremity Ischemia   107

Chapter 91

Brachiocephalic Vessel Reconstruction   107

Chapter 92

Upper Extremity Revascularization   108

Chapter 93

Raynaud's Syndrome: Vasospastic and Occulsive Arterial Disease Involving the Distal Upper Extremity   108

Chapter 94

Neurogenic Thoracic Outlet Syndrome   108

Chapter 95

Arterial Complications of Thoracic Outlet Compression   109

Chapter 96

Subclavian-Axillary Vein Thrombosis   109

Chapter 97

Upper Extremity Sympathectomy   109

Chapter 98

Occupational Vascular Problems   109

Answers for Section XIV   111

Section XV

ARTERIAL ANEURYSMS   117
Jack L. Cronenwett

Chapter 99

Overview   117

Chapter 100

Abdominal Aortic and Iliac Aneurysms   117

Chapter 101

Endovascular Treatment of Aortic Aneurysms   117

Chapter 102

Ruptured Abdominal Aortic Aneurysms   118

Chapter 103

Thoracoabdominal Aortic Aneurysms   118

Chapter 104

Aortic Dissection: Perspectives for the Vascular/ Endovascular Surgeon   119

Chapter 105

Lower Extremity Aneurysms   119

Chapter 106

Upper Extremity Aneurysms   120

Chapter 107

Splanchnic Artery Aneurysms   120

Chapter 108

Infected Aneurysms   120

Answers for Section XV   122

Section XVI

ARTERIOVENOUS FISTULAS, VASCULAR MALFORMATIONS, AND VASCULAR TUMORS   131
Robert B. Rutherford

Chapter 109

Overview[*]

Chapter 110

Diagnostic Evaluation of Arteriovenous Fistulas and Vascular Anomalies   131

Chapter 111

Arteriovenous Fistulas of the Aorta and Its Major Branches   132

Chapter 112

Traumatic Arteriovenous Fistulas   132

Chapter 113

Vascular Tumors and Malformations in Childhood   132

Chapter 114

Surgical Management of Vascular Malformations   133

[*] Asterisks denote chapters without questions.

Chapter 115

Endovascular Treatment of Vascular Anomalies   133

Chapter 116

Primary Tumors of Major Blood Vessels: Diagnosis and Management   133

Answers for Section XVI   135

Section XVII

ARTERIOVENOUS HEMODIALYSIS ACCESS   143
Anton N. Sidawy

Chapter 117

Strategies of Arteriovenous Dialysis Access   143

Chapter 118

Venous Transpositions in the Creation of Arteriovenous Access   143

Chapter 119

Management of Thrombosed Dialysis Access   144

Chapter 120

Nonthrombotic Complications of Arteriovenous Access for Hemodialysis   144

Answers for Section XVII   145

Section XVIII

THE MANAGEMENT OF SPLANCHNIC VASCULAR LESIONS AND DISORDERS   149
James M. Seeger

Chapter 121

Physiology and Diagnosis of Splanchnic Arterial Occlusion   149

Chapter 122

Treatment of Acute Intestinal Ischemia Caused by Arterial Occlusions   150

Chapter 123

Diagnosis and Treatment of Nonocclusive Mesenteric Ischemia   150

Chapter 124

Chronic Mesenteric Ischemia   150

Chapter 125

Intestinal Ischemia Caused by Venous Thrombosis   151

Chapter 126

Portal Hypertension: Surgical Management of Its Complications   152

Answers for Section XVIII   153

Section XIX

THE MANAGEMENT OF RENOVASCULAR DISORDERS   159
Kimberley J. Hansen

Chapter 127

Renovascular Disease: An Overview*

Chapter 128

Renal Artery Imaging and Physiologic Testing   159

Chapter 129

Renal Artery Fibrodysplasia and Renovascular Hypertension   159

Chapter 130

Atherosclerotic Renovascular Disease and Ischemic Nephropathy   159

Chapter 131

Endovascular Treatment of Renovascular Disease   160

Chapter 132

Open Surgical Repair of Renovascular Disease   160

Chapter 133

Renal Artery Aneurysms and Arteriovenous Fistulae   160

Chapter 134

Acute Renovascular Occlusive Events   160

Answers for Section XIX   162

*Asterisks denote chapters without questions.

Section **XX**

MANAGEMENT OF EXTRACRANIAL CEREBROVASCULAR DISEASE 167
William C. Krupski

Chapter **135**

Fundamental Considerations in Cerebrovascular Disease 167

Chapter **136**

Diagnostic Evaluation and Medical Management of Patients with Ischemic Cerebrovascular Disease 167

Chapter **137**

Anatomy and Angiographic Diagnosis of Extracranial and Intracranial Vascular Disease 168

Chapter **138**

The Role of Noninvasive Studies in the Diagnosis and Management of Cerebrovascular Disease 168

Chapter **139**

Indications, Surgical Technique, and Results for Repair of Extracranial Occlusive Lesions 169

Chapter **140**

Carotid Angioplasty and Stenting 169

Chapter **141**

Vertebrobasilar Ischemia: Indications, Techniques, and Results of Surgical Repair 169

Chapter **142**

Endovascular and Surgical Management of Extracranial Carotid Fibromuscular Arterial Dysplasia 170

Chapter **143**

Aneurysms of the Extracranial Carotid Artery 171

Chapter **144**

Uncommon Disorders Affecting the Carotid Arteries 171

Chapter **145**

Complications Following Carotid Endarterectomy and Perioperative Management 172

Answers for Section XX 173

Section **XXI**

THE MANAGEMENT OF VENOUS DISORDERS 183
Peter Gloviczki

Chapter **146**

Introduction and General Considerations[*]

Chapter **147**

Pathophysiology and Natural History of Acute Deep Venous Thrombosis 183

Chapter **148**

Clinical and Diagnostic Evaluation of the Patient with Deep Venous Thrombosis 183

Chapter **149**

Prevention and Medical Treatment of Acute Deep Venous Thrombosis 184

Chapter **150**

Catheter-Based Interventions for Acute Deep Venous Thrombosis 184

Chapter **151**

Surgical Thrombectomy for Acute Deep Venous Thrombosis 184

Chapter **152**

Vena Caval Interruption Procedures 184

Chapter **153**

Superficial Thrombophlebitis: Diagnosis and Management 185

Chapter **154**

The Pathophysiology of Chronic Venous Insufficiency 185

Chapter **155**

Classification and Clinical and Diagnostic Evaluation of Patients with Chronic Venous Disorders 185

Chapter **156**

Nonoperative Management of Chronic Venous Insufficiency 186

[*] Asterisks denote chapters without questions.

Chapter 157

Varicose Veins: Treatment by Intervention Including Sclerotherapy   186

Chapter 158

Management of Perforator Vein Incompetence   187

Chapter 159

The Surgical Treatment of Deep Venous Valvular Incompetence   187

Chapter 160

Surgical Treatment of Chronic Occlusions of the Iliac Veins and the Inferior Vena Cava   188

Chapter 161

Endovascular Treatment of Chronic Occlusions of the Iliac Veins and the Inferior Vena Cava   188

Chapter 162

Endovascular Treatment of Vena Caval Occlusions   189

Chapter 163

Evaluation and Management of Malignant Tumors of the Inferior Vena Cava   189

Chapter 164

Surgical Treatment of Superior Vena Cava Syndrome   189

Answers for Section XXI   191

Section XXII

THE MANAGEMENT OF LYMPHATIC DISORDERS   203
Peter Gloviczki

Chapter 165

Lymphedema: An Overview   203

Chapter 166

Lymph Circulatory Dynamics, Lymphangiogenesis, and Pathophysiology of the Lymphovascular System   203

Chapter 167

Clinical Diagnosis and Evaluation of Lymphedema   204

Chapter 168

Nonoperative Management of Chronic Lymphedema   204

Chapter 169

Surgical Treatment of Chronic Lymphedema and Primary Chylous Complications   204

Answers for Section XXII   205

Section XXIII

EXTREMITY AMPUTATION FOR VASCULAR DISEASE   209
Mark R. Nehler

Chapter 170

Amputation: An Overview   209

Chapter 171

Lower Extremity Amputation: Indications, Patient Evaluation, and Level Determination   209

Chapter 172

Lower Extremity Amputation: Technique and Perioperative Care   210

Chapter 173

Lower Extremity Amputation: Perioperative Complications   210

Chapter 174

Functional Outcome and Natural History of Major Lower Extremity Amputation   211

Chapter 175

Upper Extremity Amputation   211

Chapter 176

Revascularization versus Amputation   211

Answers for Section XXIII   213

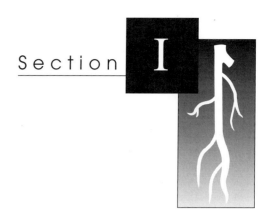

BASIC CONSIDERATION FOR CLINICAL PRACTICE

STUDY QUESTIONS

■ QUESTIONS FOR CHAPTER 1

Question 1-1

Chronic extremity swelling:

A. Demonstrates "pitting" edema only when cardiac in origin.
B. Is completely relieved by extremity elevation only when it is of venous origin.
C. Most commonly involves both extremities to a similar extent.
D. Does not significantly involve the feet and toes.
E. Is associated with pigmentation and cicatricial changes around the ankle only with chronic venous insufficiency.

Question 1-2

Chronic leg ulcers:

A. Are almost always caused by arterial or venous insufficiency.
B. Are helped to heal by dependency, which improves the distal perfusion.
C. Are not associated with pain unless secondarily infected.
D. Can almost always be diagnosed as to origin by physical examination alone.
E. Have an unpredictable spontaneous healing potential.

Question 1-3

Extremity pain of vascular origin:

A. Is difficult to diagnose by history.
B. Is usually associated with leg cramps if nocturnal.
C. Must be of arterial origin if it is precipitated by exercise.
D. Is significantly affected by leg elevation.
E. Is a harbinger of limb loss if a vascular reconstructive procedure is not successfully performed.

■ QUESTIONS FOR CHAPTER 2

Question 2-1

A patient presents with ½ block right thigh claudication of 6 months duration. There is a bruit in the right hypochondrium and a diminished right femoral pulse, suggesting a right iliac stenosis. Which of the following would be the most important in deciding against offering percutaneous transluminal angioplasty (PTA)/stenting of a right iliac stenosis?

A. Patient is retired, is not required to walk to work.
B. Patient has not had a trial of pentoxifylline.
C. The patient failed to persist with exercise therapy.
D. The absence of rest pain or ischemic foot lesions.
E. A right ankle-brachial index (ABI) of 0.45 and a left ABI of 0.55.

Question 2-2

After 9 months of treatment a 54-year-old rancher is referred with persistent 1 block right thigh claudication. Vascular laboratory studies show a right ABI of 0.70 and a left ABI of 0.95, and duplex scan demonstrates only a right iliac stenosis. Which of the following would be least important in convincing you to now proceed with PTA/stent of the right iliac stenosis?

A. The absence of angina.
B. Risk factors (hypertension, smoking, hyperlipidemia) have been well controlled with patient compliance.
C. The patient cannot tend to his ranch.
D. Exercise therapy was not successful.
E. Cilostazol (Pletal) increased walking distance from only half of a block to one block.

Question 2-3

A sedentary 76 year old attends a health fair where he is found to have a blood pressure of 150/95 and bilateral ABIs of 0.40. He has no rest pain or foot lesions. Your advice is sought. Which of the following is/are *not* appropriate initial management options?

A. Control of hypertension.
B. Obtain a lipid profile.
C. Referral to a podiatrist.
D. Stent any discrete proximal lesion to reduce the high risk of limb loss.
E. None of the above.

■ QUESTIONS FOR CHAPTER 3

Question 3-1

In comparing the reported results of two different institutions' experience with carotid endarterectomy, which of the following factors is most likely to influence early outcomes?

A. Length of stay in the intensive care unit and hospital.
B. General versus local/regional anesthesia.
C. Community versus university hospital.
D. Disease severity.
E. Patch versus non-patch.

Question 3-2

In comparing the 5-year patencies of two randomized groups of above-knee femoropopliteal bypasses performed with prosthesis (n = 21) and reversed saphenous vein (n = 22) over the same time internal, which method, if any, would be a/the proper method for comparing 5-year patencies?

A. Percent patent at the cutoff point for analysis (5 years after beginning the study).
B. Percent patent 5 years after bypass.
C. A 5-year patency estimate by the Life Table Method.
D. A 5-year patency estimate by the Kaplan-Meier method.
E. Any of the above (number of bypasses and time frame are equivalent).

Question 3-3

At follow-up after infrainguinal bypass, which of the following is not acceptable as sole criteria for reporting patency?

A. Palpable pedal pulse.
B. Patency observed at operation (e.g., graft removal for infection).
C. Patent by Duplex scan.
D. Patent by arteriography.
E. Persistent elevation of the ABI at the postoperative level of improvement.

■   QUESTIONS FOR CHAPTER 4

Question 4-1

Which answer is *not* correct?

In maintaining a vascular database one must:

A. Frequently back up the database.
B. Enter data in a timely fashion.
C. If using a commercial product, keep up with the latest versions of the software.
D. Proofread the entries.
E. Hire an assistant or consultant sufficiently expert in software programming and design to be capable of modifying the design of the database to suit your changing needs.

Question 4-2

A computerized database consists of:

A. Fields.
B. Queries.
C. Reports.
D. Relationships.
E. All of the above.

Question 4-3

Which answer is *false?*

A vascular registry:

A. Is a clinical and research tool.
B. Could be as simple as a collection of basic demographic data on index cards.

C. Requires computerization.
D. Can be used to compare surgeons' outcome data.
E. Requires dedication to data entry and maintenances.

■   QUESTIONS FOR CHAPTER 5

Question 5-1

Which of the following statements about lower extremity ischemia is correct?

A. ABI correlates well with the severity of symptoms reported by the patient.
B. After surgery for claudication, improvement in patient symptoms correlates well with increase in ABI.
C. There are no survey tools for patient reporting of general health that are useful in patients with lower extremity arterial occlusive disease.
D. Graft patency and increased ABI are sufficient for the assessment of patient outcome after treatment of lower extremity arterial occlusive disease.
E. Patient reported outcomes regarding physical function, role function, perceived health, and pain may be worse after vascular reconstruction despite the presence of a patent graft.

Question 5-2

Which of the following statements about the Short Form (SF)-36 is *not* true?

A. The SF-36 is specific for peripheral arterial disease (PAD) and may be used to track changes in patient's walking ability.
B. This survey tool, easily completed by patients, reliably indicates status of and changes in perceived health, psychologic well-being, role limitations caused by physical health problems, role limitations caused by emotional health problems, physical function, social relations, pain, and fatigue.
C. The eight domains of the SF-36 are both independently and collectively useful to track changes in patient status.
D. Physical function, role function, and pain scores are affected by PAD but are not specific for it.
E. The SF-36 is a validated and reliable patient assessment tool that has been broadly applied to patient populations with a wide variety of disease states.

Question 5-3

Which of the following would *not* benefit from extended patient outcomes assessment, including the use of a general health measure?

A. Analysis of the benefits of endovascular aortic aneurysm repair compared with open aneurysm resection.
B. Office-based assessment of patient improvement after vascular intervention.
C. Comparison of structural problems with aortic endovascular grafts.
D. Evaluation of the long-term benefits of tibial artery angioplasty.
E. Documentation of the benefits of treating patients with ruptured abdominal aortic aneurysms (AAAs).

■ QUESTIONS FOR CHAPTER 6

Question 6-1

Reporting standards recommend uniform practices for reporting the diagnosis and treatment of diseases in scientific journals, as opposed to practice standards, which recommend standards of care for those diseases. Each of the following is a component of reporting standards *except*:

A. Clinical classification of disease.
B. Criteria for improvement, deterioration, and failure.
C. Exclusion criteria for specific recommended treatment.
D. Categorization of operations and interventions.
E. Complications encountered with grades for severity or outcome.

Question 6-2

A 65-year-old man with 1 block claudication undergoes angioplasty and stenting of the superficial femoral artery. Six months later, elevated velocities are noted on duplex examination of the intervened area. Angiography is again performed demonstrating an area of in-stent restenosis, which is successfully treated by percutaneous angioplasty. This intervention should be reported as maintaining:

A. Clinical success.
B. Primary patency.
C. Assisted primary patency.
D. Secondary patency.
E. Tertiary patency.

Question 6-3

A bypass graft or otherwise reconstructed arterial segment may be considered patent when certain strict criteria are met. For scientific reports that require precise documentation, the following are considered an adequate assessment of patency *except*:

A. Palpable pulses recorded at a clinic visit.
B. Arteriography.
C. Duplex scan.
D. Maintenance of the achieved improvement in the appropriate segmental pressure index.
E. Direct observation of patency at operation or postmortem examination.

ANSWERS AND DISCUSSION

■ ANSWERS AND DISCUSSION FOR CHAPTER 1

Answer 1-1: E

Discussion 1-1

A. Pitting edema is typically produced by cardiac failure but is also present when edema is produced by severe hypoproteinemia.

B. Edema resulting from heart failure, as well as venous edema, can be relieved by extremity elevation, and to a great extent both dissipate overnight; however, in the former setting, the mobilization of fluid may produce orthopnea, paroxysmal nocturnal dyspnea, and nocturia.

C. Congestive heart failure frequently causes bilateral edema, whereas lymphedema is usually unilateral and most cases of chronic venous edema are either unilateral or at least asymmetric. Even cardiac edema is not usually symmetric.

D. Lymphedema typically begins with the toes and feet. It may progress to involve the ankles and leg in ascending fashion but not without involving the feet and toes. Cardiac edema and other orthostatic edema can also involve the feet to a degree, but venous edema almost never does.

E. Venous edema, and sometimes edema of heart failure, produces pigmentation from the breakdown of extravasated red blood cells, but only venous edema progresses, in the chronic state, to produce subcutaneous fibrosis and cutaneous atrophy in response to the extravasated red blood cells and plasma proteins. Therefore chronic venous edema is ultimately associated with second cicatricial changes and pigmentation. In the late stages of lymphedema ("elephantiasis") areas of pigmentation may develop, particularly around ankle folds, but the skin becomes hypertrophic and the subcutaneous tissues remain full because of various sizes of "lakes" of accumulated lymph. Therefore, only chronic venous edema produces contraction and scarring of the subcutaneous tissues around the ankle.

Answer 1-2: D

Discussion 1-2

A. Chronic leg ulcers are usually of arterial, venous, *or neuropathic* origin (example of latter: diabetic foot ulcers).

B. Dependency may help the healing of superficial arterial ulcers and at least relieve associated ischemic pain, but the healing of venous ulcer is aided by elevation, not dependency.

C. Neurotrophic ulcers are often not painful, whereas ischemic ulcers, whether infected and uninfected, are usually associated with ischemic "rest" pain. Venous ulcers may not be painful but usually are, and the more painful the venous ulcer, the greater the likelihood of secondary infection.

D. The underlying cause of chronic leg ulcers is usually apparent from location, appearance, and associated physical signs (e.g., absent pulses, signs of chronic venous insufficiency, or detectable neuropathy). Arterial and neuropathic ulcers are usually located on the foot, although any bony prominence or pressure point is susceptible to the latter, and the latter are painless. Venous ulcers are usually located near the malleoli or at least in the "gaiter" distribution, and the surrounding area shows signs of chronic venous insufficiency (e.g., pigmentation, subcutaneous fibrosis, and cutaneous atrophy). The chronically ischemic foot typically is "skeletonized," that is, has atrophy of the skin, its appendages (dry with absent hair), and subcutaneous fat.

E. The healing potential of leg ulcers can be predicted on the basis of noninvasive testing (e.g., segmental pressures, plethysmography, and capillary oxygen tension) and the ability to control the underlying cause (e.g., venous hypertension for venous ulcers, focal pressure points for neuropathic ulcers, and, for ischemic ulcers, the feasibility of revascularization options).

Answer 1-3: D

Discussion 1-3

A. Extremity pain of vascular origin is usually so characteristic that it can be readily suspected even before physical examination. The nature and location of the pain and the effect of exercise, rest, or elevation offer immediate clues.

B. Nocturnal leg cramps are often mistakenly attributed to vascular disease but in fact are much more common in elderly patients without vascular disease. The leg cramps associated with arterial disease come on with exercise and are relieved by rest and therefore are not present at night, with the patient recumbent and at rest. Critical limb ischemia is commonly associated with ischemic rest pain of the *foot* at night rather than nocturnal leg cramps.

C. Leg pain or discomfort brought on by exercise and relieved by rest is typical of arterial occlusive disease, and this is called claudication. However, severe venous outflow of obstruction, severe enough to produce a rapid increase in venous hypertension with exercise, is called venous claudication. This rarer form of vascular leg pain produced by exercise and relieved by rest can be identified not only by associated evidence of venous disease but also by the induced pain not being *promptly* relieved by stopping the exercise, as is the case with arterial claudication.

D. Pain caused by venous hypertension, the unifying effect of chronic venous insufficiency, is relieved by leg elevation. The rest pain of critical limb ischemia is precipitated by, or made worse by, leg elevation, and claudication does not occur during leg elevation (no exercise, no leg pain). Therefore, extremity pain of vascular origin, whether arterial or venous is affected, one way or another, by elevation.

E. Most extremity pain of vascular origin can be treated without an operation and without risk of limb loss; the pain, at rest, of critical limb ischemia, with or without ulceration/gangrene, is the only major exception to this. Painful claudication is greatly ameliorated by exercise programs and cessation of smoking, with only approximately a 5% risk of limb loss within 5 years, and well over 90% of chronic venous insufficiency can be controlled by elastic stockings and frequent leg elevation in compliant patients.

■ ANSWERS AND DISCUSSION FOR CHAPTER 2

Answer 2-1: E

Discussion 2-1

A. Retired patients should not be categorically disqualified for an otherwise appropriate intervention. They might thus be denied a long anticipated active retirement (e.g., hunting, fishing, golfing), which is disabling in itself. Other considerations are more important.
B. Pentoxifylline might improve claudication but not enough to relieve the disability. Most pharmacotherapy for claudication is unlikely to more than double the claudication distance, that is, allow the patient to walk more than 1 block.
C. An attempt at this conservative approach is normally recommended, but failure to persist with exercise therapy is not uncommon and may depend more on patient attitudes than insufficient benefit.
D. Although rest pain or ischemic lesions are accepted as mandatory indications for intervention, disabling claudication can be an appropriate indication if conservative therapy does not succeed for whatever reason, as long as atherosclerosis risk factor control is also instituted. The proposed intervention must also offer a favorable benefit:risk ratio.
E. A right ABI of 0.45 and a left ABI of 0.55 indicate bilateral, almost equally severe occlusive disease, not just an isolated right iliac stenosis. Bilateral runoff disease is likely with these low ABIs. *Unilateral* iliac PTA/stent would not be the appropriate intervention.

Answer 2-2: A

Discussion 2-2

A. This degree of claudication may mask angina. Relatively early-onset atherosclerosis with multiple risk factors suggests the likelihood of coronary disease. This should be investigated before proceeding with a PTA/stent of the iliac stenosis.
B. Institution of risk factor control is an important part of management.
C. The patient's claudication is still disabling and interfering with his livelihood.
D. A trial of exercise was made.
E. The relief of claudication has not been adequate for the patient's needs.

Answer 2-3: D

Discussion 2-3

This patient has subcritical ischemia. This discovery provides an opportunity to institute risk factor control so A and B are appropriate.

He is sedentary so may not have experienced claudication, but such patients can proceed to critical ischemia be-

cause of relatively minor foot trauma, such as incurred from cutting nails. Preventative foot care, including having nails trimmed by a podiatrist, could avoid this, so C is also appropriate.

It is tempting to prevent progression to limb loss with a low-risk endovascular procedure, but D is not appropriate *initial* management in this elderly man. Noninvasive testing to demonstrate the underlying lesions would be justified and would help if there was acute progression. Control of hypertension could bring on rest pain and justify intervention.

■ ANSWERS AND DISCUSSION FOR CHAPTER 3

Answer 3-1: D

Discussion 3-1

A. Programs to shorten hospital stay and reduce intensive care unit observation time postoperatively, in response to managed care pressures, have been shown *not* to impact outcomes.
B. The expected benefits of local/regional anesthesia, reduced postendarterectomy blood pressure swings, and shortened intensive care unit stay, have been difficult to prove statistically, but there have been no significant differences between the two in postoperative mortality and stroke.
C. Hospital/surgeon volume may make a difference, but the setting of university versus community hospital has not made a difference.
D. Greater disease severity, in terms of clinical stage (asymptomatic, transient ischemic attack, completed stroke, acute stroke—in that order), lesion severity (degree of stenosis/ulceration), and disease in collateral pathways (contralateral carotid, vertebral), has a major impact on outcomes, as do patient risk factors (not listed).
E. Patching has been shown to produce better outcomes than primary closure, but not to the degree of severity of disease or patient risk.

Answer 3-2: D

Discussion 3-2

Answer A would give the highest patency rate, by including a number of recent cases still patent and answer B would give the lowest patency rate, counting only those patent after 5 years had passed since bypass. Both the Life Table and Kaplan-Meier methods are accepted methods of estimating patencies at a given point in time after bypass when analyzing cases undergoing operation (entered) at different times over the study period, but the Life Table Method (C) is not valid for smaller numbers of cases (<30) so the Kaplan-Meier estimate (D) would be preferred in analyzing this small study.

Answer 3-3: A

Discussion 3-3

Arteriographic patency (B) used to be the gold standard, and although this is still valid, it cannot be justified for periodic follow-up. To avoid such use of arteriography, noninvasive laboratory evidence became accepted as objective evidence of patency, in this case a persistently elevated ABI. (E) Although an elevated ABI is still acceptable, the wide availability of duplex scan (C), with its frequent use in graft surveillance, has made it the preferred method, supplanting the pressure index. Duplex or some other imaging technique (e.g., magnetic resonance angiography [MRA]) is required to confirm patency if the ABI has decreased, even if it remains 0.10 above the preoperative level. Occasionally an infected graft has to be removed, and its visualized patency at operation (B) is also accepted. A palpable pedal pulse (A) may suffice for personal clinical follow-up, but it has been found to be unreliable when performed in clinic follow-ups, and a note in the chart to this effect is *not acceptable* for reporting on patencies. Furthermore, vein bypass grafts remaining patent in the face of severe runoff disease (e.g., only peroneal artery runoff) may not have a palpable pedal pulse.

■ ANSWERS AND DISCUSSION FOR CHAPTER 4

Answer 4-1: E
Discussion 4-1

(A) Frequently backing up the data and (B) entering it in a timely fashion are essential to prevent loss of data or incorrect data entry. Similarly, one must (D) proofread the entries to prevent "garbage in, garbage out." (C) Commercial products frequently upgrade software, and this can be beneficial. New versions are designed to keep up with changing needs and are user friendly enough to allow categoric changes, such as updating disease and procedural codes, including disease severity scoring, and so forth. Therefore, in most cases, expert software designers (E) are not necessary once a database has been constructed.

Answer 4-2: E

All of the responses are parts of a computerized database.

Answer 4-3: C
Discussion 4-3

A. A vascular registry is a valuable research tool but it is also useful in clinical practice.
B. Such a database can be developed without the use of a computer; however it will be limited in its use.
C. A computerized registry is an important practice tool but its *computerization is not necessary* (see B). It does require the commitment of considerable time and effort to maintain the quality of the data to allow meaningful analysis, but computerization, in the long run, saves time when it comes to data retrieval and analysis.
D. It can be used to compare surgeons' outcome data. Of course, this requires the cooperation of the surgeons involved, and entering their data in the same manner on the same database.
E. Dedication to data entry and maintenance, committing the time and effort involved, is probably the most difficult part for busy surgeons.

■ ANSWERS AND DISCUSSION FOR CHAPTER 5

Answer 5-1: E
Discussion 5-1

A. Numerous studies have documented that the symptoms experienced by a patient are not directly related to the ABI. A patient with a relatively low index may have no sense of claudication or rest pain, whereas a patient with only a moderate decrease in index may experience a significant limitation in ambulatory abilities.
B. Numerous studies have documented that technically successful interventional treatment of claudication may not correlate with improvement in quality of life as reported by the patient.
C. Although the SF-36 is a generic health care measure and not specific for lower extremity arterial occlusive disease, it has been standardized and used reliably for the detection in changes in patient-reported general health of claudicants.
D. Neither graft patency nor ABI index can reliably predict patient outcomes after intervention for lower extremity arterial occlusive disease, especially with regard to walking distance and improvement in general health.
E. As noted in several studies, careful assessment of patient outcomes using a combination of clinical and patient-reported parameters have indicated that successful lower extremity revascularization may not lead directly to an improvement in the patient's quality of life.

Answer 5-2: A
Discussion 5-2

A. Although the SF-36 can be used to track changes in the general health of patients with PAD, it is not specific for PAD. Other survey tools, such as the Walking Impairment Questionnaire and the Rose Questionnaire, provide a specific assessment of lower extremity arterial occlusive disease, especially for claudicants.
B. There are eight domains, or areas of questions, in the SF-36 that provide an excellent indication of patient-reported general health status.
C. Each of the domains of the SF-36 have been proven valid and reliable and, therefore, can be used independently to track specific changes in patient general health, such as pain or physical function. Single questions cannot be extracted from the survey and used alone to track changes.
D. The SF-36 domains of physical function, role function, and pain have been noted in several studies to be affected by PAD, especially claudication. These domains can be used to track changes in patient outcome after treatment.
E. The power of the SF-36 lies in the fact that it has been extensively used in broad patient populations with a variety of disease states and has been demonstrated to be valid and reliable.

Answer 5-3: C
Discussion 5-3

A. Because patient recovery to full health and activity is a goal of all vascular intervention, the use of a patient-reported general health assessment is of great benefit.

Such comparisons have led to the documentation that, by 3 months after treatment, patients who have undergone open aneurysm repair have general health scores similar to those who underwent endovascular repair.

B. Because patients can complete the SF-36 form easily at the time of office visits, this general health tool provides excellent information about the progress or deterioration experienced by the patient since the last visit.

C. Because extended patient outcomes assessment attempts to further define the benefits or adverse events experienced by patients who interact with the health care system, they are of little use in analyzing problems that do not directly involve patients.

D. For each pioneering application of technology, the initial focus of clinicians is on the technical feasibility and success. These have little to do with the patient benefit from the procedure. Defining patient benefit requires the inclusion of patient-reported outcomes.

E. Treating ruptured aortic aneurysms or other life-threatening emergencies is frequently associated with high mortality rates. The efforts and high costs of such procedures can be best demonstrated through the use of extended outcomes assessment. For example, Joseph and colleagues clearly documented that patients who survived treatment of ruptured aortic aneurysm had quality of life scores equivalent to age-matched control norms.

■ ANSWERS AND DISCUSSION FOR CHAPTER 6

Answer 6-1: C
Discussion 6-1

Vascular surgery *reporting standards* are intended to allow publications in scientific journals regarding vascular disease in its management to be reported in a uniform fashion and thus make them more comparable. As such they include (A) uniform classification of diseases, (B) criteria for determining and reporting patency, and for gauging the degree of change (improvement/deterioration and failure/success) associated with both conservative and interventional treatments. Factors known to affect outcome are listed, and reporting should be correlated with these. (D) Operative interventions are categorized, and (E) complications associated with them are not only categorized but also graded in terms of severity. Disease severity scoring is included in some recommendations (venous disease, AAAs), and a run-off scoring system is included for lower extremity arterial disease. In contrast, *practice standards or guidelines*, a number of which have also been endorsed by the Society for Vascular Surgery, focus on recommended indications for intervention relative to known risk factors, suggesting the number of those who may most benefit versus those whose benefit is questionable or negligible, and therefore (C) should be excluded from consideration.

Answer 6-2: C
Discussion 6-2

A. While continued clinical improvement with symptom relief may result from this secondary intervention, "clinical success" is no longer accepted in standardized reporting practices because it depends on subjective assessment, e.g., relief of symptoms presuming continued patency. All estimates of patency are based on objective criteria (see Question 6-3, below).

B. Once a secondary procedure is performed to preserve or restored patency, primary patency is lost.

C. If that procedure is performed *before* the reconstructed or bypassed segments have occluded it qualifies to be included under assisted primary patency.

D. This distinguishes it from secondary patency, which also includes procedures performed after occlusion which preserve patency. In fact, to qualify for secondary patency at least one anastamosis and more than half of the length of the original bypass graft must be retained by the secondary reconstruction

E. The term tertiary patency is not an accepted means of reporting patency. It has been suggested to apply to multiple procedures performed to preserve or restore flow across an occluded arterial segment regardless of the number of prior procedures that may have failed but has no place in standardized reporting practices.

Answer 6-3: A
Discussion 6-3

A. Palpation of pulses distal to a reconstruction or bypass obviously has clinical utility, but it is *not* sufficient to establish patency, and for estimating patency rates, in reports in scientific journals.

B. In the past, arteriography was the gold standard but serial arteriography to confirm patency had obvious drawbacks and was not acceptable for this purpose in most practices. However it may still be used in cases of questionable patency in which other methods have not been conclusive and there has been clinical deterioration. Thus it is a valid criterion.

C and D. To get around the problem of avoiding serial arteriography, standards were set to allow (D) segmental limb systolic pressure measurements distal to the reconstructed or bypassed segments to be used as an objective assessment of patency. However, now that (C) Duplex scan is widely available and used regularly in graft surveillance, it is the preferred method of confirming patency for published reports.

E. Occasionally, as in removing an infected graft that is still patent, patency can be confirmed by direct observation at subsequent surgery. Similarly, a graft proved to be patent at the time of autopsy is also acceptable.

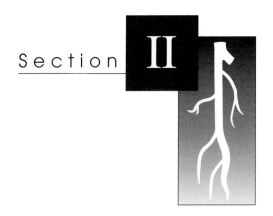
BASIC VASCULAR SCIENCE

STUDY QUESTIONS

■ QUESTIONS FOR CHAPTER 7

Question 7-1

The most common clinically significant anomaly of the vascular system is:

A. Patent ductus arteriosus.
B. Variations in the blood supply to the kidney.
C. Anomalies of the left renal vein.
D. Popliteal entrapment syndrome.
E. Persistent sciatic artery.

Question 7-2

Characteristic findings of a complete persistent sciatic artery are:

A. Port wine staining.
B. Lower leg edema with enlarged varicosities.
C. Palpable distal pulses with non-palpable femoral pulses.
D. Associated popliteal entrapment syndrome.
E. Aneurysm of the proximal thigh.

Question 7-3

Popliteal entrapment syndrome is characterized by all of the following *except*:

A. Medial deviation of the popliteal artery.
B. Lateral deviation of the popliteal artery.
C. Associated claudication at an early age.
D. Causes aneurysm and thrombosis of the popliteal artery.
E. Frequently, a similar anomaly in the contralateral leg.

■ QUESTIONS FOR CHAPTER 8

Question 8-1

The response to injury hypothesis of atherosclerosis states that the *initial* event in the formation of atherosclerotic plaque involves dysfunction of the following cell type:

A. Vascular endothelial cell.
B. Vascular smooth muscle cell (SMC).
C. Macrophage.
D. Platelet.
E. T lymphocyte.

Question 8-2

Which peptide growth factor causes endothelial cell proliferation and has been found to promote the growth of new blood vessels in the myocardium and the peripheral circulation?

A. Platelet-derived growth factor.
B. Transforming growth factor (TGF)-β.
C. Vascular endothelial growth factor (VEGF).
D. Insulin-like growth factors (IGFs).
E. Epidermal growth factor.

Question 8-3

Which of the following types represents the mature, complicated atherosclerotic lesion that is responsible for the majority of morbidity and mortality from atherosclerosis?

A. Types I and II.
B. Type III.
C. Type IV.
D. Type V.
E. Type VI.

■ QUESTIONS FOR CHAPTER 9

Question 9-1

According to Poiseuille's law, the pressure gradient in an idealized flow model is inversely proportional to the:

A. Mean flow velocity.
B. Length of the tube.
C. Fluid viscosity.
D. Fourth power of the tube radius.
E. Volume of flow rate.

Question 9-2

Which of the following statements about the collateral circulation is *false*?

A. Collateral vessels are preexisting pathways that enlarge when the parallel major artery becomes stenotic or occluded.
B. Exercise reduces venous volume in the lower limb, and this is the method by which exercise stimulates collateral development.

C. An abnormally increased pressure gradient across a collateral bed may stimulate development of collateral pathways.
D. The vascular resistance of the collateral bed is relatively fixed or constant when the major artery is widely patent.
E. The midzone of the collateral bed consists of small, intramuscular branches.

Question 9-3

Which of the following is *not* a function of the calf muscle pump?

A. It lowers the venous pressure in the dependent lower limb.
B. It reduces venous volume in the exercising lower limb.
C. It prevents venous reflux in the lower limb during exercise.
D. It increases venous return to the right heart.
E. It minimizes edema in the dependent lower limb.

■ QUESTIONS FOR CHAPTER 10

Question 10-1

What hemodynamic factors are not important in plaque deposition?

A. High shear stress.
B. Low shear stress.
C. Flow stasis.
D. Oscillation of shear.
E. High tensile stress.

Question 10-2

What are thought to be *not* important in AAA pathogenesis?

A. Lipid deposition.
B. Inflammation.
C. Extracellular matrix deposition.
D. Necrosis.
E. All of the above.

Question 10-3

What else in addition to plaque contributes to the hardening and narrowing of the arteries?

A. Fatty substances and cell waste products.
B. Scar tissue and cellular buildup.
C. Calcium.
D. Fibrin deposition.
E. All of the above.

■ QUESTIONS FOR CHAPTER 11

Question 11-1

A 65-year-old man presents to his physician with claudication, and duplex imaging shows common iliac stenosis. The patient is brought to the interventional suite and undergoes iliac angioplasty with a good result. He returns in 6 months with recurrent stenosis in the area of the previously angioplasty. What is the most likely cause of the stenosis after angioplasty in this patient?

A. Elastic recoil.
B. Neointimal hyperplasia.
C. Remodeling in response to pressure from the balloon.
D. In situ thrombosis.
E. Dissection.

Question 11-2

A 70-year-old man with rest pain has a successful femoral-posterior tibial bypass to an acceptable recipient vessel, using saphenous vein. Duplex imaging after completion revealed no evidence of technical defects. Twelve months later the vein graft on surveillance is shown to have developed a stenosis in the body of the graft. The most likely cause of the stenosis is:

A. Intimal hyperplasia.
B. A retained valve if the technique was in situ.
C. Atherosclerosis.
D. Cicatrix at an area of focal injury during preparation of the vein.
E. Inflammatory response to vibrations caused by blood flowing past a reversed valve.

Question 11-3

A 60-year-old man with bilateral claudication has both a right and a left superficial femoral angioplasty followed by immediate stenting. He develops restenosis in both treated areas. Which of the following statements explains the difference (if any) in the stenosis caused by angioplasty and that related to stenting?

A. The stenosis after angioplasty and stenting are both caused by intimal hyperplasia only.
B. The stenosis caused by angioplasty is caused by intimal hyperplasia and negative remodeling, whereas the stenosis in a stent is caused by intimal hyperplasia following thrombosis in the stent interstices.
C. The angioplasty stenosis is caused by intimal hyperplasia, whereas that in the stent is caused by negative remodeling.
D. Stenosis is caused by intimal hyperplasia and negative remodeling, in both cases.
E. The stenosis caused by angioplasty is caused by intimal hyperplasia only, whereas the stenosis associated with stenting is caused by trapped thrombus that becomes organized into fibrous tissue and then proliferates.

■ QUESTIONS FOR CHAPTER 12

Question 12-1

Of the following methods, which may *not* be used to directly assess gene transcription in cells?

A. Northern blot analysis.
B. Enzyme-linked immunosorbent assay.
C. In situ hybridization.
D. Reverse transcriptase-polymerase chain reaction.
E. All of the above (can *not* be used).

Question 12-2

Processing of polypeptide chains into functional proteins may involve:

A. Cleavage of amino terminal peptides in proteins destined for export.
B. Addition of carbohydrate moieties.
C. Cross-linking of individual polypeptide chains.
D. Macromolecular folding assisted by proteins known as chaperones.
E. All of the above.

Question 12-3

Which of the following approaches may *not* be included in therapeutic manipulation of gene expression?

A. RNA interference.
B. Competitive inhibition by monoclonal antibodies.
C. Antisense oligonucleotides.
D. Transcription factor (TF) decoy molecules.
E. None, i.e., all approaches may be included.

ANSWERS AND DISCUSSION

■ ANSWERS AND DISCUSSION FOR CHAPTER 7

Answer 7-1: A
Discussion 7-1

A. Patent ductus arteriosus is the most common clinically significant vascular anomaly. Failure of the ductus arteriosus to obliterate results in a major hemodynamic shunt from the thoracic aorta to the pulmonary system.
B. The blood supply to the metanephros (future permanent kidney) arises from caudal and cranial segmental arteries that disappear one by one as the metanephros ascends, leaving one segmental artery on each side that becomes the main renal arteries. However, given this embryology, there can be considerable variation in the arterial supply to the kidney, and accessory renal arteries are not uncommon.
C. A retroaortic left renal vein may develop if the anterior vein of the paired renal veins regresses and the posterior vein persists. In addition, both anterior and posterior veins may persist, forming a circumaortic left renal vein. These can cause surgical misadventures if encountered unexpectedly during AAA repair. In addition, approximately 20 cases of fistula between the retroaortic left renal vein and the aorta, usually at the posterior neck of an AAA, have been reported (see also Chapter 111).
D. Popliteal entrapment syndrome does not occur frequently and is commonly the result of early migration of the medial head of the gastrocnemius or late development of the popliteal artery (see also Discussion 7-3). There are five types (see also Chapter 86).
E. Persistent sciatic artery is a rare syndrome that occurs if the primitive sciatic system fails to regress in response to failure of the iliofemoral arterial pathway to develop and take over as the main arterial supply to the lower extremity. The anatomic course of this persistent artery leaves it vulnerable to compression trauma and may lead to aneurysm formation and thrombotic complications.

Answer 7-2: C
Discussion 7-2

A. Port wine staining occurs in venous malformations such as Klippel-Trenaunay syndrome but not persistent sciatic artery.
B. Edema and varicosities are associated with venous malformations or primary or secondary chronic venous insufficiency.
C. If the persistent sciatic artery is complete and there is poor or no development of the external iliac system then the patient will not have palpable femoral pulses but will have palpable popliteal or pedal pulses.
D. It is unlikely to have these two rare abnormalities occur in the same individual. They are not linked by related embryologic events.
E. Aneurysms associated with persistent sciatic artery occur in the buttock; their location is superficial and subject to compression trauma.

Answer 7-3: B
Discussion 7-3

Normally the popliteal artery develops before the medial head of the gastrocnemius migrates to its attachment on the medial femoral condyle. However, if the artery develops late or the medial head migrates early, then the artery will be displaced (A) *medially* (not laterally as in answer B) and become impinged against the femur, which can lead to (C) claudication, with onset at an early age (late teens/twenties typically) as well as (D) aneurysm formation and thrombosis of the popliteal artery. (E) This anomaly occurs frequently enough bilaterally that it should be sought in the contralateral limb wherever one leg presents clinically. MRI/MRA is the best way to make the diagnosis *and* identify the specific anatomy type.

■ ANSWERS AND DISCUSSION FOR CHAPTER 8

Answer 8-1: A
Discussion 8-1

A. All of the elements represented in the answers are believed to play a role, but the response to injury hypothesis postulates that endothelial cell dysfunction is the *initial event* in the cascade leading to the formation of atherosclerotic plaques. The endothelial cell performs many normal physiologic functions including the following: providing a nonadherent and nonthrombogenic luminal surface, modulating the coagulation system, acting as a permeability barrier that controls the flow of fluids and molecules between the plasma and arterial wall, modulating vascular tone, producing and secreting numerous growth factors and cytokines, and oxidizing lipoproteins. Abnormalities in one or more of these endothelial functions occur early in atherogenesis.
B. Vascular SMCs are normally located in the media and migrate to the intima where they accumulate, contributing to the development of atherosclerotic lesions, but this is *not* the initial event. The migration of vascular SMCs is controlled by the release of various chemotactic agents from endothelial cells, platelets, macrophages, and other vascular SMCs. They are responsive to more than 20 different growth factors and ultimately comprise a significant portion of atherosclerotic plaque.
C. Macrophages are prominent in all atherosclerotic lesions, particularly in early stages. They are the primary inflammatory mediator cells of atherogenesis and function as scavengers presenting antigens to T lymphocytes. Monocytes, attracted by adhesion molecules and chemotactic factors produced by endothelial cells (the initiator, in response to injury), migrate to the subendothelial space, becoming macrophages. Early in atherogenesis these cells take up oxidized low-density lipoprotein and become foam cells.

D. The adherence and aggregation of platelets to the endo-thelial surface, in response to its injury/dysfunction, occur early in the development of atherosclerosis and increase as the lesion progresses, but it is *not* the initial event. Thrombosis is the result of platelet adherence to irregular endothelial surfaces. Platelets also play a role in stimulating the progression of atherosclerotic lesions and are known to produce and secrete a number of growth factors and vasoactive substances.

E. T lymphocytes are present in all atherosclerotic lesions in large numbers, but their precise role in atherogenesis has not been fully determined. They adhere to atheroscle-rotic lesions and produce chemotactic agents and cyto-kines that attract and activate both macrophages and vas-cular SMCs.

Answer 8-2: C (the functions of the other factors are also explained)

Discussion 8-2

A. Although originally derived from platelets, platelet-derived growth factor has been found in a variety of cells, including vascular SMCs, fibroblasts, and endothelial cells. Platelet-derived growth factor is a potent mitogen that causes proliferation of vascular SMCs. It also affects tissue remodeling by increasing collagen synthesis and stimulating secretion of collagenase. It is a potent vaso-constrictor in a concentration-dependent fashion and has a chemotactic effect on vascular SMCs, fibroblasts, and neutrophils.

B. There are at least five members in the TGF-β family, numbered from 1 to 5. These growth factors can both stimulate and inhibit cell differentiation and prolifera-tion. The type of action exerted by TGF on a particular cell depends on multiple factors, such as the type of cell and the stage of its differentiation. TGF-β1 may also interfere with the growth and proliferative effects of other growth factors. TGF-βs play a role in stimulating extracellular matrix protein synthesis and accumulation in bone and other tissues. TGF-βs interact with multiple growth factors in the proliferation of cells of vascular origin.

C. VEGF, a peptide growth factor that causes endothelial cell proliferation, has been found to promote the growth of new blood vessels in the myocardium and the periph-eral circulation. Angiogenesis after successful gene transfer of VEGF complementary DNA in rats using an adenovirus vector was reported in 1997. Intramuscular injection of naked plasmid DNA encoding for the 165-amino acid VEGF isomer induces formation of new blood vessels in patients with chronic ischemia. Recent studies have demonstrated the potential efficacy of intra-myocardial gene therapy with VEGF.

D. IGFs have metabolic effects similar to those of insulin. In addition, they stimulate the proliferation of endothelial and vascular SMCs. IGF-I has been found to induce an-giogenesis in a rabbit corneal model.

E. Epidermal growth factor is a mitogenic factor that stimu-lates the proliferation and migration of endothelial cells.

EGF has been shown to induce tube formation by endo-thelial cells, an important step in angiogenesis. It is also an arterial vasodilator.

Answer 8-3: E

Discussion 8-3

A. Early type I and II lesions are the only lesions found in children, but may also occur in adults. They range from microscopic lesions consisting of increased cellularity and lipid accumulation to macroscopic fatty streaks.

B. Type III lesions are intermediaries between early lesions and the mature atheroma (type IV lesions). They contain characteristic pools of extracellular lipid droplets dis-persed among the layers of vascular SMCs. These lipid pools are located beneath the layered macrophages and foam cells, disrupting the coherent layer of vascular SMCs. The presence of these lipid pools signifies the progression of type II to type III lesions.

C. Type IV lesions, sometimes called atheromas, are charac-terized by a well-defined collection of extracellular lipid within the intima, known as the "lipid core." Type IV lesions are frequently eccentric in location, cause a visi-ble thickening of the arterial wall, but usually do not result in a significant narrowing of the arterial lumen and do not produce symptoms.

D. Type V lesions are characterized by the formation of prominent new fibrous connective tissue, which forms the fibrous cap. Type V lesions are seen starting in the fourth decade of life and can cause significant narrowing of the arterial lumen producing symptoms.

E. Type VI lesions are also known as the complicated le-sions and are responsible for the majority of morbidity and mortality from atherosclerosis. Type VI lesions occur when a type IV or V lesion undergoes disruption of the intimal surface, such as with plaque ulceration or hemor-rhage into a plaque. Type VI lesions may be the source of emboli or may cause arterial thrombosis, resulting in life-threatening or limb-threatening symptoms.

■ ANSWERS AND DISCUSSION FOR CHAPTER 9

Answer 9-1: D

Discussion 9-1

Poiseuille's law describes the viscous losses existing in an idealized situation. It applies only to steady (nonpulsatile) laminar flow in a straight cylindric tube with rigid walls and is related inversely to the fourth power of the radius of the wall (D). As the diameter of the conduit is reduced, there is little effect on the pressure gradient until a certain degree of narrowing is reached beyond which further reductions cause the pressure gradient to increase precipitously.

Answer 9-2: B

Discussion 9-2

Arterial stenosis results in (C) increased resistance, which is the stimulus for collateral development around the involved segment as a compensation for this obstruction. Collateral beds are divided into the following: stem arteries; mid-zone collaterals; which (E) consist of small intramuscular arteries and reentry arteries. These vessels are (A) preexisting pathways that enlarge when a stenosis or occlusion a parallel main artery. (D) The resistance within a collateral bed always exceeds that of the major artery whose function it has replaced. (B) Venous volume changes have nothing to do with collateral development.

Answer 9-3: C
Discussion 9-3

The calf muscle pump compresses the intramuscular and surrounding veins and forces blood cephalad toward the heart, thereby (D) increasing its venous return. Its action also (A) reduces venous pressure and (B) reduces venous volume in the exercising extremity. These in turn can (E) reduce edema. However, (C) it is the venous valves, not the calf muscle pump, that prevent retrograde flow or reflux.

■ ANSWERS AND DISCUSSION FOR CHAPTER 10

Answer 10-1: A
Discussion 10-1

Endothelial cells are aligned and overlapped in the direction of the wall shear stress. In areas with (B) low or reduced shear and where the direction of the shear oscillates during the pulse cycle (D), the orientation of these cells is distorted and the pattern of overlap is disrupted. This creates high tensile stress (E). In the arterial tree at bifurcations and branchings there may be eddies of relatively slow flow or stasis (C). Atherosclerotic plaques tend to form first and most rapidly at sites of decreased shear. It is believed that the opposite, (A) high shear stress, may even be protective.

Answer 10-2: E
Discussion 10-2

AAAs are thought to arise from a degenerative process. Lipid deposition, inflammation, extracellular matrix deposition, and necrosis (A–D) are all believed not to play a role in its pathogenesis. Therefore E is the correct answer.

Answer 10-3: B
Discussion 10-3

All of the other factors (A, C, D) discussed play a role in plaque formation, but only (B), scar tissue and cellular buildup are factors that contribute to the hardening *and* narrowing of the arteries.

■ ANSWERS AND DISCUSSION FOR CHAPTER 11

Answer 11-1: B
Discussion 11-1

Recurrent stenosis after 6 months is most likely the result of (B) neointimal hyperplasia. Subsequently there may be

some negative remodeling (C) but the balloon produces a shearing stress as well as direct pressure that can dilate the thinner rim away from the characteristically eccentric plaque. The former creates a separation of the plaque in the same plane used in endarterectomy, and this allows the plaque to be remodeled by the expanding balloon and contributes in a major way to lumen enlargement. Elastic recoil (A), frank dissection (E), and even in situ thrombosis (D) can occur, but these are usually acute events occurring around the time of the angioplasty and may even lead to early technical failure.

Answer 11-2: A
Discussion 11-2

(A) Intimal hyperplasia is the universal response of a vein graft to insertion into the arterial circulation and results from both the migration of SMCs out of the media into the intima and the proliferation of these SMCs. It is the most common cause of stenosis at this time. (B) A retained valve in an in situ bypass can lead to narrowing as can (D) scarring in response to injury, but these are much less common. (E) Vibrations and disturbed flow have been demonstrated around the valves in ex vivo studies of reversed veins, but their causal relationship to vein graft stenoses remains conjectural at this point. Occasionally, atherosclerosis (C) can develop in vein grafts, but a mature (type IV or higher) stenotic lesion would not appear this early.

Answer 11-3: B
Discussion 11-3

After balloon angioplasty, there can be thrombus formation, intimal hyperplasia development, elastic recoil, and negative remodeling, but intimal hyperplasia and negative remodeling contribute to later narrowing. In contrast, after stent placement, elastic recoil and negative remodeling are eliminated and thrombus formation followed by intimal hyperplasia developments are the main contributors to in-stent restenosis.

■ ANSWERS AND DISCUSSION FOR CHAPTER 12

Answer 12-1: B
Discussion 12-1

A. Northern blot analysis is a technique used to detect and quantify specific RNA sequences.
B. Enzyme-linked immunosorbent assay allows for the accurate measurement of protein antigens in solution and is *not* used to directly assess gene transcription in cells.
C. This technique allows for the in situ (within cells or tissues) detection of specific nucleic acid sequences, complementary to labeled probes.
D. Polymerase chain reaction is an in vitro mechanism for synthesizing specific DNA sequences by repetitive cycles of template denaturation, primer annealing, and extension of annealed primers and is a powerful tool for amplification of DNA.
E. Eliminated by answer B.

Answer 12-2: E

Discussion 12-2

The final amino acid sequence specifies the three-dimensional (3D) shape of the resultant protein. This change in configuration involves specialized proteins known as chaperones. Although chaperones are required for (D) correct folding of proteins, these proteins do not supply any information that influences this process. They appear to bind to unfolded or partially folded proteins and stabilize them, which prevents incorrect folding or inappropriate aggregation of these structures. After folding, the proteins may undergo further chemical modifications, which greatly expand the total possible number of variants and heterogeneity from a single gene.

Posttranslational modifications of proteins include proteolytic changes (B), glycosylation (A), and lipid attachment. Proteolytic modifications involve cleavage and subsequent cross linkage (C) of polypeptide chains. Such alterations to the structure of proteins are often required before translocation across certain membranes (which includes lysosomes, mitochondria, chloroplasts) or into the plasma membrane. Signal sequences are specific amino-terminus cleavage sites that allow for the processing of premature polypeptides such as prohormones to be cleaved into mature forms by specific cellular enzymes. This cleavage process is important for formation of certain enzymes or hormones from larger precur-

sors. In short, all of the listed (E), and many other processes are involved.

Answer 12-3: B

Discussion 12-3

A. A new approach to inhibit specific gene expression has been elucidated on the basis of the intracellular effects of double-stranded RNA molecules. This phenomenon, termed RNA interference, yields effective and specific silencing of the targeted gene, usually in a transient fashion.

B. Monoclonal antibodies are *not* used for manipulation of gene expression.

C. Antisense oligodeoxynucleotides (ODNs) are designed to have a base sequence and are complementary in terms of Watson-Crick binding to a segment of the target gene. They are generally 15 to 20 bases in length, which confers specificity to the target messenger RNA. This binding of ODNs to mRNA either results in enzymatic degradation of the mRNA or prevents the translation of RNA into its protein product.

D. TF decoys are double-stranded ODNs designed to mimic the chromosomal binding sites of the target TF. Once delivered to a cell, the decoy binds to the available TF, competitively inhibiting the TF-promoter interaction, and thereby preventing the subsequent activation of target genes.

E. Answer C eliminates E.

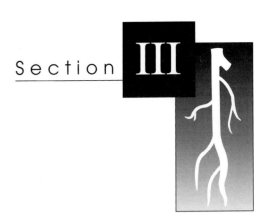

Section **III**

THE VASCULAR DIAGNOSTIC LABORATORY: BASIC TECHNIQUES

STUDY QUESTIONS

■ QUESTIONS FOR CHAPTER 13

Question 13-1

Which of the following is *least* important in qualifying a physician to work as a test interpreter in a vascular diagnostic laboratory (VDL)?

A. Understanding the diagnostic criteria for each study.
B. Being familiar with the testing procedures.
C. Understanding the clinical principles of vascular disease.
D. Knowing the principles and the limitations of the equipment.
E. Being fellowship trained and fully certified in vascular surgery.

Question 13-2

Which of the following is *not* commonly expected of technologists working in a VDL?

A. Graduating from a 2-year, curriculum-approved training course of the Society of Vascular Ultrasonographers.
B. Having practical knowledge of the relevant anatomy and physiology of the vascular tree.
C. Having practical knowledge of the common vascular diseases and their symptoms.
D. Having an understanding of the physical principles and limitations of the techniques and equipment being used.
E. Becoming a Registered Vascular Technologist (RVT).

Question 13-3

VDLs should regularly determine the accuracy of their own test results through a formal quality assurance program. Which of the following does *not* help to ensure this need is satisfied?

A. Use of a duplicate test process in which two or more people examine the same patient without knowledge of previous findings.
B. Duplication of the equipment and strict application of the diagnostic criteria of published validations of the diagnostic test.
C. Comparison of the final interpretation of a study against a "gold standard."

D. Use of clinical outcomes (e.g., healing of ulcers, amputations at the predicted level) as quality control surrogates in the absence of a suitable gold standard study.
E. Confirm test accuracy against a reference standard whenever diagnostic criteria are combined or modified.

■ QUESTIONS FOR CHAPTER 14

Question 14-1

In which of the following clinical situations would the measurement of toe pressure be more valuable than measurement of ankle pressure?

A. A diabetic patient with a chronic nonhealing foot ulcer and an ABI of 0.7 on the affected side.
B. A patient with intermittent claudication and a positive exercise treadmill test.
C. A patient who requires amputation at the below-knee level for extensive necrotic forefoot lesions extending to the ankle.
D. A patient being followed after a femoral-tibial in situ saphenous vein bypass graft.
E. A nondiabetic patient with ischemic rest pain and an ABI of 0.2 on the affected side.

Question 14-2

A potential source of error in the measurement of arterial systolic pressure in the lower limb using a pneumatic cuff and Doppler flow detector is:

A. Use of a Doppler device with a low transmitting frequency (i.e., 5 MHz).
B. Changing the site of Doppler flow detection distal to the cuff.
C. Use of a cuff that is narrow relative to the diameter of the limb at the site of measurement.
D. Use of a pulsed Doppler instrument rather than a continuous-wave device.
E. Presence of chronic venous insufficiency combined with arterial occlusive disease.

17

Question 14-3

In pulse volume plethysmography, which of the following statements is *true* regarding the dicrotic wave of the pulse volume recording (PVR)?

A. It only appears in the presence of significant occlusive lesions proximal to the recording site.
B. Absence of this feature has important diagnostic significance.
C. It is a normal component of the rapid upstroke that occurs with systole.
D. It correlates with the presence of primary vasospasm in the affected extremity.
E. It represents the reverse-flow phase of the normal peripheral arterial pulse.

■ QUESTIONS FOR CHAPTER 15

Question 15-1

A patient with CEAP (clinical, etiologic, anatomic, and pathophysiologic) class 4 findings (dermatofibrosis, pigmentation but no ulceration) reports a history of great saphenous stripping. No deep venous reflux is found on duplex examination, but several incompetent perforators are noted. Which parameter measured by air plethysmography will best help to determine whether the patient's symptoms are caused by venous insufficiency?

A. Venous volume.
B. Venous filling index (VFI).
C. Ejection fraction.
D. Residual volume fraction.
E. Valve closure time.

Question 15-2

A 56-year-old woman with CEAP class 5 finding (active venous ulceration) is found to have abnormal valve closure times in the popliteal vein and greater saphenous vein. Air plethysmography is performed, and all parameters are abnormal. A vascular surgeon decides to proceed with greater saphenous vein removal without correction of the popliteal reflux. Postoperatively, air plethysmography is repeated. Which parameter most closely correlates with symptomatic improvement after venous corrective surgery?

A. Venous volume.
B. VFI.
C. Ejection fraction.
D. Residual volume fraction.
E. Valve closure time.

Question 15-3

What information does air plethysmography add to the diagnosis and treatment of venous disease after duplex reflux mapping has been performed?

A. Additional information on the anatomic sites of disease.
B. Confirmation of valvular incompetence at a specific site or level.
C. Quantitative measurement of the hemodynamic severity of the venous reflux identified by duplex mapping.
D. Determination of potential for surgical correction of valvular incompetence.
E. Identification of the cause of the venous disease.

■ QUESTIONS FOR CHAPTER 16

Question 16-1

For determination of the diagnostic threshold for a 70% internal carotid artery stenosis by duplex scan, which of these criteria would be the most appropriate?

A. Peak systolic velocity of 230 cm/sec or greater, as recommended by a consensus of known experts in a peer-reviewed journal.
B. Stenosis calculation of 70% determined by electronic caliper measurement on power Doppler images of the stenotic region compared with normal distal segment of internal carotid artery.
C. Peak systolic velocity of 325 cm/sec or greater based on correlation of duplex data to multiplaner cerebral angiograms published by an nationally recognized expert in the field.
D. Peak systolic velocity of 290 cm/sec or greater based on correlation of cerebral angiograms and duplex results performed in one's own laboratory.
E. Avoid absolute peak velocity thresholds in favor of a ratio of internal to common carotid peak systolic velocities of 4.0 or greater.

Question 16-2

Renal duplex ultrasound is an excellent screening technique to help distinguish patients with renovascular hypertension from the much larger cohort of patients with essential hypertension. Which of the following duplex criteria has been evaluated extensively in the peer-reviewed literature and found to best identify a 60% or greater renal artery stenosis?

A. Peak systolic velocity greater than 180 cm/sec.
B. Hilar acceleration time greater than 100 msec.
C. Renal acceleration index less than 3.78 kHz shift/sec.
D. Peak systolic velocity equal to or greater than 200 cm/sec or a ratio of renal peak systolic velocity to aortic peak systolic velocity of 3.5 or greater.
E. Intraparenchymal resistive index >80.

Question 16-3

A mesenteric arterial duplex examination interrogates the superior mesenteric artery (SMA) and records a peak systolic velocity of 260 cm/sec and an end-diastolic velocity of 35 cm/sec. The celiac artery origin cannot be identified, but the common hepatic and splenic arteries are well seen. The common hepatic is studied carefully and found to contain retrograde blood flow. Blood flow direction in the splenic is normal. The proper interpretation of these examination findings is:

A. Technically inadequate examination; duplex results are uninterpretable.
B. Duplex results in the SMA indicate presence of a hemodynamically significant stenosis. Celiac cannot be identified.
C. Duplex velocities in the SMA are normal. Celiac cannot be identified.
D. Duplex velocities in the SMA are normal. Celiac origin not identified. Retrograde blood flow direction in the common hepatic artery indicates presence of a severe stenosis or occlusion of the celiac.

E. Duplex findings indicate a single celiacomesenteric artery origin.

■ QUESTIONS FOR CHAPTER 17

Question 17-1

The primary ultrasound finding associated with the diagnosis of acute deep venous thrombosis (DVT) is:

A. With B-mode scanning, incompressibility of the vein in longitudinal view.
B. With B-mode scanning, incompressibility of the vein in cross-section.
C. The presence of a color "bruit."
D. Decreased caliber of the vein.
E. An echogenic thrombus within the lumen of the vein.

Question 17-2

Compared with venography, duplex ultrasound is *least* accurate for which of the following:

A. Diagnosis of "proximal" (ileo-femoral-popliteal) lower extremity DVT in symptomatic patients.
B. Diagnosis of proximal lower extremity DVT in asymptomatic patients.
C. Diagnosis of calf DVT in symptomatic patients.
D. Diagnosis of calf DVT in asymptomatic patients.
E. Diagnosis of axillosubclavian venous thrombosis.

Question 17-3

In patients with angiographically identified pulmonary emboli, what percentage (of the following ranges) will have duplex ultrasound-detectable lower extremity venous thrombosis?

A. 0.0%–5%.
B. 10%–20%.
C. 40%–50%.
D. 70%–80%.
E. 90%–100%.

ANSWERS AND DISCUSSION

■ ANSWERS AND DISCUSSION FOR CHAPTER 13

Answer 13-1: E

Discussion 13-1

As valuable as it is, vascular surgery fellowship and certification (E) are not essential criteria for serving as an interpreter in a VDL. Other vascular specialists who have obtained the necessary background training and knowledge in vascular disease and its diagnosis may serve adequately. In fact, in a number of institutions, radiologists, neurologists, and vascular internists commonly serve in this role. However, it is necessary that such individuals understand (C) the clinical principles of vascular surgery, particularly the applied hemodynamics, (D) have knowledge of the operating principles and limitations of the equipment used in the laboratory, and (B) be familiar with the actual testing procedures themselves. Obviously an interpreter must understand (A) the diagnostic criteria for each study. In addition, although hands-on technical skills are desirable and many VDL physicians have certified themselves as RVTs, this level of technical knowledge and skill is not essential for the role of study *interpreter* in a VDL. This is more important for those playing greater roles in the VDL (e.g., serving as its director or a trainer of new technologists).

Answer 13-2: A

Discussion 13-2

There remains great variability in the knowledge and experience of technologists practicing in the field, and some laboratory staff have simply been taught the mechanics of conducting specific examinations. Formal preliminary training is valuable, and there are excellent preliminary training experiences, the curriculum of which may be approved by one or another professional society, but none are required to the exclusion of others. Therefore, A is not a prerequisite, if in fact such a course exists. The goal for all technologists, regardless of their training background, is to (E) confirm their knowledge and skills by becoming an RVT. Clearly this encompasses (B) knowledge of the relevant anatomy and physiology of the vascular tree, (C) an understanding of the common vascular diseases and their symptoms, and (D) an understanding of the physical principles and limitations of the techniques and equipment being used.

Answer 13-3: B

Discussion 13-3

(B) Duplication of the equipment and strict application of the diagnostic criteria of published validations of a particular diagnostic test do not ensure the same accuracy. A standard assumption is that if one duplicates the equipment and adopts published criteria, the clinical accuracies achieved will be similar to those quoted in the literature. This does not recognize the inherent problem in many noninvasive procedures, namely, that their accuracy is heavily operator dependent. This can be examined by (A) use of a duplicate test process

in which two or more technologist/operators examine the same patient without knowledge of previous findings. There should be carefully developed written protocols with periodic observations to ensure that each technologist adheres to them. For the laboratory as a whole, final interpretations should be compared against (C) the best available "gold standard," usually angiography or some other accepted imaging or physiologic study. Suitable gold standards are not always available, so the use of outcomes (e.g., ulcer healing) (D) may serve this need in some settings. (E) Whenever diagnostic criteria are combined or modified one must confirm test accuracy against a reference standard.

■ ANSWERS AND DISCUSSION FOR CHAPTER 14

Answer 14-1: A

Discussion 14-1

The toe pressure is valuable when it can provide information that the ankle pressure cannot. This is most common in diabetic patients in whom calcification of distal arteries renders them incompressible at the ankle level, resulting in erroneous/false high ankle pressure estimates. They are also of value in predicting healing of lesions in the forefoot and toes. The patient in question A is most likely to benefit for both those reasons, because diabetic patients can develop neurotrophic foot ulcers that will not heal despite adequate circulation and these must be distinguished from ulcers that will not heal because of associated ischemia. The patient in question E is a nondiabetic patient without a foot lesion and with an ABI compatible with rest pain. Therefore, a toe pressure would be of little additional value here. The patient in question B with claudication and a positive exercise treadmill test has no need for a toe pressure, and the patient in question D, with the in situ bypass, could be followed by ABI but should also have periodic duplex scan surveillance of the bypass itself. Finally, the patient in question C, requiring a below-knee amputation, would only benefit from a toe pressure if there was some consideration that the foot lesions might heal, but once extensive necrosis has progressed above the forefoot level to the ankle, the patient's foot could not be salvaged and a below-knee amputation would be needed. Calf pressure or plethysmography might help to ensure healing at the below-knee level if the ankle pressure was low (e.g., <50 mm Hg).

Answer 14-2: C

Discussion 14-2

In measuring segmental systolic pressures at various levels in the extremities, the Doppler probe is simply used to detect flow distal to the cuff as it is deflated (B). It is the level of the cuff rather than the distal placement of the Doppler that is important. As long as the Doppler probe can detect the return of "flow" (velocity) it can serve this purpose, therefore A and D are not significant considerations. Chronic venous insufficiency does not affect systolic arterial pressure or the measurement of segmental limb pressures other than the presence of a large ankle ulcer might make it difficult to apply an ankle cuff (E). But the cuff must be of an appropriate size relative to the girth of the limb segment being studied (C), and just as one observes that obese patients can be mistakenly thought to be hypertensive because their pressure has to be measured with an average cuff, so can thigh pressures be artificially high if measured with a regular width cuff. Thus, C is the correct answer. Sometimes this artifact is accepted in using two standard width thigh cuffs placed at the upper and lower thigh level, rather than one wide thigh cuff (to better delineate between iliac and femoral occlusive disease), but this must be standardized in each laboratory allowing for an upper thigh pressure that may be 25% higher than normal.

Answer 14-3: E

Discussion 14-3

The resting extremity is a low-flow, high-resistance circulation and as such is characterized by an end-systolic flow reversal. This is not only clearly seen on velocity tracings obtained by Doppler or Duplex scan but also may be detected on the plethysmographic or pulse-volume recordings. It is *not* related to a rapid systolic upstroke. Therefore E is correct and C is wrong. It may appear in tracings of patients without any occlusive disease, but would not be seen distal to occlusive disease (A is wrong). However, it may not be seen in some healthy patients, and therefore its absence is of little diagnostic significance (B is wrong). Increased vascular resistance, short of vasospasm, may accentuate the flow reversal in proximal velocity tracings, but flow with vasospasm is so impaired it would not be detected plethysmographically, rather one might have a diminished or flattened pulse-volume tracing, especially at the digital level (D is incorrect).

■ ANSWERS AND DISCUSSION FOR CHAPTER 15

Answer 15-1: D

Discussion 15-1

Ambulatory venous pressure (AVP) is the venous measure that most closely correlates with clinical severity of chronic venous disease. However, measurement of the AVP requires invasive monitoring that is not practical for routine use. Plethysmography allows the noninvasive measurement of venous function. The first four answers reflect plethysmographic techniques.

A. The venous volume is a measure of the total capacitance of the limb's venous system. This number is used in the other values obtained but is not a hemodynamic measure by itself.
B. The VFI measures the speed of refilling of the veins when the limb is placed in the dependent position. This value is most useful in the evaluation of the significance of axial reflux down the deep or superficial veins. It is less useful in measuring the significance of incompetent perforators, which this patient has and which may cause CEAP class 4 clinical findings.
C. The ejection fraction measures the volume of blood ejected from the limb by a single calf muscle contraction. Although a measure of calf muscle pump function, it is less useful than the residual volume fraction (see D) that measures the efficacy of repeated calf muscle contractions.
D. The residual volume fraction measures the fraction of the venous volume remaining in the limb after 10 calf contractions. This parameter has been reported as the measure correlating most closely with the AVP. The residual volume fraction determines the efficacy of the calf muscle pump and is usually impaired by significant incompetent perforators. This is why D is the correct answer.
E. Valve closure time is an anatomic measure obtained using duplex ultrasonography, *not* by a plethysmographic technique. It is increased/prolonged in patients with significant deep venous reflux, but no deep venous reflux was found on duplex examination in this patient.

Answer 15-2: B

Discussion 15-2

The nature and relative value of these test parameters have already been partly discussed in relation to question 1. The correct answer here is B. The VFI measures the speed of limb refilling when the limb is placed in a dependent position. This parameter has been found to correlate closely with CEAP clinical class and postoperative symptoms after venous surgery. If the VFI improves and moves into a normal range after surgery, greater than 90% of patients remain asymptomatic 5 years after surgery. When there are multiple sites of venous insufficiency, it is unclear whether correction of superficial disease alone will result in symptom improvement in individual patients. The VFI allows determination of whether the surgical procedure results in a significant enough hemodynamic improvement to produce (predict) a long-term reduction in symptoms.

Answer 15-3: C

Discussion 15-3

Air plethysmography provides no information on (A) the anatomic sites of venous reflux or (B) the quality (reflux/obstruction) of individual venous segments. It provides (C) hemodynamic information that, considered together, summarizes the overall effect of dysfunctional veins on the drainage of blood from the limb. It is analogous to the ABI in that it provides no information on the anatomic sites of arterial disease but gives a quantitative measure of the overall severity of occlusive disease in the limb. It does *not* identify the cause of the venous disease (E) or its potential for surgical correction (D).

■ ANSWERS AND DISCUSSION FOR CHAPTER 16

Answer 16-1: D

Discussion 16-1

Although (B) power Doppler images are improving with each new generation of duplex scanner, the weight of published evidence suggests that Doppler-derived velocity measurements still constitute the most accurate means to estimate a stenosis. Velocity-based choices A, C, and E have all been recommended in the peer-reviewed literature and *may* constitute reasonable interpretation options in laboratories in which no internal validation studies have been performed. Answer D is the best choice for a laboratory in which actual correlations with cerebral angiograms have been performed because the results take into account the laboratory-specific variables. In addition, a peak systolic velocity of 290 cm/sec is well within the published range of velocities believed to represent accurate duplex thresholds for a 70% internal carotid artery stenosis.

Answer 16-2: D

Discussion 16-2

Hilar acceleration time (B) and renal acceleration index (C) are indirect means to assess for renal artery stenosis. Although easier to perform than direct arterial duplex, the accuracy of these two measures has been assessed only by a small number of authors. They are not considered first-line studies. Peak systolic velocity of 180 cm/sec (A) has been correlated as indicative of "any degree" of renal artery stenosis in one widely cited article, but it has *not* been recommended as indicative of a 60% or greater stenosis. Intraparenchymal resistive index greater than 80 (E) has predictive value indicating renal bypass or stenting is unlikely to result in improved renal function or better blood pressure control because of the presence of intrinsic renal disease but does *not* correlate with a 60% or greater renal artery stenosis. The correct answer is D. Several well-respected authors have published retrospective and prospective studies indicating that peak systolic velocity of 200 cm/sec or greater and/or renal aortic peak systolic velocity ratio of 3.5 or greater both demonstrate excellent accuracy for identifying a 60% or greater renal artery stenosis.

Answer 16-3: D

Discussion 16-3

An important concept in duplex scanning is notation of technical adequacy. If either the technologist or the interpreting physician believes the examination is lacking from a technical perspective, that should be noted, as stated in A. In this case, although the celiac origin was not identified, there is clearly enough information to offer information of value.

The SMA velocities are normal according to data reported in contemporary publications, so B is incorrect. This being true, the correct answer is D rather than C because reversed blood flow direction in the common hepatic artery has been demonstrated to be an accurate predictor of severe celiac stenosis or complete occlusion. In this case, because the celiac could not be identified, there would be a significant likelihood that it is occluded. Velocities near threshold in the SMA suggest collateral supply to the celiac distribution.

There is nothing in this study to indicate a single celiac-omesenteric origin (E), an anomaly with approximately 1% prevalence.

■ ANSWERS AND DISCUSSION FOR CHAPTER 17

Answer 17-1: B

Discussion 17-1

There are a number of findings compatible with an ultrasound diagnosis of acute DVT. Acute DVT results in *enlargement* of the vein lumen, which contains an *echolucent* thrombus, the opposite of incorrect answers D and E, respectively. It is chronic venous thrombotic occlusion that is associated with echogenic thrombus and a decreased vein caliber (as well as extensive collaterals around the thrombosed vein). The primary means of diagnosis, and the most reliable, is (B) incompressibility of the vein using B-mode scanning with the vein in cross-section. The vein is obviously also not compressible in longitudinal view (A); however, confirmation of incompressibility is much more difficult in longitudinal section because the transducer may roll to the side of the vein and give a false impression of incompressibility or compressibility of the vein. Because there is no flow through the thrombosed vein, there will be an absence of color, not a color "bruit" (C).

Answer 17-2: D

Discussion 17-2

Sensitivities and specificities for diagnosis of proximal lower extremity DVT in both (A) symptomatic and (B) asymptomatic patients exceed 90%. Diagnosis of upper extremity venous thrombosis with duplex techniques is less well documented than for lower extremity venous thrombus. However, available studies suggest sensitivities and specificities of approximately 90% using duplex techniques to diagnose upper extremity venous thrombosis, including axillo-subclavian vein thrombosis (E). Duplex is less accurate for diagnosis of calf DVT. In modern series, in (C) symptomatic patients with calf DVT, diagnosis may be possible but with an accuracy significantly less than that for more proximal DVT. However, it is in the setting of (D) calf DVT in asymptomatic patients where duplex ultrasound is least accurate (has the lowest sensitivity and specificity) for the diagnosis of DVT.

Answer 17-3: C

Discussion 17-3

Although most pulmonary emboli arise from the deep veins of the lower extremities, there are no good data to support ultrasound as an *initial* diagnostic test for suspected pulmonary embolism. The yield of positive findings is relatively low in this setting, just less than 50%, supporting the suspicion that thrombi that might have been found in the legs now reside in the lungs. Thus, answer C represents the range of positive findings to be expected in cases of documented PE. In one cited comparison with pulmonary angiography, in patients with suspected pulmonary embolism, the sensitivity and specificity of a lower extremity venous duplex were only 44% and 86%, respectively, for DVT.

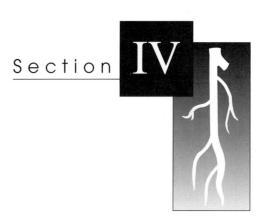

Section **IV**

VASCULAR IMAGING: BASIC TECHNIQUES AND APPLICATIONS

STUDY QUESTIONS

■ QUESTIONS FOR CHAPTER 18

Question 18-1

A 78-year-old diabetic man with non-dialysis–dependent chronic renal insufficiency is found to have a 6.5-cm infrarenal AAA and bilateral high-grade renal artery stenosis. A preoperative CO_2 arteriogram was obtained that confirmed high-grade bilateral osteal renal arterial lesions and a patent inferior mesenteric artery. The patient received four injections of approximately 40 cc of CO_2. Shortly after the procedure, he experienced abdominal pain. Physical examination revealed ecchymosis over the puncture site, but no appreciable hematoma. The abdomen was benign other than moderate diffuse mid-abdominal tenderness. The most likely cause of this patient's abdominal pain is?

A. A normal reaction from CO_2 angiography.
B. Mesenteric ischemia.
C. Aortic dissection.
D. Renal arterial spasm after CO_2.
E. Abdominal pain related to groin hematoma.

Question 18-2

Regarding gadolinium arteriography, which of the following statements is *true*?

A. Gadolinium arteriography is a valuable Food and Drug Administration (FDA)-approved option for arteriography in patients with renal insufficiency.
B. In contraposition to iodinated dye contrast agents, gadolinium high-ionic high-osmolar preparations are better suited for renal preservation.
C. Maximal doses of gadolinium should be similar to the doses used with iodinated dye contrast agents.
D. There is no nephrotoxicity associated with the use of gadolinium.
E. Gadolinium image quality is superior to that obtained by CO2 but inferior to that obtained by iodinated contrast.

Question 18-3

A 65-year-old, non-insulin–dependent diabetic woman with a high-grade right internal carotid artery stenosis and mild

baseline renal insufficiency underwent a diagnostic arteriogram with iodinated contrast employing carotid catheterization through a femoral artery access. Metformin was also given. Selective images of the right carotid system demonstrated tandem stenotic lesions of the carotid bulb and middle cerebral artery (M1 segment). The patient tolerated the procedure well; however, 4 hours after the procedure she experienced somnolence, nausea, and diarrhea. The patient was difficult to arouse, but she was able to follow commands and had a nonfocal neurologic examination. The lower extremities were warm and well perfused. Carotid duplex examination demonstrated patent carotid arteries without interval change. Computed tomography (CT) scan of the head demonstrated no acute intracranial hemorrhage or stroke changes. The most likely diagnosis in this patient is?

A. Transient neurologic attack from iatrogenic air embolization.
B. Distal cerebral plaque embolization from catheter and wire manipulation.
C. Idiosyncratic allergic reaction to the dye contrast.
D. Cerebral edema secondary to direct contrast agent hyperosmolar cytotoxicity.
E. Lactic acidosis from concomitant use of metformin.

Question 18-4

Which one of the following is a standard recommended radiographic filming projection?

A. Aortic arch with 10 degrees of left anterior oblique.
B. Renal arteries with 15 degrees of right anterior oblique.
C. Iliac bifurcation with 20 degrees of ipsilateral anterior oblique.
D. Femoral arteries with 20 degrees of ipsilateral anterior oblique.
E. Tibial trifurcation with 10 degrees of contralateral anterior oblique.

■ QUESTIONS FOR CHAPTER 19

Question 19-1

In Kistner's standard venographic classification, a grade 2 reflux means:

A. Reflux through the upper femoral veins, but not reaching the popliteal vein.
B. Reflux all the way into the calf veins and through the perforators.
C. Reflux down to a competent popliteal vein with no reflux beyond that level.
D. Popliteal valvular incompetence and leakage of contrast into the calf veins.
E. Iliac vein reflux but a competent highest femoral vein valve.

Question 19-2

Pretreatment for contrast allergy before venography includes all the listed medications *except*:

A. 50 mg of prednisone by mouth 13 hours, 7 hours, and 1 hour before the study.
B. 50 mg of diphenhydramine hydrochloride (Benadryl) 1 hour before the examination.
C. 25 mg of ephedrine 1 hour before the examination.
D. 0.5 mg of atropine 30 minutes before the examination.
E. All of the above are appropriate pretreatment.

Question 19-3

The correct name of the main deep vein of the leg between the popliteal vein and the saphenofemoral junction according to the currently correct terminology is the:

A. Femoral vein.
B. Superficial femoral vein.
C. Common femoral vein.
D. Deep femoral vein.
E. Long saphenous vein.

■   QUESTIONS FOR CHAPTER 20

Question 20-1

A "voxel" is correctly described by which one of the following:

A. A computer term meaning a visual display of digital information.
B. The smallest digital image data unit that has coordinates both in x and y axes.
C. A collection of digital images displayed as a whole.
D. A discrete spatial digital volume component made from a series of two-dimensional pixels.
E. 10^3 pixels.

Question 20-2

Regarding the use of 3D image processing, all of the following are true *except*:

A. It presents comprehensive anatomic information using computerized rotatable objects.
B. It reduces clinical interpretation time by creating intuitively obvious images.
C. It reduces interobserver error by creating a consistent archived image that facilitates measurements in three dimensions.
D. It improves visualization of the tissues by color coding each voxel in a standard preset way based on the density of the pixels.

E. It allows clearer focus on specific anatomic structures by subtraction of other structures in the same area.

Question 20-3

Disadvantages of surface rendering display images do *not* include:

A. An overly high radiodensity threshold that can yield a falsely high impression of vessel stenosis.
B. Use of serial images for quantitative measurement may produce errors.
C. Greatly increased computing power requirements compared with other image processing methods.
D. Vascular calcification may be difficult to separate from radiocontrast.
E. The necessary post-processing expertise for surface rendering does not exist in most institutions.

■   QUESTIONS FOR CHAPTER 21

Question 21-1

CT scanning is *least* useful for evaluating which of the following types of pathology?

A. Pulmonary embolus.
B. Aortic dissection.
C. Horseshoe kidney.
D. Duplicate vena cava.
E. Bypass graft patency.

Question 21-2

A patient returns for routine imaging 1 month after endovascular repair of his AAA. Contrast-enhanced CT indicates areas of lighter density (different from thrombus density) within the aneurysm sac. What condition would *not* cause this appearance?

A. Calcific plaque or calcification developing within the thrombus.
B. "Beam-hardening" or scatter caused by adjacent metallic stent.
C. Type I endoleak.
D. Contrast remaining in the sac from the time of his endovascular repair procedure.
E. Motion artifact.

Question 21-3

CT *without* contrast is *most* important in which of the following cases?

A. Traumatic aortic injury.
B. Pulmonary embolus.
C. Intracranial hemorrhage.
D. Aortic dissection.
E. Aortic aneurysm.

Question 21-4

A patient with an AAA is being evaluated for possible endovascular repair. On a contrast-enhanced CT, which of the following scan parameters is *most* important in determining the patency of small branch vessels such as accessory renal arteries or the inferior mesenteric artery?

A. Use of delayed-contrast technique.
B. Slice thickness (beam collimation).
C. Type of scanner.
D. Rate of contrast injection.
E. Emitter power (kVp and mA).

■ QUESTIONS FOR CHAPTER 22

Question 22-1

Magnetic resonance angiography (MRA) can generate arteriographic images:

A. With the use of non-nephrotoxic contrast agents.
B. Without the use of contrast agents.
C. That may contain artifacts producing false information.
D. A, B, and C are all true.
E. A and B are true but C is not.

Question 22-2

MRA is useful for which of the following vascular beds?

A. Renal artery.
B. Carotid artery.
C. Lower extremity arteries.
D. Aortic arch.
E. All of the above.

Question 22-3

Which statement regarding *lower extremity* MRA is incorrect?

A. Runoff vessels are not as well seen as with conventional contrast arteriography.
B. Both time-of-flight and contrast-enhanced techniques have been used with success.
C. Limb salvage is facilitated by the ability of MRA to detect patent runoff vessels that are not seen by contrast arteriography.
D. MRA may be used as the sole preoperative imaging modality for planning peripheral revascularization procedures.

E. MRA has been demonstrated to be a cost-effective imaging modality for planning peripheral vascular surgery.

■ QUESTIONS FOR CHAPTER 23

Question 23-1

Which of the following statements is *not* true of the use of intravascular ultrasound (IVUS) during endovascular surgery?

A. It does not eliminate the need for fluoroscopy.
B. It reduces the amount of contrast used for an endovascular procedure.
C. It reduces the fluoroscopic time.
D. It has difficulty visualizing vessel orifices.
E. Color flow imaging with IVUS does not show actual flow velocities.

Question 23-2

During AAA endovascular repair, IVUS is a useful tool for dealing with which of the following:

A. Type I endoleaks.
B. Type II endoleaks.
C. Type III endoleaks.
D. Type IV endoleaks.
E. Type V endoleaks.

Question 23-3

Which of the following *correctly* describes the use of IVUS in the management of thoracic aortic dissections, or its limitations?

A. The proximal entry point can be readily identified, but not the distal entry point.
B. Flow through the false, as opposed to the true, lumen cannot be determined.
C. Blood flow through branch vessels cannot be readily determined at the time of an interventional procedure.
D. During an interventional procedure, the IVUS catheter could perforate the aortic wall and thus must be advanced over a guidewire.
E. The relationship of branch vessels to the false lumen and dissection flap can not be determined.

ANSWERS AND DISCUSSION _____

■ ANSWERS AND DISCUSSION FOR CHAPTER 18

Answer 18-1: B

Discussion 18-1

CO_2 angiography is a valuable alternative to iodinated contrast medium is selected patients with renal insufficiency. Although rare, complications from CO_2 may potentially be serious.

A. Abdominal pain is not a normal reaction to this study.
B. Patients with large AAAs are at increased risk for gas trapping embolization to the mesenteric vessels because of the larger requirement of gas to displace a larger volume of blood and potential delayed clearance. This complication can be avoided by limiting the amount of CO_2 injection, spacing out the injections, frequent patient repositioning to favor gas clearance, and fluoroscopic reimaging before the next injection to confirm gas clearance.
C. Complications of an aortic dissection would present with a significantly different clinical picture.
D. CO_2 is usually well tolerated and has not been associated with vasospasm of renal or any other branch of arteries.
E. Groin hematoma was not apparent, but retroperitoneal hemorrhage from a high puncture can show little evidence of groin hemorrhage, but usually this presents with hypotension and if there is pain it is not mid-abdominal, as in this case.

Answer 18-2: E

Discussion 18-2

In selected patients, both CO_2 and gadolinium provide a valuable alternative for patients in whom iodinated dye contrast agents would not be well tolerated, such as patients with renal insufficiency and significant allergic reactions to iodinated contrast agents. However, these advantages of gadolinium arteriography are not absolute and are dose related.

A. Although gadolinium is FDA approved for magnetic resonance imaging, gadolinium-enhanced angiography is not approved and must be considered an off-label application.
B. Gadolinium can cause nephrotoxicity by hyperosmolarity, so high-ionic, high-osmolar preparations are *not* better suited for renal preservation than iodinated dye preparations.
C. The maximal FDA recommended intravenous doses are 0.3 to 0.4 mmol/kg, which is *not* similar to doses used with iodinating agents.
D. Gadolinium may cause nephrotoxicity by direct cellular toxicity as well as hyperosmolarity.
E. In general, the image quality of gadolinium is superior to the one from CO_2 but inferior to the one obtained by iodinated contrast agents.

Answer 18-3: E

Discussion 18-3

The time presentation (4 hours later) and absence of focalized clinical, sonographic, and radiographic findings go against a cerebrovascular event. Both (A) air embolism and (B) plaque embolism from catheter manipulation would produce immediate focal cerebral ischemic symptoms; (C) idiosyncratic reactions to iodinated agents do not present with this clinical picture; and (D) cerebral edema secondary to hyperosmolar toxicity is very unlikely and would develop in a different time frame and without diarrhea. The described clinical picture is consistent with (E) symptomatic lactic acidosis related to the concomitant use of metformin, common in this setting. Therefore, E is the correct answer.

Answer 18-4: D

Discussion 18-4

Different oblique angiographic projections allow visualization of the vessel origins so that orificial lesions are not underrecognized.

A. In general, a greater degree (15–20 degrees) of left anterior oblique projection, with the head hyperextended and rotated toward the right side will display the aortic arch vessels well.
B. The renal arteries are usually well displayed with an anteroposterior projection or mild *left* anterior oblique angulation.
C. The origin of the internal iliac artery is best displayed with a *contralateral* oblique view.
D. The profunda femoris is best seen with a 20-degree ipsilateral anterior oblique projection (correct answer).
E. The anterior tibial arteries are best displayed with *ipsilateral* anterior obliquity.

■ ANSWERS AND DISCUSSION FOR CHAPTER 19

Answer 19-1: C

Discussion 19-1

The use of specific classification criteria for venous reflux in the lower extremity is essential to evaluating clinical reports on the management of chronic venous insufficiency. The system developed by Kistner et al. has intuitive simplicity and stratifies radiographic findings with anatomic features that correlate with the adverse effects of venous hypertension. It should be understood that clinical reports of treatments for valvular insufficiency that do not classify both the pre- and posttreatment anatomic status are likely to be uninterpretable or misleading. The Kistner venographic classification requires retrograde femoral venography with the patient tilted to a head-up angle on an angiogram table. Grading reflux from 1 to 4 is based on how far down the leg veins the contrast reaches from above. In grade 1, there is only (A) reflux into the upper femoral veins. In grade 2, there is complete femoral reflux but a competent popliteal valve prevents contrast from refluxing into the calf veins, so answer C is correct. In grade 3 reflux, there is reflux down past an incompetent popliteal valve and into competent calf veins. In grade 4 there is reflux (usually rapid) all the way down through the popliteal vein and into the calf veins, which are also incompetent. Answers B and D differ only in that perforators are also visualized as refluxing in B, but this technique of retrograde venography is not an appropriate method for studying perforator vein incompetence. Finally, in regard to answer E there are no valves in the iliac veins in the majority of patients. Therefore, retrograde flow in the iliac vein (as might be seen in venography using contralateral catheter access through the common femoral vein) stopping at a competent highest common femoral vein is a normal finding.

Answer 19-2: D

Discussion 19-2

True contrast allergy is less common than a presumptive diagnosis of it that is not based on specific criteria. But when diagnostic criteria are met, pretreatment with agents known to be preventive of allergic reaction: (A) prednisone, (B) Benadryl, and, to enhance vasomotor tone, (C) ephedrine, are known to be beneficial. (D) Atropine is not known to have a benefit in the prevention of physiologic response to contrast allergy, making this the correct, and E a wrong answer.

Answer 19-3: A

Discussion 19-3

The venous segment described formerly was identified by the now-abandoned term (B) superficial femoral vein. It was used to distinguish it from the (D) deep femoral vein, although both of these veins are part of the deep venous circulation of the leg. But confusion arose because many physicians who were not knowledgeable about the anatomy of leg veins regarded thrombosis when described as occurring in the "superficial femoral vein" as being of little consequence because that name associated it with the superficial venous system, and thus it was not considered and treated as a DVT. Consensus panels producing guidelines for venous disease classification recognized this and published revised nomenclature to eliminate confusion by naming this deep vein segment, between the popliteal vein and the (C) common femoral vein, the "femoral vein," so A is the correct answer. Even though this vein is paired in approximately one third of normal subjects, the name remains the same. The saphenous vein is a superficial vein, but there are two saphenous veins that are called the greater and lesser saphenous veins in North America and the long (E) and short saphenous veins in much of Europe and the rest of the world. The same terminology consensus has settled this confusion as well, but currently, acceptance of these latter changes has been limited.

■ ANSWERS AND DISCUSSION FOR CHAPTER 20

Answer 20-1: D

Discussion 20-1

Voxel processing of medical images results from a discrete tissue volume, sampled at an arbitrary constant interval, re- sulting in a dataset comprised of a series of two-dimensional images, so answer D is correct. The picture elements comprising that original dataset are made up of pixels having x and y coordinates, *but* a voxel is the smallest digital unit having x, y, and z coordinates. Thus, answer B is wrong. Another way of saying this is to describe the voxel as a point surrounded equally by the smallest units in the x, y, and z coordinates. Thus, a voxel itself is not two dimensional, but a dataset created by the computerized "stacking" of the two-dimensional images, the result existing in computer memory as a solid block of data, as "voxels." A voxel is not (A) a computer term meaning a visual display of digital information, nor is it simply (C) a collection of digital images displayed as a whole. The number of pixels in a voxel is not fixed at any multiple of pixels, like (E) 103 pixels.

Answer 20-2: D

Discussion 20-2

Answers A, B, C, and E are all correct because they each accurately describe functional advantages of 3D postprocessing that characterize its use and clinical value. (D) Color coding of different tissues or structures (e.g., bone, blood, and plaque) is done, during postprocessing, to enhance visualization and interpretation, but not in this manner, i.e., *not* based on pixel density.

Answer 20-3: C

Discussion 20-3

The principle advantage of surface rendering display image processing is that it uses only a reduced dataset to produce the resultant image. Although the 3D appearance of surface rendering can be enhanced by adding "ray-casting" algorithms during processing, it does *not* contain the anatomic detail of volume rendering. Answers A, B, C, and D are true, in that they describe known disadvantages of surface rendering. Answer E is the correct answer (not a disadvantage) because the necessary imaging expertise now widely exists. In addition, expertise in such postprocessing techniques can be accessed by transmitting the data to medical imaging corporations or institutions where the necessary expertise does exist to perform this and other postprocessing techniques. They can return the resultant images in a reasonable time frame for local clinical decision-making.

■ ANSWERS AND DISCUSSION FOR CHAPTER 21

Answer 21-1: E

Discussion 21-1

Pulmonary embolus (A) can be detected by spiral CT by contrast bolus and rapid image acquisition, even in patients without clinically suspected disease. CT may be more accurate and more specific than ventilation-perfusion scans. CT has become the study of choice in most cases of thoracic aortic dissection (B). Left-sided or duplicate vena cava (D) or retro-aortic renal veins can be easily seen on axial CT images, and the important anatomic variations of horseshoe kidney (C) such as isthmus thickness and blood supply can be evaluated. Bypass graft patency (E) is better evaluated by diagnostic ultrasound together with physical examination, making this the *least* useful CT scanning application.

Answer 21-2: D

Discussion 21-2

Calcified plaque is commonly seen within the aneurysm sac as a more radiodense structure (A). Beam hardening, scatter artifacts, and averaging artifact from metal components of endografts (because of the extreme density of metal) can cause a similar "bright" or dense appearance in adjacent low-contrast thrombus (B). An endoleak of any kind can be detected by density difference caused by the inflow of contrast-containing blood (C). Motion artifact is capable of producing density differences because of "averaging" or distortion within the aortic sac image that require interpretation to exclude other causes (E). Contrast used for procedural guidance would not appear as a density difference within the excluded sac after 1 month (D, correct answer).

Answer 21-3: C

Discussion 21-3

The amount of intracranial hemorrhage and its effects can be evaluated adequately by noncontrast CT scanning. Intracranial hemorrhage appears as a bright density on a noncontrast scan, and contrast from intravenous agents can actually make interpretation more difficult unless a separate noncontrast study is obtained first. Therefore C is the correct answer. All of the other choices (A, B, D, and E) are far better detected and fully evaluated by the use of CT with contrast agents.

Answer 21-4: B

Discussion 21-4

Immediate renal and mesenteric arterial branches of the abdominal aorta are filled with contrast simultaneously with the aorta, so A is incorrect. The type of scanner (C) is relatively unimportant compared with other factors listed. Although the rate of contrast injection (D) affects the radiodensity of flowing blood, the usual protocol of contrast injection in abdominal CT scanning allows visualization of aortic branches, and the power settings of the scanner (E) have relatively minor effects on renal artery visualization. Visualization of small arteries such as the inferior mesenteric or accessory renal arteries is greatly influenced by (B) CT slice thickness. Increased slice thickness compromises the ability to detect small structures such as accessory renal arteries because of volume averaging artifact, but decreased slice thickness helps and B is therefore the correct answer.

■ ANSWERS AND DISCUSSION FOR CHAPTER 22

Answer 22-1: D

Discussion 22-1

MRA is a noninvasive arteriographic imaging modality. It can produce arteriographic images without the use of contrast agents (B) by exploiting the magnetic properties of flowing blood (time-of-flight angiography). More recently, gadolinium contrast agents, which are non-nephrotoxic (A), have been used through peripheral venous injection to enhance the quality of angiographic images. The selective method of fat suppression will actually result in suppression of the water signal instead. Thus, a vessel that is entirely patent may appear entirely occluded. Other potential artifacts exist, depending on the MR techniques used in an individual examination, that require understanding to interpret. Thus C is also true, making D, not E, the correct answer.

Answer 22-2: E

Discussion 22-2

MRA has been useful as a screening test for renovascular disease, particularly with the use of contrast enhancement. MRA has been shown to be accurate for the diagnosis of carotid and lower extremity occlusive disease and to be extremely helpful in the diagnosis of aortic dissection. Because all of the above are useful MRA applications, E is the correct answer.

Answer 22-3: A

Discussion 22-3

MRA often detects patent runoff vessels that are "occult" to contrast arteriography. These vessels have been successfully used for targets in peripheral bypass procedures, facilitating limb salvage. (A) MRA is at least as accurate as contrast arteriography for runoff imaging, as demonstrated by a number of multicenter trials and institutional reports. The statements in B, C, D, and E are all factually correct descriptions of current MRA use.

■ ANSWERS AND DISCUSSION FOR CHAPTER 23

Answers 23-1: D

Discussion 23-1

IVUS is a useful adjunct to many endovascular procedures. However, (A) fluoroscopy is still needed to visualize guidewire and device positioning and deployment. The amount (ml) of contrast agent (B) and the amount (time) of fluoroscopy exposure (C) can be greatly reduced by pre-evaluation with IVUS imaging. IVUS can readily (D) locate the orifices of important vessels, such as renal arteries and hypogastric arteries without the use of fluoroscopy or contrast, and thus is valuable in the endovascular repair of AAAs. Once the vessel orifice is located with IVUS, the location can be verified and referenced to a radio-opaque scale behind the patient. Therefore statement D is *not* true and is the correct answer. This ability will also reduce fluoroscopy time and contrast usage. Some newer fluoroscopy systems also allow for "pulse mode" imaging. The pulse mode can reduce the fluoroscopic time by a factor of 4, and creates an image that is very adequate for the pre-evaluation with IVUS. Finally, although Duplex scanning has been commonly used as a guide for bedside IVC filter placement, it has limitations, particularly in obese or distended patients. IVUS does not share these limitations and is being increasingly used in the

ICU (intensive care unit) setting, e.g., for multiple trauma patients.

Answers 23-2: A
Discussion 23-2

IVUS is a useful tool to confirm previously measured aortic and iliac diameters and lengths during endovascular AAA repair. After the device is deployed, it can also be used to evaluate device apposition at the proximal and distal fixation points. This may help to eliminate (A) Type I endoleaks. (B) Type II and (D) IV endoleaks are not readily seen on IVUS because of the initial endograft porosity and air. However, *after* the graft has had time to become incorporated, color flow IVUS may become a useful tool for evaluation of (C) type III and IV endoleak. However, this would be an invasive procedure and most likely limited to use during a secondary intervention. (E) Type V endoleak is not included in current reporting standards. It was once used in relation to "endotension," but the latter is now considered as AAA sac pressurization in the absence of demonstrable endoleak.

Answer 23-3: D
Discussion 23-3

Although skilled interpretation is necessary for achieving the benefits of IVUS in both defining the anatomical extent of dissection and in guiding interventional procedures, it can be readily applied to managing thoracic aortic dissection. In this regard, it does not have the limitations suggested in A, B, C, and E; but D is correct:

A. Both the proximal *and distal* entry points can be identified.
B. Flow through the false lumen *can* be identified.
C. Blood flow through branch vessels *can* be determined at the time of an interventional procedure.
D. During an interventional procedure, in this setting, the IVUS catheter could potentially perforate the aortic wall and for this reason should always be advanced over a guidance (correct answer).
E. Not only can flow through branch vessels be identified, but the relationship of these branch vessels to the false lumen and dissection flap *can* be determined.

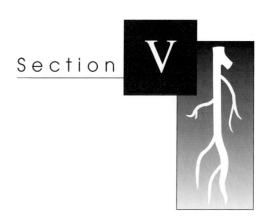

ARTERIAL DISEASES: BASIC CONSIDERATIONS

STUDY QUESTIONS

■ QUESTIONS FOR CHAPTER 24

Question 24-1

Unfavorable changes in atherosclerotic plaques predisposing to their instability include all of the following *except*:

A. Macrophage infiltration within the cap of the plaque.
B. Cytokine production by round cells within the plaque.
C. An extensive lipid core.
D. Fibrous tissue transformation.
E. Hemorrhage into the plaque.

Question 24-2

The core of a typical type 4 plaque mainly contains:

A. Fibrin and fibrinogen.
B. Inflammatory cells.
C. Collagen.
D. Cholesterol oleate and free cholesterol.
E. Foam cells.

Question 24-3

The earliest lesions of atherosclerosis usually are characterized by:

A. Endothelial denudation.
B. Breaks in the internal elastic lamina.
C. Adventitial vascular infiltration.
D. Increased intimal lipid containing macrophages.
E. Focal fibrin deposition.

■ QUESTIONS FOR CHAPTER 25

Question 25-1

Which of the following is inconsistent with the diagnosis of Buerger's disease?

A. A 24-year-old woman.
B. Repeated episodes of superficial thrombophlebitis.
C. Lower extremity ischemic ulceration.
D. Severe hypertension.
E. Occlusion of the ulnar artery demonstrated on an Allen test.

Question 25-2

Which of the following is most important in the treatment of patients with Buerger's disease?

A. Use of calcium channel blocker.
B. Cilostazol.
C. Abstinence from tobacco use.
D. Fish oil supplementation.
E. Anticoagulation.

Question 25-3

A 30-year-old man presents with ischemic ulcers on three of his fingers. He does not smoke cigarettes. Urine nicotine and cotinine levels confirm no tobacco exposure. He has never had deep or superficial thrombophlebitis. All of his immunologic blood test results are normal as is his sedimentation rate. The echocardiogram is normal. His occupation is as an accountant, and he has no hobbies. An arteriogram shows a normal aortic arch and normal arteries down to the wrist bilaterally. He has bilateral ulnar artery occlusions, multiple digital artery occlusions, and several areas of "corkscrew collaterals." Which of the following diagnostic possibilities is completely consistent with this clinical scenario?

A. Cocaine arteritis.
B. Thromboangiitis obliterans.
C. Takayasu's arteritis (TA).
D. Giant cell arteritis.
E. Radiation-induced arteritis.

■ QUESTIONS FOR CHAPTER 26

Question 26-1

Which of the following best distinguishes Takayasu's arteritis (TA) from atherosclerosis?

A. Process begins with destruction of the elastic component of the media.
B. More commonly affects men than women.
C. Always presents before 45 years of age.
D. Frequent association with hypertension.
E. Elevated erythrocyte sedimentation rate (ESR).

Question 26-2

In the United States, the most common clinical manifestation of TA is:

A. Cerebral ischemia.
B. Temporal headache.
C. Upper extremity arterial insufficiency.
D. Pulmonary hypertension.
E. Mesenteric ischemia.

Question 26-3

A 37-year-old woman presents with left arm ischemia caused by a long, tapered stenosis of the proximal left subclavian artery. The carotid arteries are not involved, but the ESR is mildly elevated. Each of the following may be appropriate treatment options *except*:

A. Prednisone.
B. Methotrexate.
C. Carotid-subclavian bypass with polytetrafluoroethylene graft.
D. Axillo-axillary bypass.
E. Subclavian endarterectomy.

■   **QUESTIONS FOR CHAPTER 27**

Question 27-1

A 38-year-old woman presents with a 2-year history of significant diastolic hypertension refractory to three antihypertension medications. She has no family history of hypertension and no systemic manifestations of atherosclerotic occlusive disease, and she does not smoke. She undergoes diagnostic arteriography. What is the most likely finding on the study?

A. Smooth focal stenosis of the right main renal artery.
B. Ostial stenoses associated with diffuse aortic atherosclerosis.
C. String of beads appearance affecting the right main renal artery.
D. Aortic hypoplasia associated with ostial renal artery stenoses.
E. Normal-appearing renal arteries.

Question 27-2

The cause of medial fibrodysplasia seems gender related. The factor that is *not* associated with its occurrence is:

A. Hormones associated with the reproductive cycle.
B. Oral antiovulants (the "pill").
C. Unusual physical stresses on the involve arteries that are greater in women than men.
D. Mural ischemia.
E. Tissue hypoxia.

Question 27-3

Renal artery medial fibrodysplasia is a complex nonarteriosclerotic disease that is most often encountered in women aged less than 50 years. Which of the following is also *true* for this condition?

A. It accounts for slightly less than half of dysplastic renal arteries.

B. It commonly regresses after menopause.
C. It extends from the main renal artery into segmental arteries in 25% of cases.
D. It rarely is associated with intracranial aneurysms.
E. It is associated with vertebral fibrodysplasia in 85% of cases.

■   **QUESTIONS FOR CHAPTER 28**

Question 28-1

A previously healthy 30-year-old woman with a history of migraine headaches is admitted to the hospital with pain, numbness, and cyanosis of both lower extremities. Examination reveals absence of all pulses distal to the femoral level. Further history revealed she had taken Cafergot the day before for intractable headaches. What is the treatment of choice to alleviate this patient's severe lower extremity ischemia?

A. Heparin.
B. Clopidogrel.
C. Nifedipine.
D. Cilostazol.
E. Nitroprusside.

Question 28-2

Which one of the following diseases is not a cause of ascending aortic aneurysm?

A. TA.
B. Turner syndrome.
C. Marfan syndrome.
D. Tertiary syphilis.
E. Polyarteritis nodosa.

Question 28-3

Concerning TA, what is the most useful test to determine disease activity?

A. Proteinase 3/antineutrophil cytoplasmic antibody.
B. Myeloperoxidase/perinuclear immunofluorescence pattern.
C. Cryoglobulins.
D. Antinuclear antibody.
E. Estimated sedimentation rate (ESR).

Question 28-4

Pulmonary artery aneurysms are most commonly associated with which one of the following diseases?

A. Behçet's disease.
B. TA.
C. Polyarteritis nodosa.
D. Ehlers-Danlos syndrome.
E. Pulmonary thromboembolism.

Question 28-5

Which of the following is not a characteristic of Behçet's disease?

A. Oral aphthous ulcers, uveitis, and pathergy.
B. Predisposition to unusual venous thrombosis.
C. Arterial aneurysms, often multiple.

D. Pulmonary artery aneurysms, commonly found.

E. Diagnostic serologic blood tests.

Question 28-6

An elevated sedimentation rate should increase suspicion of an uncommon arteriopathy in all but which one of the following cases?

A. A 10-year-old child with severe arterial hypertension.

B. A 20 year old with a newly diagnosed murmur of aortic valve incompetence.

C. A 60 year old with abdominal pain, weight loss, and AAA with a thickened wall on CT scan.

D. A 40-year-old man with severe coronary, carotid, and peripheral artery disease in the absence of cardiovascular risk factors. The skin shows peculiar yellow papules across lines of flexion.

E. A young child with coronary artery aneurysms.

Question 28-7

An 18-year-old student undergoing a routine school physical examination is found to have unsuspected severe aortic valve incompetence. A cardiac echocardiogram shows an enlarged aortic root measuring 6 cm. Which one of the following clinical features is the least likely to be present?

A. Arachnodactyly and abnormally long arms and legs.

B. Pectus carinatum or excavatum.

C. A systolic murmur of mitral valve regurgitation.

D. Lens dislocation.

E. Easy bruising.

Question 28-8

Which one of the following is not true of the underlying disorder in Marfan syndrome?

A. It has autosomal dominant inheritance.

B. It is caused by a mutation in the fibrillin-1 gene.

C. It is caused by a mutation in the gene for type 111 procollagen.

D. In 25% of cases it is caused by a spontaneous mutation.

E. The diagnosis is based on the Ghent clinical criteria.

Question 28-9

A 70-year-old nonsmoker presents with aching discomfort in both arms with activity. On examination, subclavian pulses are normal with absence of brachial and more distal pulses bilaterally. The blood test shows anemia with hemoglobin of 10 g/dL, elevated alkaline phosphatase, and elevated C-reactive protein. What is the most likely diagnosis in this patient?

A. Thoracic outlet syndrome.

B. Thromboangiitis obliterans.

C. Temporal (giant cell) arteritis.

D. TA.

E. Atherosclerosis obliterans.

■ QUESTIONS FOR CHAPTER 29

Question 29-1

The development of AAA in an individual is generally associated with several known epidemiologic risk factors.

 Of the following, which factor is *not* associated with an increased risk of development of aneurysmal disease?

A. Tobacco smoking.

B. Diabetes.

C. Age greater than 75 years.

D. Family history of infrarenal AAA.

E. Hypercholesterolemia.

Question 29-2

Patients who have AAAs are at an increased risk of development of certain other peripheral aneurysms. Aneurysmal degeneration of all the following arteries, *except* which one, is found with increased frequency in patients with infrarenal AAA:

A. Common iliac artery.

B. Superficial femoral artery.

C. External iliac artery.

D. Hypogastric artery.

E. Popliteal artery.

Question 29-3

All of the following histopathologic and biochemical features are characteristic of AAAs *except*:

A. Chronic transmural inflammation.

B. Decreased elastin content.

C. Increased production of matrix metalloproteinases (MMPs).

D. Medial SMC proliferation and hypertrophy.

E. Intimal atherosclerosis.

ANSWERS AND DISCUSSION

■ ANSWERS AND DISCUSSION FOR CHAPTER 24

Answer 24-1: D

Discussion 24-1

(D) Fibrous tissue transformation, although related to stenosis, produces a more stable plaque. On the other hand, (A) macrophage infiltration has been shown to relate to cap rupture and instability, (B) plaque macrophages and lymphocytes have been shown to produce a variety of inflammatory cytokines, (C) the role of an expanding core from inception to late instability has been recently emphasized, and (E) intra-plaque hemorrhage, particularly in the carotids and coronary arteries, is associated with sudden expansion and the onset of symptoms.

Answer 24-2: D

Discussion 24-2

In the later stages of plaque formation the core is composed *mainly* of (D) cholesterol oleate and free cholesterol, as measured in biochemical studies. On the other hand, (A) variable amounts of fibrin and fibrinogen are found on plaque surfaces, (B) inflammatory cells may line the core or appear on the surface in varying amounts, and these are often seen in the adventitia, (C) collagen appears surrounding plaques, but the core by definition of the type 4 plaque consists of lipid. Later the lipid escapes. (E) Foam cells are mainly present in early type I to III plaques.

Answer 24-3: D

Discussion 24-3

The earliest lesions are (D) focal intimal accumulations of lipid containing macrophages found at particular sites in infancy and childhood. (A) Although focal endothelial changes occur, most plaques develop beneath an intact endothelium. (B) Breaks in the internal elastic lamina are associated with type II and III lesions. (C) Vascular ingrowth characterizes late lesions. (E) Fibrin deposition occurs in some lesions but is not the most common pathway to plaque formation.

■ ANSWERS AND DISCUSSION FOR CHAPTER 25

Answer 25-1: D

Discussion 25-1

A. Although there is the misconception that Buerger's disease occurs only in men, in actuality it may occur in men or women and usually presents between the ages of 20 and 45 years. In the United States and Western Europe, between 15% and 30% of all patients with Buerger's disease are women.

B. Buerger's disease affects the arteries, veins, and nerves. Approximately 40% of patients with Buerger's disease have superficial thrombophlebitis and a smaller percentage develop deep vein thrombosis.

C. The majority of patients with Buerger's disease present with ischemic ulcerations. In the largest series from the United States, 46% of patients presented with lower extremity ulcerations, 28% presented with upper extremity ulcerations, and 26% presented with both upper and lower extremity ulcerations.

D. Hypertension is usually not seen in patients with Buerger's disease. It is not part of the clinical picture one is likely to encounter.

E. An abnormal Allen test is present in more than 60% of patients with Buerger's disease and indicates involvement of the radial and ulnar artery (or the Palmer arches) distal to the wrist. Because this disease involves the small- and medium-sized blood vessels, it is common to have involvement of the blood vessels in the hands and feet.

Answer 25-2: C

Discussion 25-2

A. Use of calcium channel blockers is helpful in the management of the vasospastic component that is present in more than 40% of patients with Buerger's disease. However, it is *not* the *primary* treatment modality and should only be used as an adjunct to more definitive therapy as discussed in answer C.

B. There are no randomized trials demonstrating efficacy of cilostazol in the treatment of Buerger's disease. Cilostazol is only approved to treat the symptoms of PAD, specifically claudication. However, there are two small case series that suggest that cilostazol may be beneficial in the healing of ischemic ulcerations of the fingers or toes in patients with small vessel occlusive disease. Therefore it may be used as an adjunct to the other therapies discussed in this chapter.

C. Complete abstinence from tobacco is the only therapy that has been shown to prevent the progression of disease and prevent amputation in patients with Buerger's disease. This includes discontinuation of cigarette, cigar, and pipe smoking, and avoidance of chewing tobacco, snuff, and other tobacco products. The role of secondhand smoke is not well delineated, but most experts in the field believe that avoidance of secondhand smoke is prudent during the acute phase of the disease.

D. There is no good evidence regarding the benefits or lack thereof of fish oil supplementation, so this form of treatment cannot be recommended in patients with Buerger's disease.

E. There is no clear-cut benefit of anticoagulation in patients with Buerger's disease. Some clinicians recommend anticoagulation in patients with Buerger's disease who have undergone a distal arterial bypass to keep the bypass open. However, there is no level I evidence that this is effective in keeping the bypass open.

Answer 25-3: A

Discussion 25-3

A. Cocaine arteritis can mimic thromboangiitis obliterans in virtually every aspect. When a patient presents with features suggesting Buerger's disease yet the patient denies smoking, the first thing that should be checked is a urine nicotine and cotinine level. If this shows no exposure to tobacco, and if the immunologic test results are all normal, the next step would be to check a toxicology screen. This should include cocaine, amphetamine, and cannabis because all three of these can mimic Buerger's disease.

B. There has not been a well-documented case of Buerger's disease in a patient who has not used tobacco in some form. Although there are sporadic cases reported in patients with no tobacco exposure, these have not measured urine nicotine or cotinine, or evaluated the patient for all the other conditions that can mimic Buerger's disease. Corkscrew collaterals are not pathognomonic of Buerger's disease but may be present in small-vessel occlusive disease of any cause.

C. TA is a large artery arteritis. Involvement of the arteries of the hands or feet does not occur. This disease occurs most frequently in young women and involves the major branches that arise from the aorta.

D. Giant cell arteritis is pathologically identical to TA, and the arterial distribution is also similar. It occurs in individuals aged more than 60 years most commonly and does not involve the small vessels of the hands or feet. The temporal artery (temporal arteritis) and the major branches off the aorta are most commonly involved.

E. Radiation-induced arteritis most commonly affects the larger vessels and produces long smooth areas of narrowing. There is no history of radiation exposure, and the large arteries are normal.

■ ANSWERS AND DISCUSSION FOR CHAPTER 26

Answer 26-1: A
Discussion 26-1

A. TA is an inflammatory process that seems to begin with destruction of the elastic component of the media. The inflammatory process then extends to the outer layers of the arterial wall, giving the appearance of a "panarteritis." In contrast, atherosclerosis begins as lipid accumulation in the intima, resulting in formation of a lipid core. Lipid accumulation attracts inflammatory cells that produce cytokines locally. The inflammatory process contributes significantly to formation of advanced plaque and may be a determining factor in plaque vulnerability to sudden expansion and rupture.

B. TA is more common in women than men, but gender predilection cannot distinguish TA from atherosclerosis in a patient with arterial symptoms.

C. TA usually presents before the age of 40 years, and this was used as a major diagnostic criterion in the past. However, age is no longer used as an obligatory criterion in modern diagnostic schemes. Although atherosclerosis usually affects patients in the seventh or eighth decade of life, up to 5% may present with symptoms before the age of 45 years.

D. As many as 70% of patients with TA may have hypertension caused by renal artery stenosis or aortic coarctation. However, hypertension is also an important risk factor for atherosclerosis and therefore cannot distinguish between the two diseases.

E. The ESR has been used to monitor disease activity in patients with TA. However, up to 25% of patients with histologically active disease have normal ESRs.

Answer 26-2: C
Discussion 26-2

In the United States, TA most commonly affects the upper extremity and cerebral circulations. The left subclavian artery is most commonly involved, and upper extremity ischemia (C) is the most common manifestation. Cerebrovascular involvement (A) is the second most common manifestation of TA. Patients with TA of the carotid circulation usually present with transient ischemic attacks or stroke; temporal headaches (B) are more commonly associated with temporal arteritis. Although TA affects the pulmonary arteries in up to 50% of patients, symptomatic pulmonary hypertension (D) is rare. Mesenteric artery involvement has been reported in 20% to 30% of patients with TA, but symptomatic mesenteric ischemia (E) is substantially less prevalent.

Answer 26-3: E
Discussion 26-3

A. The ESR has been used to follow disease activity, but it is not a specific marker for the acute phase of TA. A trial of steroids may be warranted to attempt inducing disease remission. Although tapering the steroid medication is desirable, some patients may require chronic steroids to prevent recurrent disease. Further therapy may be necessary to treat limb-threatening symptoms.

B. Cytotoxic drugs may be effective in patients with active disease that does not respond to steroids and those who do not stay in remission when steroid therapy is discontinued. Among the available agents, methotrexate has been associated with fewest side effects.

C. Symptomatic patients with TA may require revascularization to prevent tissue loss or amputation. Extra-anatomic bypass with prosthetic graft is effective when the graft is sewn to angiographically and grossly normal arteries. The presence of microscopic involvement is not a contraindication to arterial reconstruction.

D. Axillo-axillary bypass may be appropriate to avoid abnormal arteries in this case.

E. Endarterectomy is a poor choice. It is inappropriate because extensive inflammation and the transmural nature of the disease process make endarterectomy technically difficult if not impossible.

■ ANSWERS AND DISCUSSION FOR CHAPTER 27

Answer 27-1: C
Discussion 27-1

The most common form of renovascular hypertension is caused by arteriosclerotic renal artery stenosis. The second most common cause is fibromuscular dysplasia, and medial fibrodysplasia accounts for the majority of this dysplastic arteriopathy. This is usually manifested by (C) a string of beads appearance on arteriographic studies. In this particular case, the fact that the patient is a young female with significant hypertension and no systemic manifestations of atherosclerotic occlusive disease suggests the diagnosis of arterial fibrodysplasia. The other arteriographic appearances (A, B, D, E) are not compatible with this most common form of renal artery fibroplasias.

Answer 27-2: B

Discussion: 27-2

Factors that have been identified as associated with medial fibrodysplasia include: (A) estrogenic hormonal influences, (C) unusual physical stresses because of stretching of the renal arteries with ptotic kidneys and similar stretching of the extracranial internal carotid arteries with hyperextension of the neck, and (D) mural ischemia because of a paucity of vasovasorum causing (E) tissue hypoxia. (B) The use of oral antiovulants has not been associated with the development of medial fibrodysplasia.

Answer 27-3: C

Discussion 27-3

(A) Renal artery medial fibrodysplasia is by far the most common form of medial fibrodysplasia, accounting for 85% of these dysplastic lesions. (B) It does *not* regress after menopause, (D) it is associated with intracranial aneurysms in *12% to 25%* of cases, and (E) it is associated with vertebral artery fibrodysplasia in *20%* of cases. (C) It does extend into the segmental renal vessels in approximately 25% of cases.

■ ANSWERS AND DISCUSSION FOR CHAPTER 28

Answer 28-1: E

Discussion 28-1

This patient has classic symptoms of ergotism with Cafergot-induced arterial vasospasm. Ergotism most commonly involves the extremities with coolness and pallor of the feet or hands, usually symmetric, associated with absent pulses. Intermittent claudication is an early feature, but ergotism can progress to critical limb ischemia with rest pain and concern for limb loss. Prompt evaluation and treatment are often necessary. An angiogram may be necessary to exclude other causes of acute arterial insufficiency such as thrombosis in situ, atheroembolism, or dissection. Vasospasm can persist for several days after stopping ergot medications. In severe cases, intravenous nitroprusside is necessary to counteract arterial vasospasm. Oral vasodilators are often not effective.

A. Although heparin anticoagulation is certainly appropriate for patients with acute arterial occlusion because of thrombosis, it will not improve the underlying vasospasm because of ergotism.
B. Clopidogrel decreases platelet aggregation and thrombosis but does not have any role in the treatment of vasospasm.

C. Nifedipine is an excellent vasodilator medication used for the prevention of digital vasospasm in primary Raynaud's syndrome but, like most oral vasodilator medications, cannot counteract severe drug-induced vasoconstriction.
D. Cilostazol is a phosphodiesterase inhibitor with vasodilator properties and may improve claudication distance in patients with chronic atherosclerotic occlusive arterial disease, but it is not useful for this patient with acute arterial insufficiency.
E. Nitroprusside is the drug of choice for severe cases of ergotism. As a direct vasodilator, it is the most effective medication to reverse ergot-induced arterial vasoconstriction. Often a 24- to 36-hour intravenous infusion is necessary because of the long-lasting arterial effects of ergot drugs.

Answer 28-2: E

Discussion 28-2

A. TA has been called "the pulseless disease" because of its propensity for producing large-vessel stenoses caused by arterial inflammation. Most angiographic studies, however, show a mixture of both stenoses and aneurysmal dilations of large arteries. TA and giant cell arteritis can also present with isolated ascending aortic aneurysm without any branch vessel stenosis.
B. The Turner syndrome is a genetic abnormality characterized by the loss of one of the two x chromosomes and results in short stature, neck webbing, and cardiovascular abnormalities including aortic root dilation.
C. Marfan syndrome is an inherited connective tissue disorder caused by a defect in the fibrillin-1 gene resulting in defective elastic tissue. Aneurysmal dilation of the ascending aorta occurs in 90% of affected individuals and always involves the aortic root.
D. Syphilis is rare today, but arterial involvement classically involves the ascending aorta. Other mycotic aneurysms can occur at any level of the aorta.
E. Polyarteritis nodosa is a vasculitis of small and medium arteries that is often associated with renal and mesenteric artery aneurysms, but typically does not involve larger arteries such as the ascending aorta.

Answer 28-3: E

Discussion 28-3

Although all of the listed tests may be useful for the evaluation of undefined vasculitis, only the ESR may be helpful as an indicator of disease activity in giant cell arteritis. It is a nonspecific indicator of inflammation. There is no specific serologic test for giant cell arteritis.

A. These antibodies are found in most patients with Wegner granulomatosis, which is a small-vessel vasculitis. Antineutrophil cytoplasmic antibodies are directed against neutrophil proteinase 3 and cause cytoplasmic immunofluorescence (antineutrophil cytoplasmic antibody).
B. Microscopic polyangiitis is associated with antineutrophil cytoplasmic antibodies directed against the neutrophil enzyme myeloperoxidase, and this causes a perinuclear immunofluorescence pattern.

C. Cryoglobulins are immunoglobulins that precipitate in the cold and occur in small vessel vasculitis secondary to lymphomas and other hematologic malignancies and chronic infections; in particular, hepatitis C-associated essential mixed cryoglobulinemia.

D. Antinuclear antibodies are associated with connective tissue disorders including lupus and mixed connective tissue disease.

E. ESR may be elevated in any inflammatory process including large vessel vasculitis and is not specific for any disease. Very high sedimentation rates usually mean one of three conditions: malignancy, infection, or vasculitis. The sedimentation rate and C-reactive protein remain the most useful blood tests to determine disease activity and response to immunosuppression for TA. Other potential indicators of vasculitis activity include positron emission tomography or CT scan that can detect increased metabolic activity of the involved arteries.

Answer 28-4: A

Discussion 28-4

A. Behçet's disease is a vasculitis of medium and large vessels and can have devastating arterial manifestations. Pulmonary artery aneurysms can occur in up to half of patients with Behçet's disease and rupture can be fatal. Pulmonary artery aneurysms are a well-recognized complication of TA but are less common then systemic arterial involvement.

B. Polyarteritis nodosum is a necrotizing vasculitis of smaller arteries and is known for causing multiple small aneurysms of mesenteric and renal arteries.

C. Ehlers-Danlos syndrome is an inherited connective tissue disorder resulting in defective synthesis of type 111 collagen. Subtype 1V (the vascular type) is associated with fragile arteries that can result in rupture and hemorrhage of any *systemic* artery.

D. Chronic thromboembolism (repeated episodes) causes pulmonary hypertension, which may cause pulmonary artery enlargement but not true aneurysms.

Answer 28-5: E

Discussion 28-5

A. Behçet's disease is known for its hallmark features of oral and genital ulcers in addition to uveitis. Sterile pustules that occur after minor trauma are a sine qua non of Behçet's disease.

B. The increased risk of venous thrombosis in Behçet's disease has been well documented in the literature and can be the initial presentation of the disease, for example, superficial thrombophlebitis or unusual types of thrombosis with superior vena cava or Budd-Chiari syndrome.

C. Large vessel involvement occurs in 5% of patients, and arterial aneurysms can be multiple.

D. The second most common site for artery involvement in Behçet's disease is the pulmonary arteries, and one third of these patients die of pulmonary hemorrhage within 2 years after diagnosis.

E. The diagnosis of Behçet's disease is made on clinical grounds, because there is no specific serologic test for this disease.

Answer 28-6: D

Discussion 28-6

The finding of an elevated ESR, although nonspecific, may alert the clinician to an unsuspected arteriopathy. In relation to the stated cases:

A. TA commonly involves the renal arteries with activation of the renin-angiotensin system causing arterial hypertension. TA may mimic intimal fibromuscular dysplasia with smooth, tapered narrowing of the renal artery, and the only indication of active vasculitis may be the elevated ESR.

B. Although this patient may have a connective tissue disease such as Marfan syndrome, other considerations need to include Reiter's syndrome and giant cell arteritis.

C. This man has an inflammatory aneurysm (inflammatory aortitis), which classically is associated with elevated ESR.

D. In children with coronary disease, one should think of Kawasaki disease, which is associated with elevated ESR when the disease is active.

E. This patient has pseudoxanthoma elasticum, with typical features of premature diffuse atherosclerosis in the setting of skin xanthomas and abnormal stretching seen across lines of flexion. This is an inherited disorder of connective tissue, and *the ESR would be normal.*

Answer 28-7: E

Discussion 28-7

Easy bruising (E) is a feature of Ehlers-Danlos, type IV, but is not a feature of Marfan syndrome, which is suggested by this case scenario and is represented by the first four answers. (A) Marfan syndrome involves the ascending aorta in almost all cases and can present with the incidental finding of an aortic diastolic murmur because of aortic root dilation. Skeletal findings of the Marfan syndrome include long fingers (arachnodactyly), longer arms than legs (arm span to height exceeding 1.05), and (B) pectus carinatum. (C) The mitral valve is commonly involved in the Marfan syndrome causing mitral insufficiency. (D) Lens dislocation is a major criteria in the clinical diagnosis. (E) Although skin stria can occur, bruising is not a feature of Marfan syndrome, but it is a feature of Ehlers-Danlos syndrome.

Answer 28-8: C

Discussion 28-8

The Marfan syndrome is (A) an autosomal dominant genetic defect caused by (B) a mutation of the fibrillin-1 gene on chromosome 15, but *not* (C) a mutation in the gene for type 111 procollagen. It is Ehlers-Danlos syndrome that results from a mutation in the COL3A1 gene that codes for type 111 procollagen. (D) In 25% of cases of the Marfan syndrome, family history is negative and a spontaneous mutation is thought to be responsible. Despite the availability of genetic testing, the FBN1 mutation may not be detectable in 34% of patients so the diagnosis of Marfan syndrome continues to be made on the basis of (E) the Ghent major and minor clinical criteria.

Answer 28-9: C

Discussion 28-9

This patient has (C) extracranial giant cell ("temporal") arteritis that typically involves the brachial artery in the arms or the superficial femoral artery in the legs. Dynamic arterial compression from (A) the thoracic outlet syndrome would produce obstruction at the subclavian artery level. (B) Thromboangiitis obliterans typically occurs in younger patients who smoke and involves more distal extremity arteries. (D) TA occurs in a younger age group and, in the upper extremity, typically involves the subclavian artery. (E) Atherosclerosis obliterans practically never involves the brachial artery.

■ ANSWERS AND DISCUSSION FOR CHAPTER 29

Answer 29-1: B

Discussion 29-1

A. Tobacco smoking is the most significant modifiable risk factor associated with aneurysm development. Of all of the cardiovascular effects of tobacco smoke exposure, the risk of development of an aortic aneurysm is increased twice as much as the others, including coronary artery disease.

B. Diabetes is certainly *not* a risk factor. In fact it has been shown to be negatively associated with the risk of aneurysm development in both men and women.

C. The risk of aneurysm development in men and women is directly proportional to age.

D. Although the specific genetic changes and the inheritance pattern remain unknown, there is a clear increased risk among relatives of individuals with aneurysm disease. This seems to be most prominent in descendants of relatives who have aneurysmal disease at a relatively young age.

E. Although age, family history, and smoking history are the most significant factors associated with aneurysm development, hypercholesterolemia and clinical evidence of obstructive arterial disease (coronary artery disease, claudication, and cerebral vascular disease) are associated with a moderately increased risk of aneurysm disease. Other significant associations include hyper-

tension, chronic obstructive pulmonary disease, and height.

Answer 29-2: C

Discussion 29-2

A and D. Concomitant aneurysms of the common and internal iliac arteries occurs in 20% to 30% of patients with AAAs.

B and E. Aneurysms within the femoral popliteal arterial segment will be present in up to 15% of patients with AAA. Further, the presence of bilateral popliteal aneurysms is associated with a 50% incidence of concomitant aortic aneurysm.

C. The external iliac artery is only rarely found to be aneurysmal.

Answer 29-3: D

Discussion 29-3

A. Infiltration of macrophages and lymphocytes into the wall of the aorta is believed to be necessary for the elaboration of the matrix degrading enzymes. Unique to aneurysms is the presence of these inflammatory cells within the media.

B. The most striking histologic feature of AAA is the near complete absence of intact elastic fibers. This is particularly remarkable given the elastin fibers' intrinsic resistance to degradation and the relatively small number of enzymes capable of degrading this durable protein.

C. Several members of the matrix MMP family of enzymes are capable of elastolysis and have been found to be increased in human aortic aneurysm tissue.

D. As a mechanism for matrix repair, SMCs conceivably could retard matrix destruction precipitated by inflammatory cells and MMPs. However, their role in aneurysmal degeneration remains unknown. It is notable, however, that these cells are significantly diminished in quality and quantity within aneurysmal tissue.

E. Intimal atherosclerosis is a constant concomitant feature of aneurysmal disease; however, its role in the development of aortic dilatation is unclear.

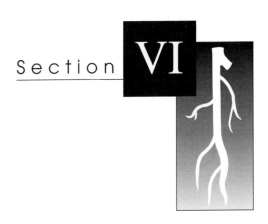
BLEEDING AND CLOTTING: FUNDAMENTAL CONSIDERATIONS

STUDY QUESTIONS

■ QUESTIONS FOR CHAPTER 30

Question 30-1

Which of the following factors is capable of initiating the activation of the *extrinsic* pathway of coagulation?

A. Tissue factor.
B. Platelet factor 4.
C. Factor VIII.
D. Protein C.
E. Factor XIII.

Question 30-2

Which of the following coagulation factors is activated by contact with surfaces and is capable of triggering the *intrinsic* pathway of coagulation?

A. Factor IX.
B. Factor XII.
C. Factor VII.
D. Factor XIII.
E. Tissue factor.

Question 30-3

Which of the following proteins is responsible for the bridging of platelet glycoprotein Ib with the damaged vascular surface?

A. Fibrinogen.
B. Collagen.
C. Factor VIII.
D. von Willebrand Factor (VWF).
E. Fibronectin.

■ QUESTIONS FOR CHAPTER 31

Question 31-1

Advantages of low molecular weight heparins over standard unfractionated heparin include all of the following *except*:

A. Greater anti-Xa and less anti-IIa activity.
B. Reduced binding to cells and plasma proteins.
C. Reduced bioavailability.
D. Subcutaneous administration.
E. Monitoring found unnecessary in most situations except in children, during pregnancy, in those with morbid obesity, and in those with renal failure.

Question 31-2

Features of warfarin anticoagulation include all of the following *except*:

A. Variable anticoagulant effect.
B. Unaffected by dietary and gastrointestinal factors.
C. Frequent drug interactions.
D. Higher bleeding rate with a variant CYP2C9 allele for hepatic cytochrome P450.
E. Anticoagulant effects need to be monitored.

Question 31-3

Which of the following statements about novel new anticoagulants is *false*?

A. Fondaparinux, a synthetic pentasaccharide, is excreted totally through hepatic metabolism.
B. Fondaparinux has a much longer half-life than heparin or low molecular weight heparin.
C. Ximelagatran, the orally available prodrug of melagatran, is a direct thrombin inhibitor.
D. Ximelagatran causes transient elevation in liver transaminases.
E. Anti-inflammatory strategies, such as selectin inhibitors, have been found experimentally to decrease thrombus formation.

■ QUESTIONS FOR CHAPTER 32

Question 32-1

The majority of the beneficial effect of thrombolysis results from:

A. The activation of fibrin-bound plasminogen rather than the activation of plasminogen in the fluid phase of blood.
B. The activation (or partial activation) of the five distinct types of physiologic plasminogen activators.
C. The release of tissue plasminogen activator (tPA) and urokinase-type plasminogen activator (uPA) from

vascular endothelium directly in contact with the thrombus thereby promoting its dissolution.

D. The activation of plasminogen to plasmin, which has a half-life of 45 minutes in the circulation.

E. The reduction of the levels of α2-macroglobulin, which is the rapid acting inhibitor of circulating plasmin.

Question 32-2

Which of the following statements regarding the physiology of the fibrinolytic system is true?

A. Plasminogen is synthesized by the vascular endothelial cells.

B. Any activation of plasminogen that occurs in the surrounding fluid phase of a thrombus is rapidly neutralized by α2-antiplasmin.

C. Plasmin's action is specific to fibrin and fibrinogen.

D. Inhibitors of tPA and uPA are derived from two sources: platelets and endothelial cells.

E. Although plasmin can break down cross-linked fibrin, non–cross-linked fibrin, and fibrinogen, its activity cannot be specifically identified in a given patient.

Question 32-3

A number of plasminogen activators have been identified and used in clinical practice. Which of the following statements is *correct* regarding plasminogen activators?

A. Streptokinase (SK) is capable of directly converting plasminogen to plasmin.

B. Urokinase has been produced from urine and cultured human kidney cells; however, because of its two-chain structure, it cannot be produced by recombinant technology.

C. Recombinant tissue-type plasminogen activator (rt-PA) preferentially activates fibrin-bound plasminogen and is inactivated primarily by plasminogen activator inhibitor (PAI)-1.

D. Tenecteplase-tPA, a bioengineered mutant of tPA, was designed specifically to improve results of catheter-directed thrombolysis.

E. Staphylokinase is a bacterial profibrinolytic agent that functions differently from SK, in that it directly activates plasminogen.

■ QUESTIONS FOR CHAPTER 33

Question 33-1

A 68-year-old man is undergoing a difficult repair of a ruptured AAA, with prolonged supraceliac clamping, and requires 10 units of packed red cells and 4 units of FFP. There is a diffuse ooze from all surgical sites. The prothrombin time (PT) and activated partial thromboplastin time (aPTT) are normal; the platelet count is 90,000, and his temperature is 34.5°C. The most appropriate next step would be to:

A. Transfuse more fresh-frozen plasma (FFP) and cryoprecipitate.

B. Pack the abdomen and return the patient to the intensive care unit for warming and further resuscitation.

C. Transfuse platelets.

D. Administer aminocaproic acid.

E. Continue searching for discrete, surgically controllable bleeding sites.

Question 33-2

Three days ago, a 37-year-old diabetic patient underwent emergent guillotine amputation of his foot because of a polymicrobial abscess with ascending erythema and crepitus suggesting tissue gas formation. He has remained in the intensive care unit requiring ventilatory support. He has now become hemodynamically unstable and developed hematochezia, bleeding from his stump, hematuria, and bloody nasogastric tube aspirates. His coagulation factors reveal a severely prolonged PT, aPTT, and thrombin time. He has a diminished platelet count and fibrinogen level. Which one of the following represents the most appropriate management of this patient:

A. Administer aminocaproic acid.

B. Administer heparin sulfate.

C. Administer FFP, cryoprecipitate, and platelets as needed.

D. Administer deamino-8-d-arginine vasopressin (DDAVP).

E. Administer recombinant activated factor VII.

Question 33-3

A 72-year-old man presents with high-grade carotid artery stenosis. His medical history is significant for von Willebrand disease (VWD). Preoperative planning would best include:

A. Perioperative administration of DDAVP.

B. Perioperative administration of cryoprecipitate.

C. Perioperative transfusion of platelets.

D. Further testing to determine the type of VWD.

E. Perioperative transfusion of VWF concentrates.

■ QUESTIONS FOR CHAPTER 34

Question 34-1

The most common genetic hypercoagulable disorder associated with a high risk of venous thromboembolism is:

A. Protein C deficiency.

B. Protein S deficiency.

C. Antithrombin deficiency.

D. Factor V Leiden deficiency.

E. Prothrombin 20210A.

Question 34-2

All of the following are acquired risk factors for venous thromboembolism *except*:

A. Prolonged immobility.

B. Pregnancy.

C. Oral contraceptive use.

D. Radiation therapy.

E. Nephrotic syndrome.

Question 34-3

A 65-year-old man, who underwent a coronary artery bypass complicated by prolonged ventilator dependence, as well as multiple episodes of septicemia and acute cholecystitis, develops a lower limb deep vein thrombosis (DVT). He is treated with unfractionated heparin. Soon thereafter, the patient presents with severe lower extremity digital ischemia and a platelet count that is 25% of normal. The patient should undergo which of the following managements:

A. Cessation of heparin and evaluation for a hypercoagulable disorder.
B. Conversion to low molecular weight heparin, workup for hypercoagulable disorder, and inferior vena cava (IVC) filter placement.
C. Cessation of heparin, institution of a direct thrombin inhibitor, and workup for hypercoagulable disorder.
D. Cessation of heparin, evaluation for anti-heparin antibody, and institution of a GIIb/IIIa receptor antagonist.
E. Cessation of heparin, placement of an IVC filter, and assay for anti-heparin antibody.

ANSWERS AND DISCUSSION

■ ANSWERS AND DISCUSSION FOR CHAPTER 30

Answer 30-1: A

Discussion 30-1

The extrinsic pathway of coagulation is activated by (A) tissue factor. This is accomplished by tissue factor complexing with factor VII. This complex is then capable of activating factor VII into VIIa. Once factor VIIa is formed, it is capable of converting factor X into Xa, which eventually leads to the formation of thrombin by converting prothrombin into active enzyme. The other factors (B, C, D, E) are not part of extrinsic pathway activation.

Answer 30-2: B

Discussion 30-2

(B) Contact with foreign surfaces (e.g., ex vivo circuits, bacterial cell walls, and uric acid crystals) leads to the activation of factor XII to XIIa. This type of contact activation is observed in septicemia, during cardiopulmonary bypass surgery, and in patients with gout. Factor XII activation can trigger the subsequent activation of factor XI to XIa. The active factor XIa then is capable of converting (A) factor IX to IXa. This eventually leads to the transformation of factor X to Xa. Factor IX (A) is part of this intrinsic pathway cascade but is not an initiator; the others (C, D, E) are either not activated by foreign surfaces or not part of the intrinsic pathway.

Answer 30-3: D

Discussion 30-3

The damaged vascular surface is capable of attracting VWF to the exposed subendothelial sites, which are rich in collagen. VWF is capable of attaching to the damaged surface. Once attached, VWF is capable of binding to platelet receptors, namely, glycoprotein Ib. Thus, the adhesion of platelets to vascular surface is mediated through (D) VWF. The other proteins listed (A, B, C, E) do not act by bridging platelet glycoprotein Ib with damaged vascular surfaces.

■ ANSWERS AND DISCUSSION FOR CHAPTER 31

Answer 31-1: C

Discussion 31-1

Low molecular weight heparins have (A) *greater* anti-Xa activity and less anti-IIa activity. Because of (B) reduced binding to cells and plasma proteins, bioavailability (C) is improved, not reduced. (D) The drug may be given by subcutaneous injection with (E) no monitoring necessary in most circumstances, leading to the possibility of outpatient therapy. Exceptions that need monitoring include renal failure (because excretion is totally through the kidneys), children, pregnancy, and the morbidly obese.

Answer 31-2: B

Discussion 31-2

Warfarin has been found to have a variable anticoagulant effect (A), which is (B) greatly affected by dietary and gastrointestinal factors that influence the availability and absorption of vitamin K. Likewise, the anticoagulant effect (C) is influenced by many different drugs. (D) Patients with genetic heterogeneity for cytochrome P450 with a variant CYP2C9 allele are more likely to bleed (3.7-fold increase). The anticoagulant effect, on the liver-produced clotting factors II, VII, IX, and X, must be monitored using the PT (E).

Answer 31-3: A

Discussion 31-3

Fondaparinux is a synthetic pentasaccharide with a long 17-hour half-life, longer than unfractionated or LMW heparin (B). It has been found to be an excellent agent for DVT prophylaxis, especially in orthopedic applications. This drug is totally excreted through the kidneys, *not the liver* (A is false). Ximelagatran, an oral direct thrombin inhibitor (C), is an agent that may potentially replace traditional oral vitamin K antagonists. Unfortunately, it causes (D) transient elevation in liver function tests. (E) Anti-selectin compounds have been found experimentally to decrease thrombus formation without augmenting bleeding potential, suggesting a new approach to antithrombotic therapy.

■ ANSWERS AND DISCUSSION FOR CHAPTER 32

Answer 32-1: A

Discussion 32-1

The most important contribution to the understanding of physiologic and therapeutic fibrinolysis was the identification of the basic mechanism of clot dissolution. This was described by Sherry and Alkjersig when they made the important observation that clot lysis occurred as a result of penetration of the clot by a plasminogen activator that then broke down plasminogen that was bound to fibrin during clotting. This explains the universal observation that intrathrombus infusions of plasminogen activators accelerate lysis compared with systemic infusion. Thus, A is correct, and C (release of tPA and uPA from vascular endothelium) is incorrect. (B) There are not five types of plasminogen activators. Two distinct types, tPA and uPA, have been identified. (D) Plasmin has an exceptionally short half-life (a fraction of a second) in the circulation (not 45 minutes [D]). (E) α2-macroglobulin is a secondary, slow-acting inhibitor of circulating plasmin. α2-antiplasmin is the primary inhibitor, which is rapid acting.

Answer 32-2: B

Discussion 32-2

A. Plasminogen is synthesized in the liver and found in human plasma and serum in an average concentration of 21 mg/dL. It is *not* synthesized by the vascular endothelium.

B. The physiologic activation of plasminogen that occurs in the fluid phase of the circulation surrounding a thrombus is rapidly neutralized by α2-antiplasmin (correct answer).

C. Plasmin's action is *not* specific to fibrin and/or fibrinogen. Plasmin cleaves protein and peptide molecules at arginyl-lysyl bonds. Therefore, in addition to fibrin and fibrinogen, plasmin hydrolyzes the coagulation factors V and VIII, components of serum complement, corticotrophin, growth hormone, and glucagon.

D. Inhibitors of tPA and uPA are derived from *many* sources: human platelets, cultured endothelial cells, human umbilical vein, hepatoma cells, liver, placenta, monocytes, and human fibroblasts.

E. Although plasmin's action on non–cross-linked fibrin is identical to that on fibrinogen in the rate of breakdown, the end products are different. BB15-42 peptide rather than BB1-42 is produced on cleavage of the BB chain of fibrin. These peptides have been used to assess specific breakdown of fibrinogen versus fibrin by plasmin. Mature fibrin contains factor XIIIa-induced intramolecular bonds, causing a slower degradation by plasmin and different end products. D-dimer is a unique derivative of a breakdown of cross-linked fibrin.

Answer 32-3: C

Discussion 32-3

A. SK converts plasminogen to plasmin *indirectly.* It must form an SK-plasminogen complex that then activates plasminogen to plasmin. However, rt-PA preferentially and directly activates fibrin-bound plasminogen. rt-PA is highly fibrin specific. It is primarily inactivated by circulating PAI-1.

B. In addition to urine and cultured human kidney cells, urokinase has been produced by recombinant technology.

C. rt-PA preferentially and directly activates fibrin-bound plasminogen. rt-Pa is highly fibrin specific. It is primarily inactivated by circulating PAI-1. Therefore, C is the correct answer.

D. Tenecteplase-tPA is a bioengineered mutant of tPA. However, it was specifically designed to be 10 times more fibrin specific than rt-PA, specifically to rapidly treat acute myocardial infarction by a single bolus, intravenous infusion.

E. Staphylokinase is similar to SK in its mechanism of action. Like SK, staphylokinase is an indirect plasminogen activator and forms a 1:1 complex with plasminogen that then activates other plasminogen molecules. Unlike the SK-plasminogen complex, the staphylokinase-plasminogen complex is rapidly neutralized by α2-antiplasmin in plasma, thereby avoiding systemic plasminogen activation and a rapid systemic fibrinolytic state.

■ ANSWERS AND DISCUSSION FOR CHAPTER 33

Answer 33-1: B

Discussion 33-1

This case features many known contributors to a perioperative bleeding coagulopathy. Prolonged supraceliac clamp may predispose to primary fibrinolysis, treatable by the transfusion of replacement factors and the use of fibrinolytic inhibitors such as (D) aminocaproic acid. However, the patient has a confounding factor that is likely contributing to the coagulopathy—a temperature of 34.5°C. Intraoperative hypothermia is usually encountered with prolonged operative time, global hypoperfusion, and intraoperative replacement with nonwarmed fluids in large volumes. As in this case, clotting tests performed with samples warmed to 37°C may be normal. Hypothermia can also cause platelet dysfunction, precipitate full-blown disseminated intravascular coagulation (DIC), and lower enzyme activity, particularly those involved in the polymerization process of platelets and fibrin. A further search for major bleeding sites (E), when none has previously been found, runs the risk of aggravating the causes of the coagulopathy, with deepening hypothermia. Therefore, the best next step is to (B) pack the abdomen and return the patient to the intensive care unit for warming and further resuscitation. Warming the patient will eliminate hypothermia as a cause of coagulopathy and allow for further assessment to identify some other underlying disorder such as DIC or primary fibrinolysis to which specific component replacement therapy (as noted previously, and represented by answers A, C, and D) can be directed.

Answer 33-2: C

Discussion 33-2

This patient has developed a coagulopathy that is likely because of disseminated intravascular coagulation (DIC). DIC is always caused by some underlying disorder, most commonly bacterial sepsis, which occurs in 30% to 50% of such patients. DIC is a continuously progressing process that can be divided into three clinical phases: compensated activation of the hemostatic system, decompensated activation of the hemostatic system, and "full-blown" DIC, the latter characterized by an extremely prolonged PT, aPTT, and thrombin time, as in this case. If antithrombin levels were measured, they would be found to be less than 50% of normal. The best treatment of DIC is directed against the inciting causative factors; early recognition can decrease its propensity to become autonomous and self-perpetuating. Once DIC is established, as in this case, clotting factors and platelets should be replaced at the rate they are consumed. This is determined by frequently monitoring laboratory values while continuing to (C) administer FFP, platelets, and cryoprecipitate, which is the correct treatment. Administration of antifibrinolytic agents, such as (A) aminocaproic acid, should seldom be used because the secondary fibrinolysis occurring during DIC is beneficial at clearing the capillaries of thrombus and thus restoring perfusion. (E) The use of recombinant activated factor VII has *not* been proven efficacious, and (B) the once popular use of heparin sulfate is no longer supported. (D) DDAVP is specific therapy for platelet disorders/dysfunction but is *not* specific for DIC.

Answer 33-3: D

Discussion 33-3

VWD is a complex disorder caused by the quantitative and/or qualitative defect of VWF. It is the most commonly inherited bleeding disorder with an estimated incidence of 1% to 2%. VWD is classified into three main types based on the deficiency of VWF. Type 1 disease is characterized by decreased amounts of VWF; type 2 disease is characterized by qualitative defects in VWF independent of the amount of factor present; and type 3 disease is characterized by the absence of VWF. Patients rarely require treatment unless they present with bleeding or are identified as having VWD preoperatively, and then the treatment depends on the procedure performed. Type 1 VWD is effectively treated with DDAVP. This medication, however, has variable effectiveness in type 2 disease and is ineffective in patients with type 3 disease. Cryoprecipitate, VWF concentrates, and platelets (C) are effective in patients resistant to DDAVP therapy. (D) Preoperative determination of the type of VWD is important in directing therapy in this patient should a problem with bleeding arise. Once the type of VWD is known, then one or more of the other responses (A) DDAVP, (B) cryoprecipitate, or (E) VWF concentrates and factor VIII/VWF concentrates may be appropriate.

■ ANSWERS AND DISCUSSION FOR CHAPTER 34

Answer 34-1: C

Discussion 34-1

Antithrombin deficiency (C) is the most common genetic hypercoagulable disorder associated with a high risk of venous thromboembolism. However, Factor V Leiden (D) is the most prevalent hypercoagulable disorder, but it does *not* have as high a risk for venous thrombosis, particularly because most patients are heterozygous for Factor V Leiden. Prothrombin 20210A (E) is the second most prevalent, but again confers less of a risk of venous thrombosis. Protein C deficiency (A) and protein S deficiency (B) are genetic hypercoagulable disorders associated with a high risk of venous thromboembolism, but their incidence is not as prevalent as the antithrombin deficiency.

Answer 34-2: D

Discussion 34-2

Radiation therapy (D) in and of itself is *not* an acquired risk factor for venous thromboembolism. Prolonged immobility (A) increases risk of stasis, and stasis can promote thrombosis. Pregnancy (B) is an acquired risk for venous thromboembolism because of the mass effect on the IVC, as well as production of prothrombic hormones. Oral contraceptive use (C) is a well-known acquired risk factor for venous thromboembolism, particularly in women aged more than 35 years and those who smoke. Nephrotic syndrome (E) is an acquired risk for venous thromboembolism because it may cause a functional protein C or protein S deficiency, because of a large-size protein loss through the kidney.

Answer 34-3: E

Discussion 34-3

This patient presents a complex case with an acute DVT and needs protection against pulmonary embolism, but the case scenario describes a person who has experienced heparin-induced thrombocytopenia (HIT) and thrombosis syndrome. This is rare; however, the patient should have (E) the heparin ceased, including all intravenous (IV) heparin flushes, an IVC filter placed to protect against pulmonary embolism, and an assay sent for an anti-heparin antibody to confirm HIT. If positive for HIT, the patient will be unable to receive heparin at any further time. Other choices are not as good. (A) Just ceasing the heparin and evaluating for a hypercoagulable disorder may reduce the risk, but the acute DVT still needs to be treated. (B) Conversion to low molecular weight heparin, although having less association with HIT, still may be a risk factor, particularly once the patient has clinical evidence thereof, and should not be done. In terms of answer C, cessation of heparin and institution of a direct thrombin inhibitor is not a wrong answer, but a workup for a full hypercoagulable disorder is not indicated at this point because the patient has evidence of HIT. (D) Cessation of heparin and evaluation for anti-heparin antibody is again part of the protocol, but use of antiplatelet antagonists has not been shown to be as efficacious as direct thrombin inhibitor or placement of an IVC filter.

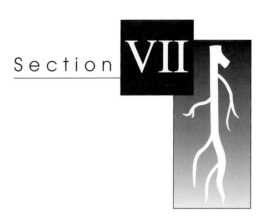

NONOPERATIVE MANAGEMENT OF PATIENTS WITH VASCULAR DISEASES

STUDY QUESTIONS

■ QUESTIONS FOR CHAPTER 36

Question 36-1

Hallmarks of the Insulin Resistance Syndrome (Syndrome X) include all of the following *except*:

A. Hypertension.
B. Increased abdominal girth.
C. Elevated triglycerides.
D. Large low-density lipoprotein (LDL) particles.
E. Low high-density lipoprotein (HDL).

Question 36-2

An 80-year-old man presents with nonlimiting claudication and a 60% right internal carotid stenosis. He is also hypertensive. Which of the following statements concerning statin medications for this patient is *false*?

A. Statins are ineffective for someone of his age.
B. Statins may reduce his overall cardiovascular mortality.
C. Statins may decrease subsequent clinical events.
D. Statins may improve walking distance.
E. Statins may stabilize plaque inflammation.

Question 36-3

A 60-year-old postmenopausal woman with mild hot flashes is noted to have bilateral 50% carotid stenosis. True statements about hormone replacement therapy (HRT) include all the following *except*:

A. HRT can ameliorate unpleasant symptoms of menopause and therefore should be prescribed for the symptomatic woman.
B. HRT can be associated with an increase in venous thromboembolic events.
C. HRT has been associated with reduced vascular graft patency.
D. HRT may be associated with reduced incidence of colon cancer.
E. HRT can increase the risk of stroke.

■ QUESTIONS FOR CHAPTER 37

Question 37-1

A 55-year-old diabetic man presents with a history of left leg claudication occurring after two blocks. He states he can usually walk through this pain and can, on most days, reach five blocks before the discomfort makes him stop and rest before going on.

Which of the following five choices is a true statement about his pain-free walking distance (PFWD) and maximal walking distance (MWD)?

A. PFWD = 5 blocks.
B. MWD = 2 blocks.
C. PFWD and MWD = 5 blocks.
D. PFWD and MWD = 2 blocks.
E. Best measured on a treadmill at a defined speed and incline.

Question 37-2

A 65-year-old male claudicant can walk 200 yards. He is a heavy smoker and 25% overweight. He is on a beta-blocker for hypertension. Appropriate advice may include the following treatment suggestions *except*:

A. Smoking cessation.
B. Initiation of a structured exercise program.
C. Dietary changes to control hyperlipidemia.
D. A trial of cilostazol.
E. Discontinuation of the beta-blocker.

Question 37-3

Which of the following statements concerning medications for claudication is true?

A. There are many medications proven to significantly improve walking distance.
B. Cilostazol may help, but it is unlikely to more than double the walking distance.
C. Trental is an effective vasodilator.
D. Side effects of cilostazol include palpitations and severe constipation.

E. Current Food and Drug Administration-approved medications include cilostazol, pentoxifylline, and naftidrofuryl.

■ QUESTIONS FOR CHAPTER 38

Question 38-1

A 65-year-old diabetic man receiving metformin and miglitol undergoes an angiogram to evaluate severe distal arterial disease. Baseline blood urea nitrogen was 35 mg/dL, and creatinine was 1.8 mg/dL. The next day his blood urea nitrogen and creatinine increased to 50 mg/dL and 3.0 mg/dL, respectively, and the CO_2 increased to 45 mmol/L. The most likely cause of these blood chemistry changes is:

A. Renal failure related to contrast alone.
B. A complication of the metformin alone.
C. A complication of the miglitol alone.
D. A complication of the contrast agent and the metformin.
E. A complication of the contrast agent and the miglitol.

Question 38-2

A 55-year-old woman is referred to the vascular surgeon for a carotid endarterectomy. After surgery she requests information on how she can prevent the "other side" from progressing. She is 5′2″ tall and weighs 165 lb. Most of the excess weight is abdominal. She does not smoke but has mild hypertension. Valid advice may include all of the following *except*:

A. Enroll in an exercise program.
B. Start a statin medication.
C. Start on antihypertensive medication.
D. Lose weight by limiting fatty foods and substituting with foods such as pasta.
E. Evaluate fasting blood glucose.

Question 38-3

Which one of the following five statements about the management of a diabetic patient is *false*:

A. Hemoglobin A1C should be checked every 6 months to monitor the effect of therapy.
B. Too aggressive therapy (glycemic control) can aggravate diabetic retinopathy.
C. Diet and exercise are integral parts of therapy.
D. Tight glycemic control has not been shown to substantially decrease microvascular complications.
E. A typical oral glucose tolerance test is performed by measurement of plasma glucose after fasting and then 2 hours after administration of 75 g oral glucose load.

■ QUESTIONS FOR CHAPTER 39

Question 39-1

A 63-year-old man with mild claudication and a family history of diabetes is found at the first office visit to have a blood pressure of 140/80 mm Hg. Correct statements about this blood pressure include all of the following *except*:

A. Diuretics may be a good first-line medication if one is to be used.
B. The patient is at risk for developing diabetes.
C. The blood pressure is elevated, but this may represent "white coat hypertension."
D. A repeat blood pressure confirming this elevation should be documented before instituting antihypertensive medications.
E. Beta-blockers are contraindicated because they worsen claudication.

Question 39-2

A 68-year-old white man with an asymptomatic 7-cm abdominal aortic aneurysm (AAA) requires open surgical repair. Preoperative evaluation discovers that his blood pressure is elevated to 188/110 mm Hg. Correct statements concerning the proper management of this patient include all of the following *except*:

A. A beta-blocker should be initiated before surgery.
B. A calcium-channel blocker is the drug of choice because the patient is not an Afro-American.
C. Surgery should be postponed until the hypertension is better controlled.
D. It is likely that at least two antihypertensive medications will be required.
E. A parenteral medication may be required if emergency surgery is required.

Question 39-3

A patient is started on an angiotensin-converting enzyme (ACE) inhibitor by her internist 1 month after a left-sided carotid endarterectomy. The vascular surgeon sees her 1 month after surgery for a routine follow-up, and her blood pressure is found to be 140/80 mm Hg. She states that she takes the medication and has noted her home-monitored blood pressure to be similarly elevated. She reports the new onset of a dry cough. True statements about her condition include all of the following *except*:

A. Her blood pressure is acceptable and probably related to the endarterectomy.
B. She still has elevated blood pressure that carries an increased cardiovascular risk.
C. Addition of a diuretic may improve her blood pressure control.
D. Changing her medication to an angiotensin receptor blocker may help her cough.
E. Changing her medication may be better tolerated than adding another medication.

■ QUESTIONS FOR CHAPTER 40

Question 40-1

Claudication can be often differentiated from pseudo-claudication by all of the following *except*:

A. Pseudo-claudication is usually bilateral.
B. Pseudo-claudication is usually more diffuse.

C. Pseudo-claudication is often relieved by bending over/forward while walking.

D. Pseudo-claudication pain may improve the further the patient walks.

E. Pseudo-claudication seldom has a burning quality.

Question 40-2

A 75-year-old man with severe ischemic cardiomyopathy is considered to be too severe a risk for the complex arterial reconstruction required for limb salvage. He has intractable rest pain in both feet, but there are no advanced skin changes. His life expectancy is measured in months. Which of the following treatment plans is most appropriate to recommend at this time?

A. Clinical optimization followed by bilateral above-knee amputation.

B. Clinical optimization followed by bilateral below-knee amputation.

C. Spinal cord stimulation.

D. Bilateral lumbar sympathectomy using mini-invasive techniques.

E. A trial of oral analgesics possibly followed by spinal cord stimulation.

Question 40-3

A 65-year-old woman with long-standing nonlimiting calf claudication, diabetes mellitus, hyperlipidemia with an elevated LDL, and hypertension is started on a statin drug. Two weeks later she presents to the emergency room with reports of increasing pain in her legs including her thighs. The pain is present all the time but is aggravated by motion. The most likely cause for her worsening symptoms is:

A. Worsening atherosclerotic stenosis in her aortoiliac arteries.

B. Diabetic neuropathy.

C. Aortic dissection caused by uncontrolled hypertension.

D. Statin-induced myositis.

E. Pseudo-claudication caused by spinal stenosis.

ANSWERS AND DISCUSSION

■ ANSWERS AND DISCUSSION FOR CHAPTER 36

Answer 36-1: D

Discussion 36-1

(D) The Insulin Resistance Syndrome, also known as Syndrome X or the Metabolic Syndrome, is characterized by *small* LDL particles that carry an increased risk for the development of atherosclerosis and cardiovascular events, so D is incorrect. The Insulin Resistance Syndrome has as its hallmarks: (A) hypertension, (B) increased abdominal girth, (C) hypertriglyceridemia, and (E) low HDL levels.

Answer 36-2: A

Discussion 36-2

(A) Statins are *effective* in reducing cardiovascular morbidity and stroke at *all ages* and may be even more effective in the elderly. (B and C) The role of statins in reducing cardiovascular morbidity is now well established, and so prescription of statins should be considered for all patients with peripheral arterial disease. (D) Although the method by which statins may increase walking distance remains to be proven, studies have shown that claudication distance can be increased by their use. (E) The reduction in event rate with statins often occurs within the first 6 months of therapy, suggesting that the effect is the result of plaque stabilization rather than an absolute reduction in cholesterol levels. This is considered to be the result of an anti-inflammatory effect on arterial plaque.

Answer 36-3: A

Discussion 36-3

Although early studies suggested that HRT might prevent atherosclerotic morbidity in postmenopausal women, recent evidence would suggest that such complications and thromboembolic events are actually increased especially in the first year after initiating such therapy. Accordingly, women with mild menopausal symptoms should try to avoid using HRT (A) unless the symptoms are severe and associated cardiovascular conditions are absent or mild. B–E are all true statements regarding HRT.

■ ANSWERS AND DISCUSSION FOR CHAPTER 37

Answer 37-1: E

Discussion 37-1

(E) Although some would suggest that the best method of evaluating walking distance is to have the patient walk a predefined walking course, environmental factors can produce variability in onset of symptoms. Also, use of such a walking test makes comparison between institutions impossible. Accordingly, walking on a treadmill at a defined speed and incline has become the standard. A–D are all incorrect. PFWD is the distance a patient can walk before developing claudication. The MWD is the distance at which the patient has to stop to relieve the claudication pain. In this question the PFWD is two blocks and the MWD is five blocks.

Answer 37-2: E

Discussion 37-2

(E) Although it has been hypothesized that beta-blockers may increase claudication, this has never been proven in controlled walking trials. (A) Smoking cessation will not necessarily increase walking distance but is an important risk-reduction measure in this high-risk patient. (B) A structured exercise program can increase walking distance. (C) Dietary control of hyperlipidemia may not control claudication but is also an important treatment adjunct that may help reduce cardiovascular morbidity. (D) Cilostazol is a medication that can improve walking distance in patients with mild claudication.

Answer 37-3: B

Discussion 37-3

(B) Patients who use cilostazol need to have realistic expectations about the benefit this drug will achieve, because few patients will become pain free and it is unlikely to "more than double" their walking distance. (A) Although many medications and herbal remedies have been proposed to reduce claudication, only a few have been shown to have any effect. (C) Trental (pentoxifylline) is *not* a vasodilator but is thought to work by increasing red blood cell deformability. (D) Cilostazol does cause palpitations, but rather than constipation, most patients will have diarrhea. (E) There are *only two* medications currently approved in the United States for the treatment of claudication: pentoxifylline and cilostazol.

■ ANSWERS AND DISCUSSION FOR CHAPTER 38

Answer 38-1: D

Discussion 38-1

(D) Although contrast agents can cause renal failure, this complication is more likely to occur when contrast is used in the diabetic patient who is also taking metformin. (B) The patient in the case study also developed significant acidosis after the angiogram. This complication is caused by the metformin. This has prompted the recommendation that metformin be stopped the day before or at least the day of the arteriographic procedure. Failure to do so can result in severe life-threatening acidosis. (C and E) Miglitol does not cause acidosis or renal failure. (A) Contrast alone is unlikely to produce this entire picture, specifically acidosis.

Answer 38-2: D

Discussion 38-2

(D) Weight loss is important. However, although fatty foods need to be limited in most diets because of their high caloric content, substitution of a diet high in carbohydrates can increase the risk of atherosclerosis by inducing or aggravating the Insulin Resistance Syndrome. Reduction in HDL levels and the production of small particle size LDL may result from such a diet. This patient is likely to be diabetic or prediabetic or have the Insulin Resistance Syndrome. Accordingly, (B) statins, (C) hypertension control, and (A) exercise are clearly important in risk modification. (E) A fasting blood glucose level is indicated as it may define her diabetic status.

Answer 38-3: D

Discussion 38-3

(D) Microvascular complications *are* reduced by tight control, and this should be the goal of therapy. (A) Because the average life span of a red cell is 120 days, the glycosylated hemoglobin A1C represents a time-averaged evaluation of blood glucose levels. This provides a simple, useful test of treatment efficacy and patient compliance and should be checked every 6 months. (B) Although tight control is important to prevent macrovascular complications, excessively tight control can aggravate diabetic retinopathy. (C) Medications are often required to treat established diabetes. However, diet and exercise remain an integral part of *any* treatment regimen. (E) The technique for performing a glucose tolerance test is standardized and is as outlined in the question.

■ ANSWERS AND DISCUSSION FOR CHAPTER 39

Answer 39-1: E

Discussion 39-1

(E) Beta blockers have not been shown to worsen claudication. (A) Diuretics are an excellent first-line medication and may also potentiate the benefit of other antihypertensives. (B) Patients with vascular disease and hypertension are at risk for becoming diabetic. (C) Some normotensive patients may seem to have increase blood pressure because of elevations caused by the anxiety associated with an office visit, the so-called "white coat by pertension." (D) One (marginal) blood pressure measurement does not constitute enough evidence to label a patient as hypertensive.

Answer 39-2: B

Discussion 39-2

(B) Calcium-channel blockers are actually beneficial in Afro-Americans because they do not respond as well to ACE inhibitors, so this statement is incorrect. (A) Beta-blockers have been proven to reduce the incidence of postoperative myocardial infarction and should be considered for all patients undergoing major vascular surgery. (C) Complication rates may be higher in patients whose blood pressure is greater than 180/110 mm Hg. It should be controlled before elective surgery. (E) In such patients, control of blood pressure can be achieved with IV medications before emergency surgery. This may be necessary but is not ideal. (D) This degree of hypertension is likely to require more than one antihypertensive agent.

Answer 39-3: A

Discussion 39-3

A. Although endarterectomy can result in alteration of baseline blood pressure, this is seldom a lasting effect and would not explain hypertension 1 month postoperatively.
B. Although the patient's blood pressure is only mildly elevated, patients with vascular disease should be maintained as near to normotensive levels as possible, otherwise their risk of subsequent cardiovascular events is increased.
C. Diuretics can have an additive effect and make increasing her ACE inhibitor unnecessary.
D. Some ACE inhibitors can cause a dry cough. This is not seen with angiotensin receptor blockers.
E. Although two medications may help control the elevated blood pressure, most patients would rather take one medication.

■ ANSWERS AND DISCUSSION FOR CHAPTER 40

Answer 40-1: D

Discussion 40-1

(D) Differentiating pseudoclaudication from vascular claudication can be very difficult especially in patients who have both conditions. However, unlike vascular claudication, pseudo-claudication *may* improve the further the patient walks. (A, B) Although vascular claudication may be bilateral, pseudo-claudication is most often bilateral and more diffuse. (C) Classically, pseudo-claudication caused by spinal stenosis is often relieved if the patient walks with a bent-over posture. (E) Vascular claudication is an aching pain and is seldom burning in quality (see also Chapter 1 for differential diagnosis of leg pain).

Answer 40-2: E

Discussion 40-2

(E) Spinal cord stimulation may be beneficial but should only be used after oral pain medication has proven to be ineffective or has resulted in complications. (A, B) Although ultimate amputation may be required for pain control, in the absence of significant skin necrosis, this should be a last resort. (C) Spinal cord stimulation may help but should only be used after attempts at pain control using oral medications have failed. (D) Lumbar sympathectomy does not completely relieve *ischemic* rest pain.

Answer 40-3: D

Discussion 40-3

(D) All of the conditions described can cause worsening pain. However, muscular pain starting soon after initiating a statin is an important warning symptom that the patient may be at risk for developing a drug-induced myositis that could prove fatal. Urgent attention should be given to this new symptom, and in most cases the statin should be withheld or withdrawn entirely.

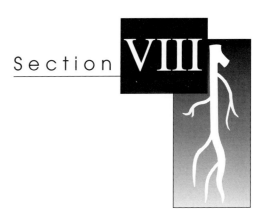

OPEN VASCULAR SURGERY: BASIC CONSIDERATIONS

STUDY QUESTIONS

■ **QUESTIONS FOR CHAPTER 41**

Question 41-1

When considering options for visceral artery reconstruction, which of the following statements is true?

A. Durability of open revascularization and angioplasty is similar.
B. Prograde visceral bypass is preferred in patients without high cardiac risk.
C. Morbidity of angioplasty and open surgical revascularization is similar.
D. Thromboendarterectomy is the most widely applicable method of open revascularization.
E. Extra-anatomic renal bypass (hepatorenal, splenorenal) is inferior to aortic-based reconstruction.

Question 41-2

The most important factor when considering thromboendarterectomy as a technique for revascularization is:

A. Patient age and comorbidity.
B. Surgeon experience.
C. Risk of infection.
D. Availability of autogenous tissue for bypass.
E. Anatomic distribution of disease.

Question 41-3

In low-risk patients, open and endovascular repair of aortic aneurysm:

A. Are associated with similar operative mortality.
B. Are associated with similar overall cost.
C. Are associated with similar durability.
D. Are equally suited to all patient groups.
E. Are associated with similar morbidity.

■ **QUESTIONS FOR CHAPTER 42**

Question 42-1

A 25-year-old man was stabbed in the right side of the neck just anterior to the sternocleidomastoid muscle. Arteriography demonstrates a carotid-jugular arteriovenous fistula. The remainder of the arteriogram is normal, but the right subcla-vian artery is noted to originate as the most distal branch of the aortic arch. Of the following, which anatomic variation is the surgeon *most likely* to encounter during cervical exploration?

A. A low-lying hypoglossal nerve.
B. A nonrecurrent laryngeal nerve.
C. A high thoracic duct.
D. A thyroid ima artery.
E. An aberrant subclavian vein.

Question 42-2

Three years after open repair of an AAA, a 65-year-old woman undergoes a right hemicolectomy for cancer. At the end of the procedure, the left colon is dusky and there are no Doppler signals obtained in the sigmoid mesocolon. The most likely explanation for this problem is interruption, during this procedure, of the:

A. Inferior mesenteric artery.
B. Ileocolic artery.
C. Left branch of the middle colic artery.
D. Arc of Riolan.
E. Left hypogastric artery.

Question 42-3

A 69-year-old man undergoes elective aortofemoral bypass for rest pain. During circumferential isolation of the left pro-funda femoris artery, the surgeon encounters brisk venous bleeding between the profunda and the superficial femoral artery branches. The most likely cause of bleeding is injury to the:

A. Profunda femoris vein.
B. Common femoral vein confluence.
C. External pudendal vein.
D. Medial femoral circumflex vein.
E. Lateral femoral circumflex vein.

■ **QUESTIONS FOR CHAPTER 43**

Question 43-1

End-to-end anastomosis:

A. Was the first anastomotic technique ever used, histori-cally.

B. Is the most common technique in aneurysm repair.
C. Is the most common technique used in arterial bypass surgery.
D. Is best performed with a single continuous suture in small-caliber vessels.
E. Can rarely be used in penetrating arterial trauma.

Question 43-2

End-to-side anastomosis:

A. Is ideal for interposition grafts.
B. Should enter the recipient vessel at a 50- to 60-degree angle.
C. Should equal the diameter of the recipient vessel.
D. Should be started at the most inaccessible point in its circumference.
E. Is not performed in long thoracoabdominal bypasses.

Question 43-3

For suturing vessels and performing anastomoses:

A. Silk sutures should no longer be used.
B. Monofilament sutures tend to break, so braided sutures should be used in prosthetic anastomoses.
C. Only interrupted sutures should be used in children to allow anastomotic growth.
D. The depth and separation (travel) of continuous suture placement should generally be equal in dimension.
E. The needle should travel "outside in on the artery, inside out on the graft" when anastomosing prostheses to arteriosclerotic arteries.

■ QUESTIONS FOR CHAPTER 44

Question 44-1

Arteriography before performing lower extremity arterial embolectomy:

A. Should focus on the affected limb, visualizing from the abdominal aorta down.
B. Does not help in operative planning and is better performed after attempting embolectomy.
C. Cannot eliminate "nonocclusive ischemia" as a potential cause of symptoms.
D. Is of significant value in identifying otherwise unsuspected secondary emboli.
E. Should not be performed through a brachial approach even if the femoral pulse is not palpable. Use contralateral femoral artery.

Question 44-2

Balloon catheter embolectomy:

A. Only requires control proximal to the catheter introduction site.
B. Should be performed using a transverse arteriotomy.
C. Uses balloon catheters 3F and larger filled with air and checked for leaks and concentricity before embolectomy is attempted.
D. Requires selection of recently improved balloon embolectomy catheters to avoid intimal injury and neointimal hyperplasia resulting from their passage.
E. Technique and the underlying disease are the most important factors contributing to intimal damage and the later development of neointimal hyperplasia.

Question 44-3

Regarding acute arterial ischemia caused by embolization:

A. It can be mimicked by nonocclusive ischemia.
B. An embolectomy specimen with a sharp rather than tapering end indicates adequate clot removal.
C. Distal back bleeding signals adequate thromboembolectomy.
D. A prominent "water hammer" pulse after arteriotomy closure is associated with complete embolectomy.
E. Intraoperative thrombolysis should not be used in conjunction with surgical thrombectomy because of the risk of bleeding at the surgical site.

■ QUESTIONS FOR CHAPTER 45

Question 45-1

Which of the following statements is *true*?

A. Endarterectomy is contraindicated in the presence of aneurysmal disease.
B. The correct plane of endarterectomy is between the intima and the media.
C. Endarterectomy has been supplanted by techniques such as arterial bypass and transluminal angioplasty.
D. Endarterectomy is contraindicated in aortoiliac occlusive disease.
E. The semiclosed technique of endarterectomy has now been abandoned.

Question 45-2

There are five types of endarterectomy: open, semiclosed, eversion, extraction, and selective. Of the following, which location is *most suitable* for endarterectomy?

A. Occlusion limited to the superficial femoral artery.
B. Occlusive lesions of the common and proximal deep femoral arteries.
C. Lesions of the innominate artery.
D. Occlusion of the external iliac artery.
E. Atherosclerotic occlusions of the aortoiliac arteries in the type 2 distribution.

Question 45-3

A 70-year-old man presents with a 6-cm AAA, three-drug hypertension, and a 90% left renal stenosis. The right renal artery is normal. Preoperative creatinine is 1.7 mg/dL. Radionuclide stress test and pulmonary function study results are normal. Proximal aortic neck is 28 mm in diameter and 10 mm in length. Of the following options, the best treatment for this patient is:

A. Open aneurysm resection with endarterectomy of the left renal artery through a retroperitoneal approach.
B. Preoperative stenting of the left renal artery followed by endovascular AAA repair with suprarenal fixation.
C. Open AAA repair with aorta to left renal artery bypass.
D. Open AAA repair with left nephrectomy.
E. Endovascular repair of AAA.

■ QUESTIONS FOR CHAPTER 46

Question 46-1

Which of the following is most important when choosing a conduit for vascular bypass?

A. Anatomic location of the bypass.
B. Risk of wound infection.
C. Indications for operation.
D. Patient comorbidities.
E. Life expectancy of the patient.

Question 46-2

The factor most important in selecting a conduit for infrainguinal bypass is:

A. Compliance.
B. Size match to artery.
C. Nonthrombogenic lining.
D. Ability to resist infection.
E. Handling characteristics at implantation.

Question 46-3

Which of the following statements is true?

A. There is no difference in the patency of autogenous and prosthetic femoral popliteal bypasses above the knee.
B. Heparin bonding has been demonstrated to improve patency of Dacron bypass grafts.
C. Cryopreserved veins are the conduit of choice for treatment of lower extremity autogenous graft infection.
D. Autogenous and prosthetic grafts have similar modes of late failure.
E. Adjuncts such as venous patching and cuffs and anticoagulation improve patency of infrageniculate prosthetic bypasses.

■ QUESTIONS FOR CHAPTER 47

Question 47-1

A 65-year-old man is undergoing saphenous vein harvesting for a femoropopliteal bypass graft. The surgeon makes a short, oblique incision in the usual location in the groin and finds that the greater saphenous vein is not in its usual location. The most common aberrant location for the thigh portion of the greater saphenous vein is:

A. Posteromedial.
B. Anteromedial.
C. Posterior.
D. Anterolateral to the usual course of the greater saphenous vein.
E. Joins the superficial femoral vein lower in thigh.

Question 47-2

In preparation of vein grafts for arterial conduits, proper handling is critical in ensuring that a minimally injured graft of good quality is implanted into the arterial circulation. Which of the following has been shown by clinical studies to be useful in minimizing vein graft injury?

A. Using a no-touch technique of harvesting.
B. Avoiding pressure distention with a syringe.
C. Minimizing vasospasm with the use of smooth muscle relaxants, such as papaverine.
D. Storing the vein in an isotonic cold solution.
E. All of the above are useful techniques in minimizing vein graft injury.

Question 47-3

A 62-year-old diabetic male, 8 months after a femoral-posterior tibial in situ saphenous vein bypass, is undergoing routine postoperative duplex ultrasound graft surveillance. Which of the following findings would suggest a critical graft stenosis because of intimal hyperplasia that would mandate immediate graft revision?

A. A peak systolic velocity of 180 to 300 cm/sec and a velocity ratio of greater than 2.
B. A peak systolic velocity of less than 180 cm/sec with a graft flow velocity of 45 cm/sec and no change in the hemodynamics (ABI).
C. A peak systolic velocity of greater than 300 cm/sec with a velocity ratio greater than 3.5 and a graft flow velocity of less than 30 cm/sec.
D. A peak systolic velocity of greater than 300 cm/sec with a velocity ratio of 2.5 and a graft flow velocity of 50 cm/sec.
E. None of the above findings mandates immediate graft revision.

■ QUESTIONS FOR CHAPTER 48

Question 48-1

A 70-year-old man, with previous bilateral saphenous vein harvesting for coronary artery bypass graft surgery, presents with a nonhealing foot ulcer. ABIs are 0.2 on the affected side. The patient has no suitable arm vein or lesser saphenous vein. The patient needs a femoral to dorsalis pedis bypass. What is the next best choice for conduit?

A. Spliced vein segments from remnants of saphenous veins.
B. Polytetrafluoroethylene (PTFE).
C. Human umbilical vein (HUV).
D. CryoVein.
E. Ringed PTFE with adjunctive fistula.

Question 48-2

All of the following are true regarding cryopreserved vessels as conduits *except*:

A. Endothelial cells (ECs) and smooth muscle cells are viable at time of implantation.
B. Early thrombosis is a problem.
C. Immune reactions are associated with thrombosis and aneurysm formation.
D. Cryopreserved veins offer a better patency than PTFE to below-knee popliteal or tibial vessels.
E. Potential roles for use include arterial homografts for infected in situ replacement and bridge therapy for children with congenital heart defects.

Question 48-3

All of the following are true regarding HUV *except*:

A. Aneurysm formation was a significant problem with the first-generation HUV grafts.
B. HUV bypasses require specific technical procedures to prevent damage to the graft and early thrombosis.
C. Patency of HUV is worse than PTFE.
D. Rate of infection is greater than saphenous vein bypass.
E. The rate of early thrombosis is decreased with postoperative use of low molecular weight dextran (LMWD) or heparin.

■ QUESTIONS FOR CHAPTER 49

Question 49-1

Which of the following represents the correct temporal sequence of most likely causes of prosthetic graft failure at these respective intervals: immediately after implantation, 1 month after, 6 months to 3 years after, and late, more than 3 years after:

A. Anastomotic myointimal hyperplasia, technical problems or hypercoagulability, thrombosis, and progression of distal atherosclerosis.
B. Technical problems or hypercoagulability, thrombosis, anastomotic myointimal hyperplasia, and progression of distal atherosclerosis.
C. Thrombosis, progression of distal atherosclerosis, technical problems or hypercoagulability, and anastomotic myointimal hyperplasia.
D. Thrombosis, anastomotic myointimal hyperplasia, technical problems or hypercoagulability, and progression of distal atherosclerosis.
E. Technical problems or hypercoagulability, progression of distal atherosclerosis, thrombosis, and anastomotic myointimal hyperplasia.

Question 49-2

Endothelial progenitor cells (EPCs):

A. Are associated with early graft failure.
B. Can be released from the bone marrow in response to ischemia and vascular injury.
C. Have no impact on spontaneous re-endothelialization.
D. Are greater in number in those who smoke.
E. Can rarely be isolated in postadolescent patients.

Question 49-3

With regard to endothelial cells (EC) seeding:

A. Animal studies have suggested that EC-seeded Dacron and expanded (e)PTFE grafts elicit decreased platelet deposition and increased patency rates, findings related to a significant reduction in anastomotic pseudointimal hyperplasia.
B. Tissue plasminogen activator has been successfully transfected into ECs through genetic manipulation, with effective expression of the agent after being seeded onto prosthetic graft surfaces.
C. The cell density of the EC lining on a normal vein is approximately 1000 ECs/mm^2. Therefore, the same density of cells is needed in a completely lined, small-caliber vascular graft for immediate confluent human EC coverage.
D. ECs adhere strongly to synthetic graft materials, and once adherent, more than 90% were retained for 24 hours.
E. For bypasses in the femoropopliteal region, equal patency rates and platelet deposition were obtained with EC-seeded ePTFE grafts and unseeded grafts after a 3-year follow-up.

ANSWERS AND DISCUSSION

■ ANSWERS AND DISCUSSION FOR CHAPTER 41

Answer 41-1: B

Discussion 41-1

(A) Open vascular reconstructions are generally more durable than angioplasty of visceral vessels, although (C) periprocedural morbidity of angioplasty is less than for open procedures. As a result, angioplasty is preferred for patients with medical comorbidities or limited life expectancy, and open revascularization may be better in younger patients in whom long-term durability is paramount. (D) Thromboendarterectomy and angioplasty are both most suitable for short lesions, whereas arterial bypass can be used for all types of lesions regardless of length (E). Extra-anatomic bypass for renal revascularization is particularly useful in older patients or those with severe atherosclerotic disease of the aorta. It has the advantage of avoiding aortic cross-clamping and is associated with less hemodynamic change than aortorenal bypass. The late results of extra-anatomic and aortic-based bypasses are similar as long as the inflow vessels are free of significant atherosclerotic disease. (B) Prograde (supraceliac) aortovisceral bypass is less prone to kinking and occlusion than retrograde bypass and is preferred in patients without cardiac problems, who can tolerate supraceliac clamping.

Answer 41-2: E

Discussion 41-2

All of these factors are of some relative importance in selecting thromboendarterectomy as a method of revascularization. (A) Because this procedure often involves more extensive mobilization than bypass it may be more risky in older patients with multiple comorbid conditions. This is particularly true when transaortic visceral endarterectomy is considered. Thromboendarterectomy avoids the need for autologous or prosthetic conduits (D) and therefore may be an attractive alternative when there is concern with infection (C). Although surgeon experience (B) is important in thromboendarterectomy, the most crucial contributing factor to success is selection of patients with a favorable distribution of disease, i.e., those with discrete disease that can be completely removed without fear of intimal flaps leading to thrombosis.

Answer 41-3: A

Discussion 41-3

Multiple prospective comparisons of open and endovascular repair of AAA in patients who were candidates for both procedures have been undertaken as part of the initial evaluation of this technology. (A) In low-risk patients, there was no statistically significant difference in mortality between the two techniques. Although there are some recent data that suggest that endovascular repair may be associated with reduced mortality compared with open repair, these are retrospective in nature. However, the remaining answers (B–E) are not true. Endovascular repair is associated with *reduced* perioperative morbidity (E), shorter hospital stay, and early improvement (3 months) in quality of life (which becomes equivalent at 6 months). These advantages come at a price. There is increased secondary intervention in patients with endografts and (B) *increased cost*, primarily because of the cost of the device and need for regular long-term follow-up to detect late endograft problems contributing to their lack of durability (C). Indications for open and endoluminal repair should be similarly applied, although "high-risk" patients (age >80 years, more than three medical comorbidities) may be better treated with endoluminal techniques provided they meet the indications for surgery. With current devices, endoluminal repair of AAA is limited by features such as neck length, arterial diameter, and aortic angulation (D).

■ ANSWERS AND DISCUSSION FOR CHAPTER 42

Answer 42-1: B

Discussion 42-1

A. The position of the hypoglossal nerve is not changed in this anatomic variation.
B. The recurrent laryngeal nerves usually arise from the vagus nerves in the chest. On the right side, the recurrent nerve loops posteriorly beneath the origin of the subclavian artery and ascends in the tracheoesophageal groove, well away from the carotid artery. When the right subclavian artery arises from the descending thoracic aorta instead of the brachiocephalic artery, the laryngeal nerve arises in the neck at the level of the carotid bifurcation and passes directly to the larynx. This "nonrecurrent" nerve is at risk for injury if the dissection is extended either medial or posterior to the carotid bulb area. A nonrecurrent laryngeal nerve occurs more frequently on the right side and has a reported incidence of approximately 0.5%.
C. The main thoracic duct is located at the base of the left neck and will not be seen during right cervical exploration.
D. Because a thyroid ima artery courses in the midline of the neck, this variation is not likely to be encountered during carotid exposure.
E. Likewise, an aberrant subclavian vein is not likely to be seen during cervical exposure (and, of importance in other operations, the aberrant subclavian artery lies deeper than usually encountered in supraclavicular explorations).

Answer 42-2: C

Discussion 42-2

The key here is the likely ligation of the (A) inferior mesenteric artery *at the time of the first operation*, the AAA repair. Because of the abundant collateral circulation between the superior mesenteric, inferior mesenteric, and internal iliac arteries, the inferior mesenteric artery can usually be safely ligated at the time of AAA repair. In such case, the circulation to the left colon relies in large part on established collaterals between the superior mesenteric and inferior mesenteric arteries, specifically through the left branch of the middle colic artery and the ascending branch of the left colic artery.

A. The inferior mesenteric artery has presumably been previously ligated (and would *not* be encountered during right hemicolectomy anyway).

B. The ileocolic artery would be taken in a right colectomy but is *not* part of this critical collateral pathway described.

C. Ligation of the left branch of the middle colic artery would disrupt the now critical collateral circuit to the left colon and may result in acute left colon ischemia (correct answer).

D. The Arc of Riolan is an important collateral between the superior and inferior mesenteric arteries and is at risk during left colectomy, but would *not* be interrupted during right hemicolectomy.

E. The left hypogastric artery is an important inflow source to the lower left and sigmoid colon, through the superior hemorrhoidal connection with the inferior mesenteric artery, but would also *not* be interrupted during a right colectomy.

Answer 42-3: E

Discussion 42-3

(E) The lateral femoral circumflex vein crosses anterior to the profunda femoris artery near its origin. Injury to this vein can occur during dissection in the "crotch" formed between the superficial and deep femoral branches. The other vessels (A–D) may be encountered during such a groin exposure, and some are close to the dissection site, but they are not so exquisitely vulnerable during this particular maneuver as the lateral circumflex vein. This vein can also be the location for arteriovenous fistulas caused by percutaneous puncture of the overlying superficial femoral artery and has been used to create a temporary arteriovenous fistula to protect venous thrombectomy and crossover venous bypass.

■ ANSWERS AND DISCUSSION FOR CHAPTER 43

Answer 43-1: B

Discussion 43-1

(A) The first vessel anastomosis was a *side-to-side* portocaval shunt performed in dogs by Nikolai Eck in 1877. Subsequently, in early clinical attempts at arterial anastomosis, the end-to-end anastomosis was commonly used because it was conceptually the simplest, and most procedures were simple repairs. (B) It is the technique routinely used for repair of aneurysms, but end-to-side anastomoses are more common in arterial bypass surgery (C). When performed as a perpendicular anastomosis in small vessels, an end-to-end anastomosis is prone to narrowing and secondary thrombosis, particularly if *continuous* suture technique is used, because of a "purse stringing" effect (D). In penetrating arterial trauma (E), where resection of the injured segment with end-to-end anastomosis can commonly be performed, the end-to-end anastomosis should be performed with techniques that avoid narrowing, for example, by using interrupted sutures, performing a triangulation technique if continuous sutures are used, expanding the anastomotic line with blood flow before

the final tying of sutures, and/or beveling the ends to produce a larger oblique suture line.

Answer 43-2: D

Discussion 43-2

A. End-to-side anastomosis is ideal for bypass grafts but *not* for interposition grafts where they would require more length and exposure and leave adjacent blind-ended cul-de-sacs.

B. Acute angled anastomoses are best, usually entering the recipient vessel at between 30 and 45 degrees. Such an angle will usually produce an opening that is twice the diameter of the donor vessel, which is ideal.

C. The recipient vessel diameter is normally as large or larger. Although matching diameters of the bypass graft and the inflow/outflow vessels seems sound in principle, the anastomotic opening, being oblique and with an acute angle of entry, needs to be much bigger.

D. One should start the anastomosis at the most inaccessible point on its circumference. Ordinarily, this is at the "heel" in acute-angle entry anastomoses but may be at the posterior midline in more perpendicular anastomoses where there is limited mobility (correct answer).

E. In repairing thoracoabdominal aneurysms, where the visceral arteries are included, these are actually implanted end-to-side, even though this is performed like a lateral (side-to-side) anastomosis. Additional bypasses (e.g., to the left renal artery) are attached to the main prosthesis by end-to-side anastomosis.

Answer 43-3: D

Discussion 43-3

A. Silk sutures are biodegradable and disintegrate with time, but they are acceptable for autogenous tissue anastomoses (e.g., portosystemic shunts), which heal before the silk loses its strength. However, prosthetic anastomoses do not heal in the same fashion and, in fact, depend indefinitely on the suture material for their strength and integrity. Using silk in this latter setting was responsible for many if not most anastomotic aneurysms up until the mid-1960s when the practice was discontinued.

B. Polyethylene monofilament sutures were observed to "fracture" in time and created problems when used to place artificial heart valves. Braided Dacron suture, coated to improve handling properties, then became popular and was used until the newer polypropylene monofilament sutures proved durable.

C. In the past, interrupted sutures were always used for anastomoses in children to allow for commensurate growth, but now synthetic absorbable monofilament suture with a suitably long half-life (e.g., polydioxanone) allows continuous suture techniques to be performed.

D. "Equal depth and travel" is a good rule in performing continuous anastomoses, although this is not always possible, particularly in aneurysm surgery.

E. The opposite, "inside-out on the artery, outside-in on the graft," is the correct method for performing such anastomoses, because penetrating atherosclerotic arteries "outside in" might lift up an intimal plaque without penetrating it, thereby leading to an intimal flap, dissection, and thrombosis when flow is restored.

■ ANSWERS AND DISCUSSION FOR CHAPTER 44

Answer 44-1: D

Discussion 44-1

A. Although visualizing the arterial tree proximal to the affected limb, up to the abdominal aorta, is important, full bilateral (rather than unilateral) lower extremity arteriography should generally be performed before performing an embolectomy (for several reasons cited next).

B. It does help in operative planning by providing important information about the occlusive event. Precise arteriographic localization of the occlusion helps the surgeon to place the incision in the optimal site. In addition, the presence of underlying atherosclerotic occlusions and/or stenoses may be identified. Unexpected inflow disease may be detected and appropriate inflow and outflow "landing sites" may be identified should a bypass be required.

C. Nonocclusive ischemia (described in the discussion of question 3) may be ruled out as a potential cause of symptoms.

D. Unsuspected additional emboli may be detected and treated. Indeed, multiplicity of occlusions in locations that are not usually sites of chronic disease is one of the most certain pieces of evidence to support embolization as the causative mechanism of the acute ischemic event.

E. Arteriography should be performed through a brachial approach in the absence of palpable femoral pulses. Crossover catheterization from the opposite femoral artery may not visualize unsuspected lesions superiorly or in the limb contralateral to the one presenting with ischemic symptoms.

Answer 44-2: E

Discussion 44-2

A. During embolectomy an adequate length of artery must be exposed to allow control *both proximal and distal* to the catheter introduction site.

B. Although a transverse arteriotomy has some advantages, a longitudinal incision may be preferentially used because it allows the embolectomy site to serve as a graft anastomotic site if a bypass is required. Meticulous closure, with or without a patch as dictated by the status of the artery, avoids the risk of luminal narrowing, which can be associated with longitudinal arteriotomy.

C. Balloon catheters 3F and larger are inflated with saline and checked for concentricity and leaks. An eccentric balloon displaces the catheter tip and body toward one side of the arterial wall and produces increased drag and friction. Air is used for inflation in smaller diameter catheters (1F and 2F) because the inflation lumen of these catheters is too tiny to permit quick adjustments in balloon size during balloon passage and withdrawal. An exception to the latter is when even small amounts of air could be hazardous, as in cerebral arteries.

D. There is a strong correlation between the shear forces applied to the arterial wall during embolectomy and the degree of intimal injury resulting in intimal hyperplasia. However, different brands of balloon embolectomy catheters have been compared regarding their potential for injury and intimal damage, and their differences are slight in this regard.

E. Freedom from underlying chronic disease and the use of proper technique, especially appropriate balloon catheter sizing and the avoidance of overdistension of the vessel, have a greater role in preventing intimal damage than the choice of any particular brand of balloon catheter (correct answer).

Answer 44-3: A

Discussion 44-3

A. Nonocclusive ischemia may occur in the lower extremities and mimic acute thromboembolism. It relates to systemic causes of decreased perfusion. The common setting is chronic peripheral arterial disease in patients with myocardial dysfunction (acute myocardial infarction or heart failure).

B. To the contrary, a smooth, tapering clot indicates adequate removal of thrombus, whereas a sharp cutoff suggests that additional thrombotic material remains.

C. Impressive back bleeding may stem from collateral vessels proximal to a residual distal thromboemboli and is not an indicator of complete thromboembolectomy.

D. The presence of a strong "water hammer" pulse actually suggests persistent distal obstruction.

E. When the distal outflow tract is occluded by clots that cannot be retrieved by mechanical means, intraoperative thrombolysis may offer a worthwhile option for revascularization. Mechanical extraction devices are first used to remove as much thrombus as possible. The inflow artery is then occluded, and boluses of a thrombolytic agent are instilled distally. After approximately 20 minutes, arteriography is performed and boluses of thrombolytic agents may be repeated until the distal bed is cleared of clot. This may resolve the ischemia of itself, or the subsequent angiogram may identify a distal vessel that can be used as a target for bypass if the ischemia has not been resolved.

■ ANSWERS AND DISCUSSION FOR CHAPTER 45

Answer 45-1: A

Discussion 45-1

Endarterectomy is applicable to a wide range of arterial pathology in many anatomic locations. Successful endarterectomy relies on establishing the proper dissection plane and the integrity of the remaining adventitia. For these reasons endarterectomy is contraindicated in the presence of aneurysmal disease (A is true). The appropriate plane of endarterectomy (B) is in the media, removing most of the inner portion of the media and leaving primarily adventitia and some fibers of the outer media. Although bypass and transluminal angioplasty have become popular in many areas in which endarterectomy is applicable, (C) they have *not* supplanted this technique, particularly at the carotid bifurcation and the origin of the deep femoral artery (E). Resurgent interest in combining semiclosed endarterectomy with distal endpoint stenting (Moll) may increase the application of this technique. Endarterectomy can be used successfully in type I aortoiliac occlusive disease and has the advantage of avoiding prosthetic material (D).

Answer 45-2: B

Discussion 45-2

All of these lesions can be treated by endarterectomy, with varying degrees of success. (A) Moll has reported good results with remote endarterectomy of lesions confined to the superficial femoral artery. Results approach those of above-knee prosthetic bypass and avoid long incisions and the use of prosthetics (B). Endarterectomy is often used in focal lesions of the common femoral artery that involve the origin of the deep femoral artery. When this is performed, it is usually accompanied by a patch closure. It may be performed with either inflow or outflow bypass. Of the options listed, this is the most suitable for endarterectomy. (C) Lesions of the innominate artery may be treated with endarterectomy; however, the technique may be limited by aortic "spillover" lesions that make clamping the inflow vessel difficult. In addition, the proximal clamp may impinge on the origin of the left common carotid artery. This limits endarterectomy in lesions that involve the origin of the innominate artery. (E) Type 2 aortoiliac diseases, which involve the external iliac and common femoral arteries in addition to the aorta and common iliac vessels, are not well suited for endarterectomy. (D) External iliac involvement is a relative contraindication to endarterectomy of the aortoiliac segment. Although external iliac arteries can undergo endarterectomy, indications are infrequent.

Answer 45-3: C

Discussion 45-3

This patient is a good surgical risk with indications for both AAA repair and left renal revascularization. Baseline elevation of creatinine in the presence of a unilateral renal stenosis suggests some degree of intrinsic renal disease. Although the anatomy would permit endovascular AAA repair, there are several features that make open repair a more attractive option in this low-risk patient. They include the following: age less than 75 years, suboptimal anatomy (both neck length and diameter), and baseline renal dysfunction. There is evidence that endovascular AAA is associated with some persistent deterioration in renal function over time, and follow-up often requires administration of contrast to detect and repair endoleaks. Suprarenal fixation could be used in an aneurysm with this anatomy, but the presence of a renal stenosis makes this less desirable.

Of the options available, option A involves endarterectomy of the renal lesion, which may be complicated in patients with underlying aneurysmal disease. Option B would be acceptable in an elderly high-risk patient, but it is not the preferred method for treatment in this case. Option C provides the best treatment for both the AAA and the renal artery lesion with excellent long-term results. Option D subjects the patient to an unnecessary left nephrectomy. Every effort should be made to spare renal parenchyma particularly in patients with baseline dysfunction. Option E does not address the renal stenosis.

■ ANSWERS AND DISCUSSION FOR CHAPTER 46

Answer 46-1: A

Discussion 46-1

All of the factors listed may influence the choice of a conduit for vascular bypass.

A. However, all of these factors are of secondary importance compared with the anatomic location of the bypass. Suprainguinal bypasses (for aortoiliac occlusive disease) and bypasses that involve large-diameter short conduits, especially in high-flow beds like the renal artery, can be better performed with prosthetic conduits. The available diameter ranges of prosthetic grafts give them some advantage over a smaller autogenous conduit in these locations. However, infrainguinal reconstructions are best performed with autologous conduits whenever possible because of the significant advantage of superior long-term patency associated with these grafts.

B. Prosthetic grafts carry a greater risk of infection than do autogenous or biologic grafts, but the risk is low enough that this is not a major determinant, rather it is the poorer patency of the former than influences the choice.

C. Indications for operation (e.g., claudication or critical limb ischemia) may influence some surgeons in selection between prosthetic or autogenous conduits (but not a primary determinant).

D and E. Increased patient comorbidities and reduced life expectancy may prompt some to eschew the extra time of dissection required for autogenous bypass in favor of a prosthetic graft, but this can only be done in above-knee femoropopliteal bypasses when there is reasonably good runoff. Time of operation is less important than ending up with the best-performing bypass conduit.

Answer 46-2: C

Discussion 46-2

All of the features are of some importance in choosing a conduit for infrainguinal bypass.

A. Mismatch in compliance between the native artery and bypass conduit promotes intimal hyperplasia.

B. Matching the size of the conduits to the size of the artery minimizes the effects of turbulent flow in the conduit and at the anastomoses.

C. However, the *most important feature* of an infrainguinal conduit is the presence of a thromboresistant inner lining. Such bypasses can be exposed to very low flows, which if they drop below the "thrombotic threshold velocity" of the graft can lead to graft occlusion. Much development research has been expended to produce prosthetic grafts with lower minimum velocity thresholds with some success, but, despite years of effort, no non-autogenous graft has been developed that approaches the thromboresistance of autogenous tissue.

D. Ability to resist infection is desirable and in some contaminated settings plays a greater role in the choice of conduit, but this is a consideration in less than 10% of cases.

E. Handling characteristics and ease of handling at implantation are important, possibly more to the surgeon than to the patient, but are even less important than compliance and size match.

Answer 46-3: E

Discussion 46-3

A. Autogenous vein is the preferred conduit for infrainguinal reconstruction. Despite several observational studies and trials that showed no statistically significant difference in patency between autogenous and prosthetic grafts in the above-knee position, in no trial has the prosthetic arm been equivalent or superior to autogenous vein in absolute patency rate. Recent trials have, in fact, shown statistical superiority of patency for autogenous vein in femoral popliteal bypass in both the above-knee and below-knee positions.

B. Heparin bonding has reduced thrombus deposition on Dacron grafts but has not improved patency in clinical trials.

C. Cryopreserved veins have been proposed for use in infected or potentially infected fields but have *not* been conclusively shown to be superior to antibiotic bonded prosthetic grafts.

D. Although patency of all grafts is influenced by anastomotic hyperplasia and progression of inflow and outflow disease, mid-graft failure is much more common in autogenous vein, occurring anywhere in the body of the graft. This is the rationale for frequent duplex follow-up of vein grafts, but not prosthetic grafts.

E. Both venous patches and cuffs, and use of anticoagulants, have been shown to improve the patency of prosthetic bypasses below the knee.

■ ANSWERS AND DISCUSSION FOR CHAPTER 47

Answer 47-1: D

Discussion 47-1

Variations in the anatomy of the saphenous vein are common. Bifurcated systems occur in 20% or more of patients. Variations in anatomy in both the thigh and the calf have prompted many surgeons to use preoperative vein mapping with duplex ultrasound to identify a suitable vein for bypass and to avoid a poorly placed incision, which may impede healing. When performed, vein mapping should be done with the patient standing or with a proximal tourniquet. Locating the vein can be done with accuracy, although defining characteristics such as true diameter and the presence of thickening or recanalization are less reliable. When the saphenous vein is not in its usual position medial to the femoral artery and vein, it most commonly courses anterolaterally. D is the correct answer.

Answer 47-2: E

Discussion 47-2

The quality of the vein conduit is the most important factor predicting the long-term success of lower extremity bypass. Considerable clinical and experimental work have demonstrated that significant ultrastructural changes occur during routine harvesting of the saphenous vein. These changes re-

sult in endothelial loss and damage to the smooth muscle layer of the vein and cause both early and late graft loss. Proper technique in harvesting vein grafts is essential and includes perivenous infiltration with papaverine to reduce venospasm, no-touch technique of vein harvesting, and distention at physiologic pressures whenever possible. Distention with a syringe under uncontrolled pressure can cause severe damage and should be avoided. The vein should be used as soon as possible, but when stored the solution should be cold and isotonic to preserve biologic function of the conduit. Thus E, all of the above, are useful.

Answer 47-3: C

Discussion 47-3

Vein graft surveillance after implantation using duplex ultrasound allows the identification and timely correction of vein graft defects. As many as 15% to 20% of vein grafts may develop lesions that require repair. Timely repair has resulted in a significant reduction in vein graft thrombosis. Intimal hyperplasia usually occurs between 3 and 24 months in vein grafts. Not all lesions must be repaired, and some may stabilize or regress with time. In determining which lesions require intervention, the surgeon depends on changes in both the ABI and graft flow velocity. Because the absolute flow velocity in a graft depends on many factors such as the inflow, outflow, and diameter of the conduit, a single parameter is insufficient to identify critical stenosis that requires repair. In general, peak systolic velocity should be as described in option C: greater than 300 cm/sec and the ratio of this peak velocity to velocity in the remainder of the graft should be greater than 3.5. There should also be a reduction in velocity of flow distal to the stenosis to less than 45 cm/sec. The values in option A suggest a mild to moderate stenosis that can be watched and may resolve with time. Although the graft flow velocity in B is low (45 cm/sec), lack of velocity elevation or decrease in ABI suggest that this low velocity may be caused by limited runoff of the tibial bypass. In option D the stenosis is more severe than in A, but the velocity ratio and distal velocity are not severe enough to warrant intervention. This patient might show progression over time and may warrant increased surveillance. Only option C meets all requirements for intervention. E is correct.

■ ANSWERS AND DISCUSSION FOR CHAPTER 48

Answer 48-1: C

Discussion 48-1

This patient has a limb-threatening situation that requires a long bypass for healing. Prosthetic grafts are a poor choice in this situation (answers B and E), even with adjunctive techniques. Little has been written about the use of (A–D) fistula to the dorsalis pedis (DP) vessel. The results of multiple spliced veins (A) are poor and become worse as the number of segments increase. Although short-term success might be expected with (D) CryoVein, its cost and the problem of late rejection with occlusion remain serious problems. Of the choices listed, (C) HUV is associated with the best long-term results and is the correct choice.

Answer 48-2: D

Discussion 48-2

Cryopreservation retains the viability of both endothelial and smooth muscle cells (A). Although this results in a true "biologic conduit," these cells become immunologic targets for host rejection. This can occur early in the form of acute thrombosis or at 12 to 18 months. (B) It may manifest as either aneurysmal degeneration or obliterative vasculitis with occlusion. (C) To date, no processing has been able to remove the antigenicity from these veins. Decellularizing cryopreserved veins may offer some promise. (D) CryoVein has *not* been proved superior to PTFE in crural reconstruction. (E) Its main advantage is in infected fields or as bridge therapy when more definitive reconstruction can be planned in the future.

Answer 48-3: C

Discussion 48-3

HUVs have been used successfully as arterial substitutes for decades. These veins were prepared by glutaraldehyde tanning to decrease antigenicity. (A) Early grafts were prone to aneurysmal degeneration over time, a problem that was corrected by altering the tanning process and covering the veins with a mesh that constrains dilation. A major objection to HUV is the technical procedures and requirements that accompany the implantation to avoid damage and early thrombosis rates. These problems have discouraged many surgeons from using this conduit routinely. (C) To the contrary, HUV patency rates exceed those of PTFE, and (D) infection rates are similar to those of autogenous saphenous vein. (E) Early thrombosis rates can be reduced with perioperative antithrombotic protocols using either heparin or dextran.

■ ANSWERS AND DISCUSSION FOR CHAPTER 49

Answer 49-1: B

Discussion 49-1

Immediate graft failure is usually the result of technical problems during surgery and mandates reexploration to restore patency, beginning with the anastomoses, but also checking for twists, kinking, or other causes of compression of the mid-graft. After technical causes have been excluded, the various hypercoagulable states must be investigated and appropriate anticoagulation initiated. Graft failure beyond the immediate postoperative period, in the first month after placement, is most commonly the result of thrombosis in the face of high distal resistance (poor runoff); the thrombosis may occur in the graft itself or ascend into the graft from a distal occlusion, but the underlying cause is usually found distally in the runoff vessels. Prosthetic grafts require a certain minimum threshold velocity to remain patent, and often antiplatelet therapy is used in an attempt to lessen this com-

plication. After 6 months, myointimal hyperplasia at the anastomosis is the most common reason for graft failure; a smooth transition rheologically (e.g., by minimizing anastomotic mismatch) and/or enhancing the creation of a confluent endothelium may lessen the proliferative response mediating this persistent problem. Late graft occlusions (>3 years after graft placement) are most commonly secondary to the progression of distal atherosclerotic disease and thus may be independent of the characteristics of the graft itself.

Answer 49-2: B

Discussion 49-2

A. EPCs have *not* been associated with early graft failure.
B. EPCs *are* released into circulation in response to certain stimuli such as ischemia and vascular trauma (correct answer).
C. Animal models have shown that they can localize to prosthetic grafts and thus may effect spontaneous re-endothelialization.
D. EPCs are depressed (not increased) in those who smoke and persons with increased cardiovascular risk factors.
E. EPCs are readily isolated from patients of all ages (thus, E is incorrect), but there seems to be an age-dependent decrease in patients *with cardiovascular disease.*

Answer 49-3: B

Discussion 49-3

A. Although animal studies have suggested that EC-seeded Dacron and ePTFE grafts increase graft patency rates and decrease platelet deposition, they have *not* shown a consistent reduction in anastomotic pseudointimal hyperplasia.
B. Tissue plasminogen activator has been successfully elicited from transfected ECs seeded onto prosthetic grafts. Genetic manipulation of vascular cells and proteonomic regulation of these genes hold future promise for improvements in prosthetic grafts (correct answer).
C. Immediate confluent EC cell coverage, at the same density as a vein graft, is *not* a reasonable goal with prosthetic grafts in humans (see also discussion of answer D). Survival of enough seeded cells to eventually reach confluence is a more feasible strategy.
D. Initially, there is a fivefold loss of seeded EC after exposure to flow. Studies on the kinetics of EC seeding showed that only 20% of initially adherent cells were lost during the first hour and 60% were lost within the first 24 hours, and this must be compensated for in the initial inoculation of prosthetic grafts. Also, ECs adhere poorly to synthetic graft materials, and adhesive proteins such as fibronectin are needed to improve cell adhesion function.
E. EC-seeded ePTFE grafts have been shown to have superior (not equivalent) patency rates and decreased platelet deposition compared with unseeded grafts at 3 years in humans.

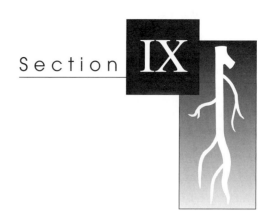

ENDOVASCULAR SURGERY: BASIC CONSIDERATIONS

STUDY QUESTIONS

■ QUESTIONS FOR CHAPTER 50

Question 50-1

Problems associated with the endovascular "mini-fellowship" training paradigm in the US include which of the following:

A. Some states require specialized licensing for such trainees.
B. The program may have a detrimental effect on the institution's traditional vascular surgical fellowship program.
C. The completion of a mini-fellowship does not guarantee that the trainee's institution will allow privileging in some or all of the endovascular modalities that were part of the program.
D. Access to adequate imaging equipment may be impeded by other specialists, at the home institution, irrespective of the training experience.
E. All of the above.

Question 50-2

Which of the following is *true* about the COCATS document?

A. It was based on a joint study by the National Institutes of Health and National Science Foundation.
B. It recommends a minimum number of diagnostic and interventional procedures to develop the skills necessary for the endovascular treatment of vascular disease.
C. It outlines the problems associated with present endograft technology in the treatment of AAAs.
D. It is a document written by the Society for Vascular Surgery outlining the indications for endovascular therapy.
E. Is the seminal work on credentialing for advanced endovascular therapies in surgery.

■ QUESTIONS FOR CHAPTER 51

Question 51-1

A patient presents for diagnostic arteriography for chronic right lower extremity ischemia after thrombosis of the right limb in an aortobifemoral bypass graft. Access is attempted through the left groin. The area is firmly scarred, and the patient is obese. Each of the following represents appropriate methods of gaining access *except*:

A. Use of a single-wall puncture needle with ultrasound guidance.
B. Use of a double-wall puncture needle.
C. Use of a 4F micropuncture system.
D. Use of a Doppler "smart" needle.
E. Consideration of a brachial artery approach.

Question 51-2

Concerning the diameter of an access system and a coaxially placed catheter, which of the following is true:

A. The listed French diameter of a guide catheter represents its inner diameter (ID).
B. The listed French diameter of a diagnostic catheter represents its ID.
C. French size may be converted to millimeters by multiplying the French value by three.
D. In building a coaxial sheath-guide system, a 6F sheath can be placed through an 8F guide catheter.
E. The listed French diameter of a sheath designates its outer diameter (OD).

Question 51-3

A patient presents with a symptomatic 95% stenosis at the origin of a heavily calcified left common iliac artery and has an asymptomatic 30% right common iliac proximal stenosis. The normal common iliac size is gauged to be 8 mm. Retrograde right and left femoral access is achieved, and kissing balloon dilation with 8-mm balloons resulted in recoil of the left iliac lesion down to a residual luminal diameter of 5 mm (~40% diameter reduction), with a 5 mm Hg resting translesion pressure gradient. An appropriate *next* step would be:

A. Placement of bilateral 8-mm balloon expandable stents in both common iliac arteries.
B. Use of a cutting balloon on the left in conjunction with a standard balloon on the right.
C. Use of bilateral drug-eluting stents in the proximal iliac arteries.

D. Placement of a 6-mm self-expanding stent in the left iliac artery and an 8-mm self-expanding stent in the right iliac artery.

E. Nothing further, because the left iliac lesion is likely to be less symptomatic now that stenosis is less than 50% of normal diameter.

■ QUESTIONS FOR CHAPTER 52

Question 52-1

Appropriate anatomic inclusion criteria for endovascular infrarenal aortic aneurysm repair include all of the following *except*:

A. A proximal neck length of 15 mm or more.
B. A proximal neck diameter of 28 mm or less.
C. A funnel-shaped proximal neck.
D. Absence of heavy calcification at the proximal attachment site.
E. Absence of circumferential thrombus at the proximal attachment site.

Question 52-2

A patient presents with a 7.5-cm aneurysm that begins 20 mm below the renal arteries, with a proximal aortic neck that is 25 mm in diameter. There is a distal aortic neck that is 25 mm in length and 25 mm in diameter. The iliac anatomy is normal. Of note, the patient is high risk on the basis of an ejection fraction of 20% and severe chronic pulmonary disease. The most appropriate treatment for this patient would be:

A. A bifurcated endograft.
B. A tube endograft.
C. An open surgical procedure with tube graft reconstruction.
D. Observation with periodic ultrasound monitoring of diameter increases.
E. An aorto-uniiliac device, landing the limb in the ipsilateral external iliac artery, placing a contralateral iliac occluder, and performing a femoral-femoral bypass.

Question 52-3

A patient underwent repair of an infrarenal aortic aneurysm and left common iliac aneurysm with a bifurcated endograft, landing the distal limbs in the right common iliac and left external iliac arteries. The proximal neck was 30 mm long, with parallel walls and a diameter of 24 mm, and without thrombus or calcification. The intraoperative completion angiogram demonstrated a small amount of retrograde filling of the aneurysm sac from a few lumbar vessels. On the 1-month postoperative computed tomography (CT) scan there is evidence of a large endoleak, located anterior to the prosthesis distally in the aortic aneurysm sac. This endoleak is likely to be:

A. A proximal type I endoleak.
B. A distal type I endoleak from the left external iliac artery.
C. A distal type I endoleak from the right common iliac artery.
D. A type II endoleak from retrograde flow from the left hypogastric artery.
E. A type II endoleak from the lumbar vessels that was visualized on the intraoperative completion angiogram.

■ QUESTIONS FOR CHAPTER 53

Question 53-1

The mechanism of action of thrombolytic agents such as urokinase or alteplase is:

A. Direct cleavage of fibrin polymer.
B. Conversion of fibrin-bound plasminogen to plasmin and subsequent digestion of the fibrin by active plasmin.
C. Conversion of prothrombin to thrombin and subsequent activation of plasminogen by thrombin.
D. Release of alpha-2 antiplasmin with subsequent digestion of fibrin polymer.
E. Conversion of plasmin to plasminogen, with plasminogen degradation of fibrin thrombus.

Question 53-2

Of the following scenarios, which represents the best application for catheter-directed thrombolysis?

A. A patient with a thrombosed popliteal aneurysm with two patent tibial arteries.
B. A patient with a localized common femoral artery embolus.
C. A patient presenting with lifestyle-limiting claudication and a superficial femoral artery occlusion.
D. Acute occlusion of a saphenous vein femoropopliteal bypass graft, occurring 12 hours postoperatively.
E. A patient with a thrombosed popliteal aneurysm and occluded proximal tibial arteries.

Question 53-3

A patient presents with occlusion of a PTFE femoropopliteal bypass graft, initially placed 3 years ago for rest pain in a patient without autogenous graft alternatives. The rest pain has recurred. The most appropriate *next* treatment for this patient is:

A. Catheter-directed thrombolysis with alteplase.
B. IV urokinase.
C. Observation, protecting the foot and allowing time for the rest pain to abate.
D. As in B, but with the addition of heparin anticoagulation.
E. Open surgical thrombectomy of the graft through a mid-thigh exposure through a transverse incision.

■ QUESTIONS FOR CHAPTER 54

Question 54-1

A patient underwent carotid artery stenting through an 8F femoral sheath, with a polyester suture femoral closure device. The patient presents on the fourth postprocedure day with low-grade fever, rubor, and a nonpulsatile mass over the groin access site. There is no associated groin bruit or thrill. The *most likely* diagnosis is:

A. A femoral false aneurysm from inadequate closure of the femoral puncture site.

B. A superficial wound infection localized to the dermal and immediate subdermal levels.
C. Deep infection involving the closure device.
D. A femoral artery to femoral vein arteriovenous fistula.
E. Inflammatory changes usually associated with large-bore femoral access with hematoma.

Question 54-2

A patient with renal artery stenosis and renovascular hypertension is treated with a stent. The procedure was performed through the right groin with a 7F sheath. A closure device was used. In the observation unit 2 hours later, the patient's blood pressure has decreased from 150/80 to 90/40, the heart rate is 120 beats/min, and the patient is nauseated and has right thigh pain. On examination, the groin access site is normal in appearance, without any sign of a hematoma. The following should be performed:

A. Immediate transport to the operating room for exploration of the common femoral access site.
B. Order blood from the bank, ensure adequate venous access, and transport patient to radiology for an emergency abdominal/pelvic CT scan.
C. Begin a neosynephrine drip to counteract the vasodilation known to be induced by diminished renin after this treatment of the renal artery stenosis.

D. Return to the angiography suite and through contralateral access perform diagnostic pelvic and femoral arteriography.
E. Administer 500 mL of neosynephrine containing IV fluids over 15 minutes, place a pulmonary artery catheter, and monitor hemodynamic parameters to guide further circulatory support.

Question 54-3

After diagnostic coronary arteriography through a 5F sheath placed in the right groin, a patient has pain and numbness lower down in the right leg. On examination, the right femoral pulse is easily palpable, but no pulses are palpable below this. The leg is cool and mottled from the mid-thigh to the foot. The most likely diagnosis is:

A. Occlusion of the common femoral artery from a catheter-related injury.
B. Embolization of atheromatous debris to the thigh and lower leg.
C. Embolization of thrombus to the popliteal artery terminus.
D. Occlusion of the iliac artery from a catheter-induced dissection.
E. Catheter-induced vasospasm.

ANSWERS AND DISCUSSION

■ ANSWERS AND DISCUSSION FOR CHAPTER 50

Answer 50-1: E

Discussion 50-1

Although endovascular mini-fellowships provide one of the most efficient mechanisms to retrain practicing vascular surgeons, there are some significant drawbacks to this training paradigm. Licensing to allow hands-on training experience is arduous in some states. The host institution must ensure that its case volume is high enough to provide adequate numbers for the traditional vascular surgical fellows as well as the mini-fellow. Last, trainees should ensure that their home institution will make access available to imaging equipment and that turf issues will not impede a rational, privileging process.

Answer 50-2: B

Discussion 50-2

The COCATS document was organized by the American College of Cardiology. It outlines training in peripheral vascular disease, diagnosis, and percutaneous intervention. Three levels of training are specified, along with suggested threshold case numbers to define competence. Although the numbers differ somewhat from those suggested by the vascular surgical and radiology societies, the overall tenor of the recommendations is similar to that published by the different societies.

■ ANSWERS AND DISCUSSION FOR CHAPTER 51

Answer 51-1: B

Discussion 51-1

A. A single-wall puncture needle is the standard choice for access in most patients. The patient has scarring and is obese, so ultrasound guidance may minimize the risk of complications and facilitate access.
B. A double-wall puncture needle is not commonly used, especially in a blind fashion to achieve access in a difficult groin. This is *not* an appropriate choice in this patient.
C. A micropuncture technique is probably the safest means of gaining femoral access in the patient with a difficult groin. Scarring may make this procedure somewhat difficult, however. In such case, ultrasound guidance may facilitate access.
D. A Doppler "smart" needle is also a good choice in the patient with difficult access.
E. A brachial approach is an appropriate option in a patient with groins used in a previous aortofemoral reconstruction, especially when the patient is obese.

Answer 51-2: D

Discussion 51-2

A. The size of a guide catheter is designated by its OD.
B. As with a guide catheter, the size designation denotes the OD.
C. French size can be converted to millimeters by *dividing* (not multiplying) the French value by three. In other words, a 6F catheter will have an OD of approximately 2 mm.
D. Because sheaths are designated by the ID and guide catheters are designated by the OD, a 6F sheath has an OD of something greater than 6F (usually ~8F). Thus, a 6F sheath requires an 8F guide catheter to build a coaxial system.
E. The size designation of a sheath represents its ID.

Answer 51-3: A

Discussion 51-3

A. This is a common scenario with heavily calcified iliac lesions. Appropriate management consists of the placement of kissing, *balloon-expandable* stents. The use of *self-expanding* stents at this location with a lesion unresponsive to balloon angioplasty is less appropriate although still chosen by some interventionalists.
B. Cutting balloons, as presently available, are not large enough to remediate the left iliac lesion.
C. There is no reason to use a drug-eluting stent in this scenario, and presently available versions are too small to use at the iliac location.
D. A 6-mm self-expanding stent is a poor choice for two reasons. First, the size choice is inappropriate for an 8-mm artery. Second, a balloon-expandable stent is a better choice in a heavily calcified lesion that responded poorly to balloon dilatation.
E. Even though the patient may demonstrate some clinical improvement with the 40% left iliac lesion (as opposed to its 95% baseline state), it is unwise to leave a patient with a resting pressure gradient after balloon angioplasty alone. The use of a stent is appropriate in this scenario.

■ ANSWERS AND DISCUSSION FOR CHAPTER 52

Answer 52-1: C

Discussion 52-1

A. A proximal neck of 15 mm is the standard threshold used for endovascular repair.
B. At least one commercially available endovascular device accommodates a proximal neck diameter of 28 mm.
C. A funnel-shaped (conical) neck is a *relative contraindication* to endovascular repair.
D. Heavy calcification at the proximal neck may increase the risk of a type I endoleak.
E. Thrombus, especially when circumferential, is considered to be a relative contraindication to endovascular repair of infrarenal aneurysms. The risk of a type I endoleak may be increased, as may the risk of embolization.

Answer 52-2: A

Discussion 52-2

A. The patient described is "high risk" in terms of associated comorbidities but would be considered an appropriate candidate for an endovascular repair. The described anatomy falls within the guidelines for commercially available devices. A bifurcated device is the best choice.

B. Tube endografts have been associated with poor durability, even in the presence of an apparently adequate distal aortic neck. Late distal type I endoleaks occur with unacceptably high frequency when such a configuration is used.

C. An open surgical procedure is inappropriate in this high-risk patient with anatomy appropriate for endovascular repair.

D. Observation is not prudent in a patient with a large aneurysm and endovascular options.

E. Although an aorto-uniiliac strategy could be applied in this patient, the distal landing zone should be in the common rather than the external iliac artery. There is no need to sacrifice the ipsilateral hypogastric artery. This option is usually applied to those with difficult distal anatomy but may also be used in ruptured AAA.

Answer 52-3: D

Discussion 52-3

A. There is no reason to believe that a distally located contrast collection is the result of a proximal type I endoleak that was not visualized on the intraoperative images, especially in the setting of an ideal proximal aortic neck.

B. Although a distal type I leak from the left external iliac artery is possible, it is not the most likely option.

C. A distal type I leak from the right common iliac artery is also possible, but not the most likely cause in this setting.

D. This patient did not undergo embolization of the left hypogastric artery. It is not surprising, therefore, that this vessel would be associated with a type II leak that fills the aneurysm sac anteriorly (correct answer).

E. Type II leaks from retrograde lumbar artery filling are most commonly located posteriorly in the sac. This endoleak was anteriorly located.

■ ANSWERS AND DISCUSSION FOR CHAPTER 53

Answer 53-1: B

Discussion 53-1

A. None of the commercially available thrombolytic agents directly degrade fibrin; they all work through the conversion of plasminogen to plasmin.

B. Both urokinase and alteplase act by converting fibrin-bound plasminogen to plasmin; the plasmin subsequently degrades fibrin polymer to fibrin degradation products.

C. Prothrombin-thrombin plays *no role* in fibrin degradation.

D. Alpha-2 antiplasmin is a natural *inhibitor* of circulating plasmin and does not degrade fibrin.

E. Plasmin is not converted to plasminogen; rather, the reverse is the direction of pathway whereby plasminogen activators, such as urokinase or alteplase, effect thrombolysis.

Answer 53-2: E

Discussion 53-2

A. Thrombolysis of this thrombosed popliteal aneurysm will accomplish little; the patient will still need an arterial reconstruction down to the patent tibial arteries, and the now open popliteal aneurysm will need to be ligated are excluded.

B. Localized common femoral emboli are best treated by a limited open surgical embolectomy, usually performed under local anesthesia.

C. *Chronic* arterial occlusions, especially those with a high likelihood of being caused by thrombosis of an atherosclerotic lesion, are not appropriate applications for thrombolysis.

D. Although patients with acute graft occlusions may otherwise be reasonable candidates for catheter-directed thrombolysis, the exception to this is the patient whose graft occlusion occurs during the *early* postoperative period. Hemorrhage at the anastomoses is common when thrombolysis is used early after graft implantation. Moreover, the cause of the occlusion is commonly a technical misadventure that will require remediation by an open surgical reoperation.

E. Popliteal aneurysm thrombosis *without* patent tibial arteries to provide open runoff for a surgical reconstruction or bypass is an appropriate indication for thrombolysis. Rather than to remove thrombus from the occluded aneurysm, however, therapy is directed at restoring patency to one or more tibial arteries to provide outflow for the vascular graft. This is the best application of those listed.

Answer 53-3: A

Discussion 53-3

A. Catheter-directed thrombolysis with alteplase or urokinase is now accepted initial therapy for a graft occlusion accompanied by the return of chronic critical ischemia. It usually achieves patency and identifies the underlying lesion responsible for the occlusion and thus directs appropriate corrective measures (e.g., balloon angioplasty, patch angioplasty, or some other reconstruction).

B. Systemically administered plasminogen activators such as urokinase or alteplase are ineffective for large peripheral thrombi, in contrast with smaller, coronary arterial thrombi.

C. The patient described has rest pain, and patients with chronic critical ischemia should undergo some form of intervention to prevent limb loss.

D. Heparin anticoagulation will not affect the graft thrombosis and is inappropriate therapy for critical ischemia when better alternatives exist.

E. Although an open surgical thrombectomy of this occluded graft can be a reasonable alternative, *it involves exposure of the anastomotic areas*, usually distally at first, to allow access to the outflow vessels to facilitate patch-angioplasty of a distal anastomotic neointimal lesion, should one be encountered, or serve as the distal site for a new bypass graft. Unlike vein grafts, the underlying lesion in PTFE graft thrombosis usually lies at one of the anastomoses, *not in the middle of the graft.*

■ ANSWERS AND DISCUSSION FOR CHAPTER 54

Answer 54-1: C
Discussion 54-1

A. A femoral false aneurysm is unlikely to present with rubor and a low-grade fever. Moreover, the mass would be pulsatile.
B. A superficial wound infection, cellulitis as described, is unlikely to be associated with a mass.
C. Deep wound infections are all too common with closure devices. The clinical scenario described is typical of such an infection.
D. An arteriovenous fistula would be associated with a bruit, and fever would be unlikely.
E. The findings are unusual, not common, and should make one suspect infection. Failure to treat this aggressively may culminate in arterial infection and disruption of the closure.

Answer 54-2: B
Discussion 54-2

A. The diagnosis is not certain, but a catheter injury may be poorly accessible from a groin exposure. Given its appearance, as long as the patient is resuscitated and relatively stable, a diagnostic imaging study (B) is warranted.
B. The most likely diagnosis is retroperitoneal hemorrhage from a high groin puncture causing hypotension and nausea. The patient should be stabilized with volume resuscitation, a diagnostic CT scan should be performed, and

the patient may need to be taken to the operating room for repair of the arterial wound.
C. Although hypotension after renal artery intervention occurs with some frequency, it should not be presumed. Hemorrhage should be excluded as the cause before treating the patient with vasopressors.
D. Although some form of percutaneous control of the arterial defect is attractive, the defect may be located such that placement of a covered stent would not be feasible. Moreover, the bleeding may not be rapid enough to visualize arteriographically. Surgical control is more appropriate in cases of retroperitoneal hemorrhage secondary to high groin access.
E. Although a fluid bolus is necessary to treat the hypotension, accurate diagnosis of the location of the hemorrhage and definitive treatment should not be delayed.

Answer 54-3: A
Discussion 54-3

A. The most likely cause of an ischemic lower extremity after femoral access is injury to the femoral artery with resultant thrombosis. A groin pulse will be present initially, until the static column of external iliac blood thromboses.
B. Atheromatous embolization characteristically produces mottling of the skin of the lower extremity, without loss of peripheral pulses.
C. Embolization to the popliteal artery terminus produces calf and foot symptoms, but the thigh should not show signs of ischemia because it is supplied by the profunda femoral artery.
D. Dissection of the iliac artery, compromising its lumen, would result in an absent or diminished femoral pulse.
E. Vasospasm, although sometimes the cause of a slightly cool extremity after angiography and catheter-guided procedures, should not be associated with the degree of ischemia described here.

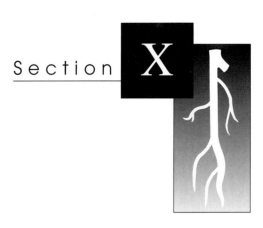

COMPLICATIONS OF VASCULAR SURGERY AND ISCHEMIA: PREVENTION AND MANAGEMENT

STUDY QUESTIONS

■ QUESTIONS FOR CHAPTER 56

Question 56-1

An elevation in the serum level of which enzyme is most specific for making the diagnosis of an acute myocardial injury after vascular surgery?

A. Creatinine phosphokinase (CPK).
B. Troponin C.
C. Troponin T.
D. Troponin I.
E. Myocardial band enzymes of CPK (CPK-MB).

Question 56-2

The most reliable indicator of myocardial injury in a postoperative vascular surgery patient is:

A. Chest pain.
B. Dyspnea.
C. Elevated cardiac enzyme levels.
D. Pulmonary artery wedge pressure.
E. Electrocardiogram (EKG) abnormalities.

Question 56-3

Which of the following interventions has been shown to be most effective in reducing perioperative cardiac morbidity among patients undergoing vascular surgery?

A. Intraoperative pulmonary artery catheter monitoring.
B. The administration of statin lipid-lowering agents.
C. Routine preoperative coronary angiography.
D. Preoperative use of antiplatelet drugs.
E. Perioperative beta blockade.

■ QUESTIONS FOR CHAPTER 57

Question 57-1

A 70-year-old man with chronic obstructive pulmonary disease (COPD) (forced expiratory volume in 1 second of 30% predicted) has developed an enlarging (now 6.5 cm) infrarenal AAA. Which of the following is a true statement regarding the risk of postoperative pulmonary complications?

A. The risk is too high in the described patient, and the patient is advised against having operative repair.
B. Preoperative antibiotics are useful in reducing the risk of postoperative pneumonia in patients with stable COPD.
C. Patients with wheezing on physical examination should have medical therapy optimized preoperatively, including 1 week of prednisone for those who do not respond to standard management.
D. Theophylline should be added routinely to the medical management of patients with severe COPD.
E. A full set of preoperative pulmonary function tests should be obtained preoperatively to help guide intraoperative ventilator management.

Question 57-2

On postoperative day 3 after thoracoabdominal aneurysm repair, an 82-year-old woman has just been extubated to 50% oxygen by face mask. Over the next 12 hours her oxygen saturation decreases from 95% to 88%. Which one of the following therapies is of proven benefit and should be used at this time?

A. Cough and deep breathing exercises, used 10 times every hour while awake.
B. Pain control with epidural anesthesia.
C. Endotracheal intubation with 100% oxygen delivery.
D. Continuous positive pressure of 20 cm should be administered.
E. Increase fractional inspired oxygen and apply noninvasive positive pressure ventilation at 10 cm inspiration/10 cm expiration.

Question 57-3

A 70-kg, 77-year-old man has developed acute respiratory distress syndrome (ARDS) 2 days after a ruptured AAA repair. He is currently on a fraction of inspired oxygen of 80%, tidal volume (TV) of 1000 mL, intermittent mechanical ventilation of 16, and positive end-expiratory pressure (PEEP) of 5 cm Hg. His arterial blood gas is pH 7.30/PaO_2 50/$PaCO_2$ 50. His condition would be best improved by the following:

A. Increase TV (e.g., to 1200 mL).
B. Increase both fraction of inspired oxygen and TV.
C. Reduce TV (e.g., to 450 mL) and increase respiratory rate while keeping plateau pressure below 30 mm Hg.
D. Increase PEEP to 15 cm and increase TV to 1200 mL.
E. Apply high-frequency oscillation ventilation.

■ QUESTIONS FOR CHAPTER 58

Question 58-1

The patient at greatest risk for contrast nephropathy after arteriography is:

A. The patient with severe hypertension.
B. The patient with normal renal function and bilateral renovascular disease.
C. The diabetic patient.
D. The patient with renovascular disease in combination with abdominal aortic aneurysm.
E. The patient with renovascular disease in combination with aortic occlusive disease.

Question 58-2

Contrast nephropathy after angiography is best avoided by the use of:

A. Acetyl cysteine before and after angiography.
B. Mannitol at the time of angiography.
C. Hydration before angiography.
D. Fenoldopam.
E. Low-dose dopamine after angiography.

Question 58-3

Pre-renal azotemia is characterized by all the following *except:*

A. Low renin output.
B. Normotension or hypotension.
C. Urine-specific gravity of 1.010.
D. Fractional excretion of sodium (FeNa) <1.
E. Low left ventricle end-diastolic volume.

■ QUESTIONS FOR CHAPTER 59

Question 59-1

Which of the following is the *least likely* cause of prosthetic graft infection?

A. Perioperative contamination from skin flora.
B. Bacteremia.
C. Mechanical bowel erosion.
D. Preoperative upper respiratory tract infection.
E. Perioperative contamination from adjacent lymph nodes.

Question 59-2

All of the following are effective strategies to minimize the development of prosthetic graft infection *except:*

A. Starting perioperative antibiotics 24 hours preoperatively.
B. Minimizing the patient's preoperative in-hospital length of stay.
C. Using a preoperative antimicrobial scrub.
D. Avoiding contact of the arterial prosthesis with the skin.
E. Paying meticulous attention to hemostasis in the surgical wound.

Question 59-3

Which of the following is the *least* appropriate strategy for treating an infected aortic graft when the responsible organism is Staphylococcus epidermidis?

A. Graft excision and in situ prosthetic graft replacement.
B. Graft excision and extra-anatomic bypass.
C. Graft excision and in situ replacement with deep lower extremity veins.
D. Antibiotics and observation.
E. Graft excision and in situ replacement with a cryopreserved conduit.

■ QUESTIONS FOR CHAPTER 60

Question 60-1

A patient with fever and back pain is noted on physical examination to have a new pulsatile mass in the abdomen. His history is significant for undergoing repair of an abdominal aortic aneurysm with placement of an aortoiliac Dacron graft 5 years previously. If you were considering the diagnosis of an infected anastomotic aneurysm, the best initial test in his evaluation should be a (an):

A. Computed tomography (CT) scan.
B. Radionuclide scan.
C. Erythrocyte sedimentation rate.
D. Aortogram.
E. Upper gastrointestinal (GI) endoscopy.

Question 60-2

If there is a prominent femoral pulse 5 years after an aortofemoral bypass, what is the *best* way to evaluate the patient for an anastomotic aneurysm?

A. Duplex ultrasound scan.
B. Magnetic resonance imaging.
C. Arteriogram.
D. CT scan.
E. Radionuclide scan.

Question 60-3

Ten years after right carotid endarterectomy with vein patch angioplasty the patient experiences an ipsilateral hemispheric transient ischemic attack. Physical examination reveals an unusually strong palpable pulse in the right neck. A duplex scan demonstrates no significant carotid stenoses on either side, although the report indicates a bulbous vessel on the right. What is the next step of evaluation?

A. Immediate surgical exploration.
B. Arteriogram.
C. Magnetic resonance angiography.

D. Transcranial Doppler.
E. CT with contrast.

■ QUESTIONS FOR CHAPTER 61

Question 61-1

Which of the following is *not* a cause for development of a graft enteric fistula?

A. Indolent graft infection.
B. Duodenal injury.
C. Mechanical erosion.
D. Bacteremia.
E. Anastomotic pseudoaneurysm.

Question 61-2

Which of the following is *least* helpful in diagnosing an aortoduodenal fistula?

A. Arteriography.
B. CT scan.
C. Upper GI endoscopy.
D. Leukocyte tagged nuclear scanning.
E. Barium upper GI series.

Question 61-3

Which of the following is the *least* effective strategy for treating the patient with an aortoenteric fistula?

A. Local aortic anastomotic and bowel repairs.
B. Graft excision, bowel repair, and extra-anatomic bypass.
C. Bowel repair and in situ graft replacement with lower extremity deep veins.
D. Bowel repair and in situ graft replacement with cryopreserved cadaveric allografts.
E. Bowel repair and aortic ligation if distal perfusion is adequate.

■ QUESTIONS FOR CHAPTER 62

Question 62-1

A patient with peroneal nerve injury who has weakness of dorsiflexion of the ankle will also have:

A. Loss of ankle jerk.
B. Weakness of eversion of the ankle.
C. Weakness of inversion of the ankle.
D. Weakness of plantar flexion of the ankle.
E. Sensory deficit on the plantar surface of the foot.

Question 62-2

A femoral nerve lesion results in all of the following findings on physical examination *except:*

A. Paralysis of the quadriceps muscle.
B. An absent knee jerk.
C. Weakness of knee flexion.
D. Loss of sensation over the anterior and medial thigh.
E. Loss of sensation over the inner aspect of the calf down to the level of the medial malleolus.

Question 62-3

Patients with neuropathy *after* an episode of acute severe ischemia may have all of the following *except*:

A. Paresthesias of the foot.
B. A feeling that the foot is cool but actually it is warm to touch.
C. Loss of mobility of the toes.
D. Sensory loss that is most often confined to the dorsomedial part of the foot.
E. Wasting of the small muscles of the foot.

■ QUESTIONS FOR CHAPTER 63

Question 63-1

Which of the following about lymphoceles is *not* true?

A. The most common site of presentation is the groin.
B. The differential diagnosis includes wound infection and hematoma.
C. Ultrasonography is a useful diagnostic test.
D. Lymphoceles in the presence of a synthetic graft must be repaired to avoid graft infection.
E. Injection of isosulfan blue is helpful in identifying the culprit lymphatic.

Question 63-2

Which of the following is the most common cause of leg edema after femoral-tibial bypass graft placement?

A. Deep venous thrombosis.
B. Superficial venous thrombosis.
C. Harvest of the saphenous vein.
D. Reperfusion hyperemia.
E. Lymphatic disruption.

Question 63-3

Which of the following is *not* an accepted treatment for chylous ascites after AAA repair?

A. Medium-chain triglyceride diet.
B. Total parenteral nutrition and complete bowel rest.
C. Repeated paracentesis.
D. Percutaneous sclerotherapy.
E. Surgical exploration and ligation of the responsible lymphatic.

■ QUESTIONS FOR CHAPTER 64

Question 64-1

After *technically appropriate* open repair for aortoiliac reconstructions, which of the following statements is *true*?

A. According to overall series, approximately 25% of men regain erectile function.
B. Most potent men become impotent.
C. Men with preoperative erectile dysfunction (ED) will regain potency.
D. Most men will have retrograde ejaculation.
E. Erectile capacity persists but in the absence of ability to achieve orgasm.

Question 64-2

Female sexual disorder (FSD):

A. Requires objective assessment of arousal and lubrication.
B. Is rare and not relevant to aortoiliac reconstruction.
C. Does not occur after hysterectomy.
D. Afflicts 10% to 20% of women.
E. Is best estimated from questionnaires.

Question 64-3

Planning aneurysm reconstruction to prevent postoperative erectile dysfunction (ED) includes:

A. Consideration of endovascular repair.
B. Study of the origins of the internal iliac arteries.
C. A nerve-sparing approach.
D. Preservation of pelvic blood flow.
E. All of the above.

■ QUESTIONS FOR CHAPTER 65

Question 65-1

A 60-year-old man, who had a below knee femoral-popliteal bypass with reversed greater saphenous vein (GSV) 16 months ago, presents in the emergency department with new-onset (<24 hours) of short-distance claudication. Duplex ultrasound confirms graft occlusion. The foot is viable with sensory and motor function intact. The patient is a smoker but does not have diabetes. The best treatment for this man is:

A. Heparin anticoagulation.
B. Pletal (Clopidigrel).
C. Open surgical thrombectomy.
D. Elective repeat bypass with another vein.
E. Catheter-directed intra-arterial thrombolysis.

Question 65-2

An 80-year-old man in atrial fibrillation required tibial-peroneal trunk and popliteal embolectomy after promptly presenting to the emergency department with an acutely ischemic leg. He had not been previously anticoagulated. In the OR, after completing the embolectomy through a femoral approach, you observe that the patient's foot is pink and warm. Posterior tibial and dorsalis pedis pulses are not palpable, but velocity signals are audible by Doppler. Pedal pulses are palpable in the contralateral foot. The patient has tolerated the procedure without other complications. Cardiac enzymes in the emergency department were within normal range. The most appropriate *next* step in your treatment should be:

A. Close the incision, maintain heparin anticoagulation, and begin warfarin.
B. Inject papaverine in the femoral artery and reexamine the foot.
C. Perform four-compartment fasciotomies.
D. Perform intraoperative arteriography to confirm the adequacy of the embolectomy.
E. Explore the distal popliteal artery to perform tibial and peroneal embolectomy under direct vision.

Question 65-3

On completion of an antegrade celiac and superior mesenteric bypass for chronic mesenteric ischemia, pulses are easily palpable in the common hepatic and distal superior mesenteric arteries. Optimal results for this patient's revascularization will be achieved if you now:

A. Reverse the heparin with protamine and close.
B. Listen with a Doppler probe to confirm good flow velocity, reverse the heparin, and close.
C. Perform a lateral aortogram in the OR to confirm technical adequacy.
D. Perform intraoperative duplex ultrasonography to confirm technical adequacy.
E. Close, leaving the patient anticoagulated.

ANSWERS AND DISCUSSION _____

■ ANSWERS AND DISCUSSION FOR CHAPTER 56

Answer 56-1: B

Discussion 56-1

(A) CPK, including CPK-MB (E), may be released from skeletal muscle as the result of surgical trauma or ischemia-reperfusion, so an elevated level postoperatively is not necessarily indicative of myocardial injury. The troponins (C, T, and I) (C and D), are normal muscle proteins involved in the calcium-regulated actin-myosin interactions. Qualitative and quantitative antibody assays of troponin T and I have been used for the clinical diagnosis of acute myocardial infarction. However, troponin C (B) is found *only* in cardiac tissue, is 13 times more abundant than CPK-MB in the myocardium, is *not* detectable in the blood of healthy individuals or in patients with renal failure as is CPK-MB or troponin T, and may remain elevated for up to 7 to 10 days in the blood after an acute episode of myocardial injury. Elevation of troponin C has been shown to be independently predictive of mortality among patients with unstable angina and non-Q wave myocardial infarctions.

Answer 56-2: C

Discussion 56-2

It has been demonstrated that symptoms (like A and B) are absent or atypical in as many as 75% of individuals experiencing myocardial ischemia after major vascular surgery. Clearly, multiple causes may be responsible for dyspnea, and chest pain is often absent. (D) An elevation in pulmonary artery wedge pressure, indicative of left heart failure, can occur in the absence of documented myocardial injury. (E) The EKG is difficult to interpret in postoperative patients and often will not exhibit classical ST segment elevations or the development of new Q waves. Therefore, (C) cardiac enzyme elevations provide the most reliable means of diagnosing myocardial injury.

Answer 56-3: E

Discussion 56-3

(A) Both prospective and retrospective studies have failed to demonstrate a measurable benefit of pulmonary artery catheter use in the patient population undergoing vascular surgery. (B) Although there is growing evidence that statin medications may benefit the patient with atherosclerotic disease through plaque stabilization, there is little evidence to suggest this has resulted in reducing perioperative cardiac morbidity to date. (C) Coronary angiography is invasive and should be reserved for patients with suspected severe coronary disease on the basis of symptoms and/or abnormal non-invasive screening tests. (D) Although antiplatelet medications have been demonstrated to reduce the incidence of cardiac ischemic events in the population at risk in general, there is little evidence to suggest that this benefit is seen in the perioperative period. (E) On the other hand, there is compelling evidence that perioperative beta blockade is associated with reduced perioperative cardiac morbidity.

■ ANSWERS AND DISCUSSION FOR CHAPTER 57

Answer 57-1: C

Discussion 57-1

(A) Despite the increased risk of postoperative pulmonary complications in patients with obstructive lung disease, there seems to be no prohibitive level of pulmonary function below which surgery is absolutely contraindicated. Clinicians should not use treatments based solely on an upcoming surgery unless they are otherwise indicated independent of the need for surgery. Multimodality treatment programs include chest physical therapy, bronchodilators, and smoking cessation. (C) Standard therapy for COPD includes use of ipratropium for patients who have daily symptoms plus the addition of inhaled β-agonists as needed for symptoms. When indicated, antibiotics and corticosteroids can reduce the risk of postoperative pulmonary complications in patients who have COPD. Unless a patient has been shown to be a nonresponder, clinicians should use systemic corticosteroids for patients who have COPD before surgery if airflow obstruction has not been maximally reduced and the patients are not at their best baseline despite other therapies, as determined by symptoms (e.g., wheezing) and peak flow. (D) Theophylline use should be reserved for patients who are not responsive to other maximal therapies. (B) There is no role for routine antibiotics before surgery; clinicians should recommend antibiotics only if a change in the chest radiograph or the character or amount of sputum suggest lower respiratory tract infection. In these cases, elective surgery should be canceled until the patient has returned to the baseline level of function. (E) There are two reasonable goals that could justify the use of preoperative pulmonary function tests: (1) identification of a group of patients for whom the risk of the proposed surgery is not justified by the benefit or (2) identification of a subset of patients at higher risk for whom aggressive perioperative management is warranted, but not as a guide to respirator therapy.

Answer 57-2: E

Discussion 57-2

Clinically significant atelectasis has been reported in 30% of patients undergoing thoracic surgery. Altered compliance of lung tissue, impaired regional ventilation, and retained airway secretions contribute to its development. Strategies to decrease atelectasis after surgery involve (A) lung expansion maneuvers and (B) pain control (epidural anesthesia); both strategies are effective in reducing pulmonary complication rates. *But*, although these are effective in prevention, this patient has impending respiratory failure and more aggressive maneuvers are needed. The lungs of many of these patients have decreased compliance, often requiring higher inspiratory pressures to achieve the same level of inflation, and are associated with an increased breathing effort. This increased breathing effort can further contribute to oxygen debt and mechanical ventilatory failure. Pulmonary edema may also be present, resulting in decreased forced residual capacity. Therefore, patients such as the one described often require positive pressure ventilation to improve gas exchange. (E) Continuous positive airway pressure (10 cm H_2O), not 20 cm (D), should be used initially, with noninvasive positive pressure ventilation added for patients with substantial hypercapnia or unrelenting dyspnea. In recent years, noninvasive positive pressure ventilation (i.e., the combination of pressure support and PEEP delivered by face mask or nasal mask) has been used increasingly to avoid endotracheal intubation in patients with acute respiratory failure. It should be used first here, rather than reintubation (C). Clinical trial evidence strongly supports its use in this setting to bring about rapid symptomatic and physiologic improvements, and these trials have documented reductions in the need for intubation, in mortality rates, and, in some studies, in hospital length of stay.

Answer 57-3: C

Discussion 57-3

ARDS is a diffuse inflammatory process involving both lungs that arises as a complication of diseases that produce a severe systemic inflammatory response. Diagnostic criteria include an acute onset, PaO_2/FiO_2 ratio less than 200, and bilateral lung infiltrates on chest radiograph, without a clinical suspicion of pneumonia, plus a normal left atrial pressure (if suspicion of an elevated left atrial pressure is present, a pulmonary artery catheter should be placed to assess wedge pressure). For example, a pulmonary capillary wedge pressure of less than 18 mm Hg in combination with the previously stated findings would be consistent with ARDS. Traditional ventilator strategies have relied on TVs in the range of 10 to 12 mL/kg (A, B, D). But delivery of such a TV into a smaller actual lung volume has significant consequences. Dependent portions of the lung, which are atelectatic, do not open with this lung volume; thus, the remaining lung has to accommodate this larger volume causing higher peak and plateau inspiratory pressures. Portions of the lung with open alveoli can become overdistended and may develop shear force stress, increased vascular permeability, loss of surfactant function, cytokine production, and further local and systemic end-organ injury. This increase in lung inflammation perpetuates the systemic inflammatory response syndrome. Strategies for managing ARDS with smaller TVs were developed from these concepts. This so-called protective mechanical ventilation is characterized by elevated PEEP, TV less than 6 mL/kg, permissive hypercapnia, and use of pressure-limited ventilator modes. Patients receiving protective mechanical ventilation compared with conventional ventilation have been shown to have a lower 28-day mortality and a higher rate of weaning. In a multicenter randomized trial involving 517 critically ill patients, the ARDS Network compared traditional ventilation TVs (12 mL/kg) with lower TVs (6 mL/kg) and found that the use of lower TVs in patients with ARDS resulted in fewer ventilator-dependent days and decreased mortality (40% conventional ventilation vs. 31% protective ventilation). Recently, the ARDS Network reported on the ALVEOLI trial, which confirmed the benefit of (C) a strategy that lowers TV and limits plateau pressure in patients with ARDS. The optimum PEEP in patients with ARDS cannot be predetermined (D). Thus, patients with

ARDS should be managed with a "protective lung ventilation strategy," which incorporates a TV of 4 to 6 mL/kg with limitation of plateau pressure to less than 35 cm H_2O, and an FiO_2 of less than 60%. Because lower TVs are used in this protective strategy, traditional goals of gas-exchange have to be modified and O_2 saturations of 88% should be accepted, and higher values of $PaCO_2$ should be expected. This is nonstandard therapy, whose use in adults should be considered when FiO_2 requirements exceed 60% and mean airway pressure is approaching 20 cm H_2O or higher. (E) "High frequency oscillation ventilation" is not appropriate here.

■ ANSWERS AND DISCUSSION FOR CHAPTER 58

Answer 58-1: C

Discussion 58-1

The nephrotoxicity of iodinated contrast agents has been recognized for many years. Renal toxicity after administration of ionic agents occurs most commonly in patients with preexistent renal dysfunction and those with (C) diabetes mellitus. The risk is much higher in patients with type I diabetes as opposed to type II diabetes. In addition, diabetic patients seem to be less likely to recover from contrast-induced renal dysfunction than nondiabetic patients. (A) Hypertension may contribute to long-term deterioration in renal function but is not a risk factor per se for contrast-induced renal failure. Likewise, although any patient undergoing contrast angiography may have acute renal dysfunction as the result of high doses of administered contrast agents, poor hydration before angiography, atheroembolization, and other risk factors, the patient with (B) normal renal function is at very low risk of this complication, even in the setting of renovascular disease and (D) aortic aneurysmal or (E) aortic occlusive disease.

Answer 58-2: C

Discussion 58-2

The duration of time that the kidney is exposed to iodinated contrast agents is a critical risk factor in the development of acute renal dysfunction after angiography. Therefore, maximizing urine flow rate during and immediately after angiography is a helpful strategy in minimizing the development of this complication, and pre-angiography hydration is very critical in this regard. (C) Studies have demonstrated that hydration with 0.45% saline is more effective in preventing contrast-induced renal dysfunction than with 0.45% saline and (B) mannitol. (A) Acetylcysteine is an oxygen free radical scavenger, and it has been suggested that administration of this agent before and during angiography may be protective of renal function. In one study the administration of acetylcysteine and hydration provided better renal functional protection during angiography than the administration of placebo and hydration. Further study is necessary to confirm these early findings. (D) Fenoldopam is a dopaminergic type-1 receptor agonist that *may* reduce the risk of acute renal failure by increasing renal blood flow and the rate of glomerular filtration. There is evidence from animal experimentation suggesting that this agent may be protective of renal function after the administration of iodinated contrast agents and after aortic surgery. Subsequent studies have not been as encouraging. Further work is necessary to determine its potential benefit in protecting patients against contrast-induced renal dysfunction. Likewise, (E) low-dose dopamine will increase renal perfusion, and this agent has been used frequently during open aortic surgery. However, its potential to prevent renal dysfunction remains largely unproven in this setting, as well as in patients undergoing angiography. Thus, A, D, and E are unproven. C has proven effective and is a standard accepted preventative measure, while B is not.

Answer 58-3: C

Discussion 58-3

Acute renal failure in the early postoperative period is most often attributable to prerenal causes. A contracted intravascular volume must be distinguished from cardiac dysfunction in selecting the proper therapy. Hypovolemia in this setting is characterized by (B) hypotension or normotension, (D) a low fractional excretion of sodium, and (E) low left ventricular end-diastolic volume. A low renin output (A) is also seen. Conversely, a cardiogenic cause would lead to fluid retention and a relatively fixed, low urine-specific gravity of 1.010 (C).

■ ANSWERS AND DISCUSSION FOR CHAPTER 59

Answer 59-1: D

Discussion 59-1

The most common cause of prosthetic graft infection is (A) bacterial contamination of the prosthesis during implantation, often from the skin or (E) adjacent lymph nodes. Although much less commonly responsible, bacterial seeding of a prosthetic graft can result from (B) bacteremia days to years after implantation. Urinary tract or pulmonary sepsis, or soft issue infection at other sites may be responsible. (C) Graft enteric erosion or graft enteric fistula formation are other common causes of aortic graft sepsis. Although (D) a preoperative upper respiratory tract infection may predispose to postoperative respiratory complications of general anesthesia, there is no evidence that it is an independent risk factor for graft infection.

Answer 59-2: A

Discussion 59-2

Prophylactic antibiotics are clearly indicated in patients in whom implantation of a prosthetic graft is anticipated. To be most effective, the antibiotics should be given just before skin incision. There is no evidence that a longer period of prophylactic antibiotic administration (such as A, 24 hours pre-op) is more efficacious. (B) Minimizing the patient's in-hospital length of stay preoperatively will reduce the likelihood of skin contamination with more virulent, antibiotic-resistant organisms. Likewise, a good antibacterial soap scrub preoperatively (C) and avoidance of prosthesis contact with the skin (D) are relevant because skin contamination is an important cause of graft infection. (E) Similarly, wound hematoma may contribute to poor wound healing and the development of wound infection, and subsequent graft infection.

Answer 59-3: D

Discussion 59-3

There is growing evidence that (A) graft excision and in situ replacement with another prosthetic conduit is a reasonable approach for the patient with proven Staphylococcus epidermidis infection. Likewise, replacement with (C) a deep lower extremity vein or (E) a cryopreserved conduit is also an acceptable option. Wide soft tissue debridement should be part of this approach. Clearly, the traditional strategy of (B) complete graft excision and extra-anatomic bypass is a very reasonable approach in this clinical setting, as it is when the infection is caused by a more virulent organism or a graft enteric fistula. Although Staphylococcus epidermidis may be a relatively low virulence organism, once the graft infection is proven and established, observation, even with antibiotics, is not acceptable in contemporary practice because the infection will ultimately progress and secondary complications may occur.

■ ANSWERS AND DISCUSSION FOR CHAPTER 60

Answer 60-1: A

Discussion 60-1

The incidence of aortic anastomotic aneurysm is relatively low, less than 5% in most series, although the incidence increases with the duration of follow-up. Infection is one potential cause, even among patients who present late. An abdominal CT scan (A) is the most reasonable *next* step in the evaluation of this patient. It can establish the presence of an aneurysm, differentiate an anastomotic from a para-anastomotic lesion, and provide some circumstantial evidence of an infectious cause. It may also demonstrate a non-vascular cause of this patient's symptoms. (B) Radionuclide imaging studies demonstrate the accumulation of leukocytes in the perigraft tissues and can provide supportive evidence for the diagnosis of an infected aneurysm, but they are not an initial step in the diagnostic workup. Likewise, an erythrocyte sedimentation rate (C) should be elevated in a chronic inflammatory state, but it is largely a screening study and there are many other potential causes of an abnormal test result. An aortogram (D) would be helpful in planning operative intervention, but this invasive test should not be performed before the diagnosis is established. (E) Upper GI endoscopy is useful in evaluating the patient with a suspected aortoenteric fistula, but it would provide little useful information in this case.

Answer 60-2: A

Discussion 60-2

A duplex ultrasound scan (A) is the most cost-effective method to confirm the diagnosis of a femoral anastomotic aneurysm. Although an MRI (B) may also demonstrate the aneurysm, and can provide additional information suggesting a possible infectious cause, it should not be the first diagnostic test in the otherwise uncomplicated case. An arteriogram (C) may be indicated before repair in the patient with occlusive disease, but it is not a reasonable initial screening study. A CT scan (D) is the *next* most reasonable test once a femoral anastomotic aneurysm is confirmed, to rule out a proximal anastomotic aneurysm because the risk factors are the same. On the other hand, in the absence of a suspected infectious cause, a radionuclide scan (E) is not indicated.

Answer 60-3: E

Discussion 60-3

The incidence of carotid patch pseudoaneurysm is·low, and well less than 1% in most series. Although many present with an asymptomatic or painful neck mass, some patients will present with a cerebral ischemic event secondary to embolization of thrombus within the lesion. (A) Immediate surgical exploration in the stable patient is not necessary here and should be deferred pending radiographic confirmation of the diagnosis. A CT scan with contrast (E) will provide excellent anatomic detail before operative repair, so that arteriography (B) or MRA (C) is not usually necessary. (D) Transcranial Doppler *may* have a role to play in evaluating symptoms in other settings but it clearly is not indicated in the workup of a carotid patch aneurysm.

■ ANSWERS AND DISCUSSION FOR CHAPTER 61

Answer 61-1: D

Discussion 61-1

Although (D) bacteremia may be responsible for a minority of prosthetic graft infections, there is little evidence that it is directly responsible for the genesis of a frank graft enteric erosion or fistula (C). On the other hand, the repetitive pulsation of the prosthesis, or an anastomotic pseudoaneurysm (E), against the wall of the third or fourth portion of the duodenum or other intestinal structures over time may lead to bowel erosion and fistula formation. This is why it is so critical to impose tissue between the graft and the adjacent duodenum at the time of graft placement. There is some evidence that this cause may be less common when aortic procedures are performed through the retroperitoneal approach. Likewise, (B) unrecognized duodenal injury at the time of graft implantation may be responsible for the early occurrence of this serious complication. Devascularization of the duodenal wall may contribute. Finally, (A) indolent infection of the prosthesis may eventually present with GI erosion.

Answer 61-2: E

Discussion 61-2

(A) Formal arteriography can provide anatomic information that may be useful for operative planning although it is very unreliable in identifying the fistula because most stable patients will have an occluding thrombus at this site. On the other hand, upper GI endoscopy (C) is very useful. It can identify other sources of upper GI bleeding, such as a duodenal ulcer or gastritis, and not infrequently it will provide evidence very suggestive of the diagnosis of the aortoduodenal fistula, such as compression of the duodenum, ulcerative bleeding, and on occasion actual visualization of the graft material. In addition, (B) abdominal CT scanning is a very useful diagnostic modality in this clinical setting. Key find-

ings include periaortic gas or fluid, a pseudoaneurysm, or bowel wall thickening. Even the seldom used leukocyte tagged nuclear scans (D), by indicating a localized inflammatory process, can be supportive of the diagnosis. On the other hand, (E) barium studies are specifically *contraindicated* if a graft enteric fistula is suspected. They rarely establish the diagnosis and complicate subsequent contrast-enhanced CT studies and angiography.

Answer 61-3: A

Discussion 61-3

(A) Local anastomotic and bowel repairs have been associated with mortality rates in excess of 60%. (B) Although graft excision and bowel repair with extra-anatomic bypass have also been associated with significant perioperative morbidity, this has been reduced in recent years by staging the extra-anatomic repair before the abdominal component of the procedure by a day or so. In situ arterial reconstruction is feasible in some patients, and either (C) deep veins or (D) cryopreserved allografts are useful in selected cases to avoid extra-anatomic bypass. In some patients in whom the aortic graft was placed for chronic occlusive disease, there may be sufficient collateral flow after aortic ligation to maintain limb viability (E). In this case arterial reconstruction may be deferred and revascularization performed later, after the septic focus has resolved.

■ ANSWERS AND DISCUSSION FOR CHAPTER 62

Answer 62-1: B

Discussion 62-1

Peroneal neuropathy presents as weakness of dorsiflexion and (B) eversion of the ankle, with preservation of (C) inversion and (D) plantar flexion, which are functions of the posterior calf muscles innervated by the posterior tibial nerve. The sensory deficit is confined to the dorsum (*not* plantar surface, E) of the foot and perhaps to the lateral calf, and the ankle jerk (A) is preserved. It is possible to confirm the diagnosis with nerve conduction studies. The most common cause is compression of the nerve at the fibular head.

Answer 62-2: C

Discussion 62-2

A femoral nerve lesion results in (A) flaccid paralysis of the quadriceps muscle, (B) an absent knee jerk, and (D) loss of sensation over the anterior and medial thigh and (E) the inner aspect of the calf down to the level of the medial malleolus. The flexors of the knee are innervated by the sciatic nerve, so knee flexion is preserved and C is the correct answer. Femoral neuropathies may result from surgery in the groin, particularly hip replacement or vascular surgery or from hematoma in the groin from iatrogenic procedures in the groin or from anticoagulation.

Answer 62-3: D

Discussion 62-3

After an episode of severe ischemia, however, it is not unusual for patients with a satisfactorily revascularized leg to continue to experience pain as the result of neuropathy. The neuropathic pain is burning and paresthetic (A) in nature, is frequently worse with rest and at night, and is unaffected or relieved by walking, in marked contrast with the pain of claudication. (B) The patient perceives the foot to be cold, although it is in fact warm. (C) The patient may have loss of mobility of the toes.

Examination no longer reveals signs of significant ischemia. Instead, the small muscles of the affected foot are wasted (E) compared with those of the normal side, and they are weak. There may be slight ankle weakness, and the ankle reflex may be depressed compared with that of the normal side. There is a unilateral *stocking* sensory loss (*not* confined to the dorsamedial foot, D), particularly to vibration sense. Unlike the findings in neuropathies caused by diabetes, uremia, drug intoxication, or alcoholism, the findings in ischemic neuropathy are asymmetric, with sensory and motor findings exclusively or prominently in the limb that was afflicted by severe ischemia.

■ ANSWERS AND DISCUSSION FOR CHAPTER 63

Answer 63-1: D

Discussion 63-1

(A) The groin is the most common site of presentation of a lymphocele. (B) The differential diagnosis of this mass includes hematoma, seroma, and frank wound infection. (C) Ultrasound is very helpful in differentiating a lymphocele from a hematoma. (D) Small lymphoceles will often resolve spontaneously, so that operative intervention is not universally required. (E) At operation, it is very helpful to inject isosulfan blue in a toe web space to help identify the responsible leaking lymphatic in the groin for ligation.

Answer 63-2: E

Discussion 63-2

Some lower extremity edema is seen in more than 50% of individuals who undergo infrainguinal bypass graft surgery. Although venous thrombosis may contribute to leg edema in some cases, the incidence of (A) deep and (B) superficial venous thrombosis after infrainguinal bypass grafting is quite low so that this is not the cause in the majority of cases. Likewise, venous return through the superficial venous system is minimal compared with the deep system so (C) that harvest of the saphenous vein per se is not a significant contributor to leg edema after bypass surgery, although lymphatic may be disrupted if this is done roughly. Although one may experience increased capillary filtration in the limb after successful arterial revascularization (D), blood flow regulation has been shown to normalize within 1 week of surgery. (E) Interruption of lymphatic channels is the most important and central cause of limb edema after infrainguinal bypass surgery.

Answer 63-3: D

Discussion 63-3

Most patients with chylous ascites after aortic surgery can be managed conservatively. (A) Oral feeding with a me-

dium-chain triglyceride diet will decrease chyle formation and allow eventual healing in many cases. With more severe chylous ascites, (B) total parenteral nutrition may be instituted to allow complete bowel rest. (C) Intermittent paracentesis may be helpful to relieve symptoms of abdominal discomfort and nausea. Failure to respond to conservative management is an indication for (E) operative exploration and closure of the injured cisterna chyli. Although (D) percutaneous sclerotherapy has been effective in managing localized lymphoceles, it has *no* role in treating chylous ascites.

■ ANSWERS AND DISCUSSION FOR CHAPTER 64

Answer 64-1: A

Discussion 64-1

(A) Results of retrospective series of aortoiliac reconstructions using appropriate techniques yield a wide range of results, but an average of approximately 25% regain erectile function. The results depend on the technique, diagnostic, and postoperative surveillance. Answer B would be true for conventional techniques not carried out with protecting potency in mind. Because of patient age, C is false, as is D, if the sympathetic chain is not interrupted. E is an exceedingly rare complication.

Answer 64-2: A

Discussion 64-2

(A) Objective measurements of FSD are now being performed. Measurement of female arousal and lubrication is more complex than observation of erection in men but can be done and are required. B, C, and E are false. (D) There are no good estimates of the prevalence of FSD.

Answer 64-3: E

Discussion 64-3

The choice of individual procedure (A) relates to (C) sparing nerves and (D) preserving pelvic blood flow which, in turn, may require studying the origins of the internal iliac arteries (B). According to survey data, endovascular repairs that preserve the internal iliac in preliminary study seem to be more favorable than open repairs in regard to ED. Thus E (all of the above) is correct.

■ ANSWERS AND DISCUSSION FOR CHAPTER 65

Answer 65-1: E

Discussion 65-1

Although all of the options described may have a role to play in the management of this patient, on balance (E) catheter-directed intra-arterial thrombolysis is the optimal approach in this setting. Although there has been considerable controversy over the years with respect to the best treatment of the patient with an acute infrainguinal bypass graft thrombosis, and although the results of thrombolysis have been somewhat disappointing in terms of long-term patency, there is evidence that the best long-term results of thrombolysis in lower extremity grafts are achieved in vein grafts that have late failure in patients without diabetes. The advantage of angiography and thrombolysis is that it allows identification of the underlying cause of the graft failure, and on the basis of the causative lesion(s) one can make a determination with respect to the role of angioplasty versus surgical revision. In the absence of biplane angiography in the OR, completion angiography after surgical thrombectomy (C) may miss important lesions in the vein graft or inflow or outflow tract. Further, thrombolysis avoids mechanical endothelial damage to the vein graft resulting from the mechanical thrombectomy. There is no question that the best long-term results in this setting will result from (D) revascularization with a new vein bypass graft, but in many cases there may be inadequate autologous vein available. Further, with an initial vein graft thrombosis, it is most reasonable to attempt salvage of the original graft. (A) Heparin should be administered to prevent thrombus propagation, but a more definitive intervention is indicated. (B) If successful revascularization cannot be achieved, Pletal can be a reasonable option for the patient with intermittent claudication, but in this scenario the goal should be salvage of the graft and complete resolution of the patient's symptoms.

Answer 65-2: D

Discussion 65-2

(D) Completion arteriography should always be performed in the stable patient, even in the presence of palpable pulses. The presence of palpable pulses would not necessarily ensure a completely successful thromboembolectomy procedure because balloon catheter thrombectomy may be incomplete or arterial injury may be caused by the procedure. There may be residual thrombus or intimal injury that can predispose to early recurrent thrombosis and that can be identified on completion arteriography. Answer A would be acceptable if the patient was unstable for any reason. However, because this patient is stable, the adequacy of embolectomy should be confirmed. Likewise, answer B is also a reasonable and low-risk maneuver to treat arterial vasospasm in the distal vessels, and that may occur in relatively normal vessels after mechanical thromboembolectomy but cannot be assumed. Answer E might be necessary if complete embolectomy is not possible from the groin, or if angiography demonstrates distal clot. Fasciotomy (C) may or may not be needed, depending on the likelihood of developing a compartment syndrome, and that clinical judgment will largely be based on the duration and severity of ischemia before successful revascularization.

Answer 65-3: D

Discussion 65-3

Some objective method should be undertaken to confirm the technical adequacy of the reconstruction. Although contrast angiography (C) is the "gold standard," it is cumbersome and difficult to perform in the OR in this setting. (D) Duplex ultrasound represents the most reasonable option, and a very accurate means of identifying technical defects in the OR. (B) Assessing the outflow vessels with a continuous wave Doppler provides a very subjective test of the adequacy of the bypass graft, whereas duplex is much more sensitive by providing real-time imaging and an objective assessment of arterial flow velocities in the imaged vessels. Whether the surgeon elects to reverse the heparin anticoagulation (A) or continue systemic anticoagulation postoperatively (E) is a matter of clinical judgment based on the patient's anatomy and other clinical factors, but this does not relate to the issue of ensuring a successful technical reconstruction.

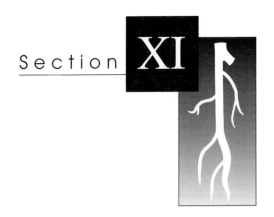

Section **XI**

ACUTE LIMB ISCHEMIA

STUDY QUESTIONS

■ QUESTIONS FOR CHAPTER 66

Question 66-1

Pertaining to the *revised* Rutherford (Society for Vascular Surgery, 1997) classification for acute limb ischemia, which of the following is true?

A. The classes are now the same as for chronic limb ischemia.
B. Class 1 ischemia includes patients with limbs that are viable and no intervention is necessary, irrespective of symptoms.
C. Class 2A ischemia includes patients with limbs that are not immediately threatened and observation is all that is necessary.
D. Class 2B ischemia includes patients with severe enough ischemia that revascularization is necessary, but the time frame for intervention is not critical and does not play a role in the technique selected.
E. Class 3 ischemia consists of limbs with irreversible ischemia where salvage is not possible and some level of amputation will be necessary.

Question 66-2

A 36-year-old previously healthy man presents with a right lower extremity femoral vein deep vein thrombosis (DVT) after a transcontinental airplane flight. A hypercoagulability screen is positive for the factor V Leiden mutation, and the patient is appropriately treated with outpatient low molecular weight heparin and then warfarin. Suddenly, 2 weeks later the patient develops simultaneous left hemiplegia and right leg ischemia. There is coolness, mottling, and sensory loss of the right leg, the right femoral pulse is very strong, but no pulses are palpable below this level. The most likely explanation for the right leg ischemia is:

A. Acute embolic occlusion of the right carotid and femoral arteries (the latter at its bifurcation) from embolization through a patent foramen ovale.
B. Acute thrombotic occlusion of the right superficial femoral artery (SFA).
C. Phlegmasia cerulea dolens caused by the progression of the right femoral DVT.
D. Acute aortic dissection.
E. Acute embolic occlusion of the right common iliac at its bifurcation.

Question 66-3

A relatively healthy 62-year-old man presents with 12 hours of intense right foot pain, now 2 years after a common femoral to posterior tibial reversed saphenous vein bypass performed for rest pain. The foot is hypesthetic and mottled, but the calf is nontender and soft. The most appropriate management of this patient would be:

A. Administration of low molecular weight heparin and outpatient follow-up in 1 week for consideration of elective revascularization.
B. Below-knee amputation for irreversible ischemia of the foot.
C. Retrograde left femoral (crossover) access for arteriography and catheter-directed thrombolytic therapy.
D. Antegrade right femoral access for arteriography and consideration of percutaneous mechanical thrombectomy (PMT).
E. Immediate operation with placement of a new femoral to posterior tibial expanded polytetrafluoroethylene (PTFE) graft.

■ QUESTIONS FOR CHAPTER 67

Question 67-1

A 76-year-old man with a history of atrial fibrillation presents with acute onset of bilateral leg pain and weakness of 2 hours duration. He has not undergone previous surgery and has no history of claudication. Heart rate is 120/min, and blood pressure is 180/90 mm Hg. His lower extremities are cool and pale with severe motor and sensory defects. Femoral pulses are absent. Of the following, which is the most appropriate *initial step* in management?

A. Systemic heparinization and urgent angiogram.
B. Systemic heparinization and immediate operative exploration.
C. Intravenous beta-blocker and urgent CT angiogram of chest and abdomen.
D. Venous duplex scan to locate the occlusion.
E. Systemic heparinization followed immediately by catheter-directed thrombolysis.

Question 67-2

Two hours after revascularization for acute ischemia, a 65-year-old man has severe pain in the involved extremity. On examination, the calf is tense with severe pain on passive flexion. Pedal pulses are not palpable but Doppler signals are audible. All of the following are likely to be identified in this patient *except*:

A. Metabolic acidosis.
B. Hyperkalemia.
C. Hypercalcemia.
D. Elevated creatinine phosphokinase levels.
E. Myoglobinuria.

Question 67-3

The most appropriate management of the patient described in the preceding question 67–2 is:

A. Elevation of extremity and administration of intravenous mannitol.
B. Measurement of compartment pressures and fasciotomies if greater than 30 mm Hg.
C. Fasciotomies, regardless of the compartment pressure.
D. Analgesia and observation provided pedal artery signals are still audible.
E. Immediate femoral arteriography with runoff to confirm adequacy of revascularization.

■ QUESTIONS FOR CHAPTER 68

Question 68-1

Which of the following would be an *unusual* presentation of a patient with atheromatous embolization?

A. Livedo reticularis on the skin of the legs and feet.
B. Blue toe(s).
C. Renal failure.
D. Normal blood pressure.
E. Weight loss and fatigue.

Question 68-2

The renal involvement in atheromatous embolization syndrome can by characterized by which of the following:

A. Accelerated hypertension.
B. Acute and chronic renal failure.
C. A delay of several days to weeks from the time of the insult to the elevation in the serum creatinine.
D. Eosinophilia.
E. All of the above.

Question 68-3

Which of the following statements is correct?

A. Atheromatous embolization most frequently presents as a spontaneous event.
B. The liver and GI tract are the most common sites involved in atheromatous embolization.
C. The kidneys almost always recover when targeted by atheroembolism.
D. Eosinophilia is pathognomonic of atheromatous embolization.
E. Patients with a disseminated atheroembolism syndrome have a 1-year mortality exceeding 50%.

ANSWERS AND DISCUSSION

■ ANSWERS AND DISCUSSION FOR CHAPTER 66

Answer 66-1: E

Discussion 66-1

A. There are two separate classification schemes for patients with acute versus chronic ischemia. The classification for chronic ischemia has six levels, although the classification for acute ischemia has only three (with a subdivision for class 2).

B. Patients with class 1 acute ischemia are viable if there is no further progression, but many will require elective or semi-elective revascularization for symptoms of lifestyle-limiting claudication or more severe symptoms.

C. Patients with class 2A symptoms (i.e., paresthesias and numbness without motor deficit) will usually require some form of intervention, albeit not always on an emergency basis.

D. Patients in class 2B (with sensory and motor deficits) always require very urgent revascularization to prevent limb loss. Although the quickest approach is usually surgical, OR availability can be a problem. Catheter-directed lysis takes time to achieve full patency, but circulatory improvement may be seen in a few hours. If the patient is already on an angio table with a catheter in place, this may be the fastest option.

E. Class 3 is defined as irreversible ischemia because it has progressed to the point where significant tissue-loss, in addition to permanent paralysis and sensory loss, is unavoidable, making this the correct answer.

Answer 66-2: A

Discussion 66-2

A. This presentation is classic for paradoxic embolization through a patent foramen ovale. The simultaneous occurrence of cerebral and lower extremity ischemic symptoms further substantiates this diagnosis.

B. There is no reason to suspect that this young, previously healthy patient should develop a thrombotic SFA occlusion; an event that most commonly develops in the setting of preexisting atherosclerotic disease. Although arterial occlusions are probably more common in patients with factor V Leiden mutation, the data remain controversial and, in contrast with DVT, arterial manifestations are relatively rare.

C. Phlegmasia would not explain this patient's cerebral neurologic event. Further, the description of the right leg is not that of a phlegmasia cerulea dolens.

D. Although an acute aortic dissection can explain simultaneous cerebral and lower extremity events, the right femoral pulse would be diminished in intensity if this were the cause of the problem.

E. An acute embolic occlusion of at the right common iliac bifurcation would be associated with a diminished right femoral pulse. In contrast, this patient's femoral pulse is strong; the "very strong" pulse suggests a "water hammer pulse," one that is classically associated with an embolus to the common femoral bifurcation.

Answer 66-3: C

Discussion 66-3

A. Heparinization alone was formerly thought to be an acceptable initial treatment for acute limb ischemia, buying time for resolution of the ischemia or elective revascularization. This approach remains controversial and may have a place in less critical acute ischemia, but definitive remediation of this severely ischemic limb is the proper treatment option in patients without prohibitive comorbidities. Furthermore, outpatient treatment with low molecular weight heparin is not appropriate for a patient with acute limb ischemia.

B. This patient has class 2B ischemia and should be offered revascularization before ischemia progresses to nerve or tissue loss. Amputation is an appropriate option only for class 3 ischemia.

C. A contralateral approach is most appropriate for the initial diagnostic arteriogram in a patient with acute limb ischemia. This offers the option to place a sheath over the aortic bifurcation and proceed with thrombolysis or other percutaneous interventions. This is the best option.

D. Ipsilateral access should *not* be chosen for the initial diagnostic study, especially in a patient for whom cannulation of a bypass graft originating from the common femoral artery may be desirable. PMT does not have proven efficacy in this setting.

E. There exists the potential to salvage this patient's saphenous vein bypass graft. The observation that it functioned for 2 years suggests that a localized stenotic lesion may underlie the acute thrombosis. The placement of a new expanded PTFE graft would be only a short-term solution, considering the patency when placed down to the tibial level, plus it deprives the patient of the opportunity to preserve a more durable autogenous conduit, with a lesser intervention.

■ ANSWERS AND DISCUSSION FOR CHAPTER 67

Answer 67-1: B

Discussion 67-1

A. The severity of this patient's ischemia (class 2B) mandates prompt operative exploration to rapidly restore lower extremity arterial perfusion and prevent tissue loss. An angiogram would add little and, of note, would need to be performed from a brachial approach.

B. Immediate operative thromboembolectomy is the most rapid means to achieve reperfusion in this patient with class 2B ischemia.

C. These two interventions will do nothing to reperfuse this patient's lower extremities.

D. A venous duplex is not indicated in this case of obvious arterial compromise.

E. Thrombolytic therapy would require many hours to achieve reperfusion. Although one might make a case for percutaneous mechanical thrombectomy, pharmacologic thrombolysis alone, is inappropriate.

Answer 67-2: C

Discussion 67-2

A. This patient has classic reperfusion syndrome, with compartment syndrome and some degree of skeletal muscle infarction, even if on a microscopic level. Release of ischemic byproducts is common in patients with severe lower extremity ischemia, and metabolic acidosis is a frequent finding.
B. Cellular ischemia results in membrane leak, potassium egress from the cell, and systemic hyperkalemia.
C. Calcium levels do not characteristically increase after ischemia-reperfusion.
D. Muscle ischemia results in leakage of creatine phosphokinase from the cells.
E. Myoglobin is released from ischemic skeletal muscle, and myoglobinuria is a common finding after ischemia-reperfusion.

Answer 67-3: C

Discussion 67-3

A. Although elevation of an extremity is appropriate for patients with very early compartment syndrome, the patient described has advanced changes and simple elevation is unlikely to be effective.
B. Clinically, this patient has a severe compartment syndrome and *compartment pressures are irrelevant*; fasciotomy is indicated.
C. The appropriate treatment for this patient is immediate fasciotomy.
D. The loss of pedal pulses or Doppler signals is one of the last events in the progression of a compartment syndrome. Continued observation will allow the muscle and nerve ischemia to progress to irreversible infarction.
E. There is no evidence that adequate reperfusion has not been achieved; rather, reperfusion has resulted in swelling and a compartment syndrome. Arteriography will result in further delay before fascial decompression.

■ ANSWERS AND DISCUSSION FOR CHAPTER 68

Answer 68-1: D

Discussion 68-1

A. Livedo reticularis is a common finding in the atheromatous embolization to the lower extremity arteries and presents as a blue-red mottling or discoloration of the skin that occurs in a netlike pattern, seen on the buttocks, thighs, or legs. It is caused by obstruction of small arteries, capillaries, or venules in the deep dermis, and when the skin is biopsied in patients with atheromatous embolization, cholesterol crystals may be seen in the dermal blood vessels. Livedo reticularis, however, is not pathognomonic of atheroemboli and has an extensive differential diagnosis including, but not limited to, other causes of intravascular obstruction (i.e., antiphospholipid antibody syndrome, cryoglobulinemia, endocarditis, and left atrial myxoma), vasculitis, and drug-induced (i.e., quinidine, quinine, amantadine, and catecholamines).
B. In the classic presentation, called the "blue toe" syndrome, it usually presents with the abrupt appearance of cool, cyanotic, and painful toes. This may occur despite the presence of palpable distal pulses, but with more extensive atheroembolism, distal pulses may be absent.
C. The kidneys are a prime target for cholesterol crystal embolization because of the enormous amount of blood that flows through the kidneys and the close proximity of the renal artery orifices to the abdominal aortic segment where atheromatous plaque is quite common.
D. The blood pressure is usually extremely high and difficult to control in atheromatous embolization syndrome because of activation of the renin angiotensin aldosterone system. Normal blood pressure is distinctly unusual in patients with atheromatous embolization.
E. Atheromatous embolization syndrome may present as a multisystem disease and mimic a necrotizing vasculitis. Patients with *disseminated* atheromatous embolization from a proximal source may present with fever, chills, malaise, and weight loss.

Answer 68-2: E

Discussion 68-2

A. Patients with atheromatous embolization may present with accelerated and difficult to control hypertension. This is the result of embolization to the small blood vessels of the kidney causing ischemia and thus activating the renin angiotensin aldosterone system. Severe and difficult to control hypertension is distinctly uncommon in acute tubular necrosis, thus helping to differentiate these two entities.
B. Atheromatous embolization may present with acute, subacute, and chronic renal failure. If there is a very large shower of embolic debris, the patient may present with acute oliguric renal failure. The patient may also present with chronic renal failure of unknown cause.
C. A more common presentation of renal failure is a delayed onset of renal failure (after the inciting event, i.e., transcatheter aortography). The patient may progress to endstage renal disease or may level off at a higher serum creatinine level than before the inciting event. This delay is the result of the foreign body reaction that occurs after significant atheromatous embolization.
D. Eosinophilia can be found in up to 80% of cases and probably is related to the generation of complement C5, which has chemotactic properties for eosinophils. The eosinophilia, however, tends to be transient and short-lived.
E. All of the above answers are therefore correct.

Answer 68-3: E

Discussion 68-3

A. The most frequent presentation of atheromatous embolization is after a catheter-based procedure such as angiography, angioplasty, and stenting of the coronary or peripheral arteries, precipitated by catheter passage and disruptive contacts with mural plaques during endovascular manipulations. Atheromatous embolization may also occur after vascular surgery, be associated with anticoagulation and thrombolysis, or occur spontaneously.

B. The skin is the most common (and visible) target site of atheroembolism. However, the brain, heart, liver, pancreas, gall bladder, bone marrow, and intestines may all be involved, although less frequently.

C. Although there are occasional cases of recovery after an episode of atheroembolic renal failure, most cases either progress to end-stage renal disease or stabilize at a lower glomerular filtration rate. This is one of the differentiating features between renal failure caused by atheroembolism and renal failure secondary to acute tubular necrosis.

D. Eosinophilia may occur early and transiently in atheromatous embolization or it may not occur at all. It is not pathognomonic of this condition, for eosinophilia can occur in many other diseases.

E. In general, the prognosis of patients with atheroembolic disease is poor, most likely related to the severe and diffuse atherosclerosis that is present in this patient population. The 1-year mortality reported in four different reported series has varied from 64% to 81%. Causes of death were multifactorial and included cardiac, central nervous system, and GI ischemia.

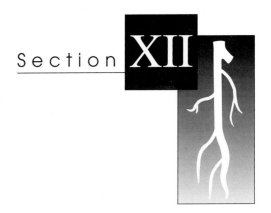

Section **XII**

VASCULAR TRAUMA

STUDY QUESTIONS

■ QUESTIONS FOR CHAPTER 69

Question 69-1

Regarding urban civilian vascular injuries, which of the following statements is correct?

A. Most vascular injuries occur in the chest and abdomen.
B. The majority are secondary to blunt trauma.
C. The most frequent cause of lower extremity vascular injury is long-bone fracture.
D. Most vascular injuries occur in the lower extremities.
E. Because of increasing automobile accidents, extremity vascular injuries are now equally divided between penetrating and blunt trauma.

Question 69-2

Regarding the clinical presentation of arterial injuries, which of the following is true?

A. Most extremity arterial injuries are accompanied by significant external bleeding.
B. Most penetrating arterial injuries in the chest present with a widened mediastinum, as seen on the anteroposterior chest x-ray film.
C. The outcome of major arterial injuries in the abdomen is dependent on both the presence of retroperitoneal tamponade and anatomic location.
D. Most blunt aortic injuries occur between the origins of the left carotid and the left subclavian arteries.
E. External bleeding from penetrating extremity trauma is best controlled by tourniquet until direct control by operative exploration.

Question 69-3

Which of the following statements is true?

A. The presence of a distal pulse rules out an extremity arterial injury.
B. Arteriovenous (AV) fistulas are commonly found soon after penetrating trauma to the popliteal vessels.
C. Complete arterial transection in penetrating trauma is usually signaled by massive bleeding.
D. An angiogram is mandatory in the evaluation of penetrating injuries in the proximity of major axial vessels, regardless of the absence of hard or soft signs.
E. The presence of hard signs of arterial injury requires operative intervention, but soft signs allow further investigation.

■ QUESTIONS FOR CHAPTER 70

Question 70-1

A young man is admitted after having been shot in the neck. On arrival he was hypotensive and taken immediately to the OR because of a large hematoma and continued bleeding. Preoperatively, the patient was conscious and moving all his extremities. The injuries include damage to the left internal jugular vein and transection of the left internal carotid artery, with brisk back bleeding. The procedure(s) of choice would be:

A. Ligate both ends of the internal carotid artery.
B. Reconstruct the internal carotid artery with a Dacron prosthetic graft.
C. Ligate both ends of the internal carotid artery under the protection of systemic heparin followed by warfarin anticoagulation.
D. Reconstruct the internal carotid artery using end-to-end anastomosis or an interposition graft of saphenous vein, followed by a completion imaging study.
E. Ligate both ends of the internal carotid artery and perform extracranial to intracranial bypass.

Question 70-2

Which of the following statements regarding acute injuries of the internal carotid artery is true?

A. Contralateral hemiparesis for more than 12 hours is a contraindication to repair of a penetrating wound of the internal carotid artery.
B. Delayed repair of a laceration of the internal carotid artery is dangerous because of the possibility of causing conversion of a bland cerebral infarct into a hemorrhagic infarct.
C. Patients with injuries of the carotid artery who are admitted with alterations in consciousness should not undergo operation until they become lucid.
D. Occlusion of the internal carotid artery as a result of a stab wound should be treated nonoperatively.
E. Repair/reconstruction is indicated, whenever technically feasible, if the artery is patent, regardless of brisk back bleeding.

Question 70-3

Patients who have sustained blunt trauma to the carotid artery from motor vehicle accidents may also have injuries of the head and neck. Which of the following statements is true?

A. Clinical features suggestive of blunt carotid trauma, consisting of contralateral hemiparesis or hemiplegia, difficulty speaking, and ataxia, are readily apparent early on, despite associated neck or head trauma.
B. Most patients who have injuries to the carotid artery caused by blunt trauma will have bruising, ecchymoses, swelling, or other obvious local signs of cervical trauma.
C. Patients with blunt trauma to the carotid artery may present with Horner's syndrome or a transient attack of cerebral ischemia or only limb paresis.
D. Hyperextension injuries of the neck often produce discrete damage to the carotid artery at the level of the third cervical vertebra.
E. The majority of patients who have had injuries to the carotid artery caused by blunt trauma will have signs of neurologic damage if a careful examination is performed initially.

■ QUESTIONS FOR CHAPTER 71

Question 71-1

Radiologic clues that suggest blunt aortic injury include all of the following *except*:

A. Wide mediastinum.
B. Double shadow of the aortic knob.
C. Increased cardiac:thoracic ratio.
D. Depression of the left main stem bronchus greater than 140 degrees.
E. Deviation of the nasogastric tube.

Question 71-2

In a reasonably stable patient with a suspected gunshot injury to the descending thoracic aorta, aortography:

A. Is mandatory.
B. Consistently locates the site injury and provides a "road map" for subsequent repair.
C. Is technically difficult in terms of catheter access and placement.
D. Should use views tangential to the apparent trajectory.
E. Is risky because nephrotoxic doses of contrast agents are often needed.

Question 71-3

Multiple incisions are used for thoracic trauma, based on the anticipated injury and need for obtaining proximal and distal vascular control. Of these, which is the most appropriate to manage blunt trauma disruption of the origin of the innominate artery from the aortic arch?

A. Left anterolateral thoracotomy.
B. Bilateral anterolateral thoracotomy crossing the sternum.
C. Right "book" thoracotomy (anterolateral thoracotomy and supraclavicular incisions joined by sternotomy).
D. Median sternotomy with cervical extension along the right sternomastoid muscle.
E. Left posterolateral thoracotomy.

■ QUESTIONS FOR CHAPTER 72

Question 72-1

Retroperitoneal hematomas caused by blunt trauma identified during an exploratory laparotomy:

A. Should all be explored.
B. Only pelvic hematomas should routinely be explored.
C. Perirenal hematomas should be explored, even if not enlarging.
D. Stable midline hematomas should all be explored to rule out major venous injuries.
E. Stable mesenteric hematomas should be explored if the bowel is dusky.

Question 72-2

Management of celiac artery injuries:

A. Includes identification of the celiac artery that originates from the abdominal aorta at the L_2 level.
B. Should not include ligation of the celiac artery because severe liver ischemia will result.
C. Should not include ligation of the celiac artery because it results in anemic infarction of the spleen.
D. May include ligation of the celiac artery, because this does not result in hepatic ischemia or splenic infarction, or contribute to later chronic mesenteric ischemia.
E. Dissection of the celiac artery trunk is relatively easy because it is surrounded by loose connective tissue.

Question 72-3

When treating iliac vascular injuries which of the following is true?

A. The ureter crosses over the origin of the external iliac artery.
B. The common iliac veins join at the L_5 level to form the inferior vena cava over the aortic bifurcation.
C. Stable hematomas pelvic (zone III) hematomas caused by *penetrating* trauma should not be explored.
D. Complex injuries to the external iliac artery in the presence of significant hemodynamic instability should be managed by ligation of the artery.
E. Temporary intraluminal shunt and "damage control" (expedient hemostasis, closure, and resuscitation) are appropriate in hemodynamically unstable patients with complex common or external iliac artery injuries.

■ QUESTIONS FOR CHAPTER 73

Question 73-1

An 18-year-old man sustains a single gunshot wound (GSW) to the right medial thigh. On arrival to the emergency department, he is in stable condition. On examination of his thigh, he has a small hematoma over the GSW entrance site and no palpable popliteal or pedal pulses. Doppler signals are present in both pedal vessels, with an ABI of 0.6. What is the most appropriate next step in the management of this patient?

A. Close observation of ABI and neurologic function for 24 hours.

B. Immediate exploration in the OR.
C. Duplex sonography of the medial thigh.
D. Lower extremity arteriogram.
E. Local exploration of the GSW to remove the bullet.

Question 73-2

A 21-year-old woman sustains a stab wound to the left arm. An angiogram demonstrates a small nonocclusive intimal flap in the mid-brachial artery. What is the most appropriate management of this "minimal" arterial lesion?

A. Resection and interposition grafting with saphenous vein.
B. Observation and discharge in 24 hours if no change in vascular status.
C. Resection and interposition grafting with PTFE.
D. Stent placement across the lesion.
E. Anticoagulation for 6 months with monthly follow-up examinations.

Question 73-3

A 26-year-old man is involved in a severe motorcycle accident. On admission, he has an obvious deformity of his right lower leg and absent pulses or Doppler signals at the ankle. Motor and sensory functions are intact. X-ray films of the lower leg show a comminuted proximal tibia fracture. Preoperative angiogram reveals an occluded infrageniculate popliteal artery. Which sequence of treatment steps is the *most* appropriate to provide optimal outcome to this patient?

A. Immediate external fixation stabilization of the fracture then repair of arterial injury.
B. Shunting of the arterial injury, external fracture stabilization, repair of arterial injury, and fasciotomy.
C. Primary amputation at the level of the fracture.
D. Repair of arterial injury and external traction stabilization.
E. Repair of the arterial injury and closed reduction under fluoroscopy with stabilization in a long-leg cast with windows for inspection of the wound and distal pulses.

Question 73-4

A patient presents 3 weeks after cardiac catheterization through the right femoral artery with reports of pain and occasional bleeding from the puncture site. His femoral pseudoaneurysm was diagnosed 1 week ago and treated with an ultrasound-guided thrombin injection. He now presents with redness over the right groin, a small area of skin necrosis, and an easily palpable pulsatile mass. The most appropriate treatment for this patient is:

A. Repeat ultrasound-guided thrombin injection.
B. Placement of a covered stent through a remote arterial access site.
C. Open surgical repair with debridement of necrotic tissue and muscle flap coverage.
D. Ultrasound-guided compression therapy.
E. Local debridement of all necrotic or infected tissue, antibiotic irrigation, and systemic administration; cover wound with moist dressings and perform delayed arterial repair after secondary wound closure.

■ QUESTIONS FOR CHAPTER 74

Question 74-1

A 21-year-old man involved in a motorcycle accident sustains significant lower extremity trauma. At the scene, significant hemorrhage is present from the lower extremity with an obvious bony deformity in the distal thigh. On examination, the patient has an open distal femur fracture with no palpable pulses or Doppler signals in the foot. He is taken directly to surgery where a suprageniculate popliteal artery injury is repaired with a saphenous vein graft and a popliteal vein transection is ligated, followed by stabilization of his distal femur fracture. The patient required a total of 10 units of blood products during the procedure. Which clinical variable is *not* associated with an increase likelihood of developing a lower extremity compartment syndrome?

A. Popliteal vein ligation.
B. Concomitant bone and vascular injury.
C. Method of arterial repair (primary as opposed to use of a graft).
D. Severe degree of preoperative ischemia as evidenced by no Doppler signals in the foot.
E. Massive blood product requirements.

Question 74-2

On evaluation 5 hours postoperatively in the intensive care unit, the same patient in question 74-1 reports persistent pain in his affected lower leg. On examination, his blood pressure is 85/40 mm Hg with a mean of 50 mm Hg. His calf and foot are warm with a 2^+ palpable pulse in the dorsalis pedis artery. There is diminished sensation over the lateral portion of the foot, and mild edema is present up to knee. Compartmental pressures are as follows: anterior, 35 mm Hg; lateral, 33 mm Hg; posterior, 27 mm Hg; deep posterior, 25 mm Hg. The most appropriate management of this patient is?

A. Administration of more pain medications.
B. Observation with repeat compartment measurements in 3 hours.
C. Immediate four-compartment fasciotomies.
D. Immediate two-compartment fasciotomies (anterior and lateral) with observation of the medial compartments.
E. Re-explore and reconstruct the popliteal vein.

Question 74-3

Three days after a lower leg four-compartment fasciotomy, a patient is found to have a persistently elevated temperature, white blood cell count, and creatinine phosphokinase level. Examination of the leg in the OR shows extensive necrotic muscle in the lateral compartment and a small area of necrosis of the gastrocnemius muscle. What is the most appropriate management of this patient?

A. Debridement of necrotic muscle and closure of the fasciotomy site.
B. Debridement of necrotic muscle and reevaluation in the OR in 48 hours.
C. Debridement of necrotic muscle and free flap coverage of the remaining anatomic defect.
D. Below the knee amputation.
E. Above knee amputation.

■ QUESTIONS FOR CHAPTER 75

Question 75-1

Sympathectomy for patients with causalgia is most appropriate when applied to:

A. Stage I disease.
B. Stage III disease with failed medical treatment.
C. State II disease with failed medical treatment.
D. Stage II disease with failed medical treatment and strongly positive response to sympathetic block.
E. Patients with any relief from sympathetic block, regardless of apparent stage.

Question 75-2

Which of the following is most helpful in the diagnosis of causalgia:

A. Positive three-phase bone scan.
B. Quantitative sweat test.
C. Positive response to sympathetic block.
D. Thermometry.
E. Bone radiography.

Question 75-3

Complex regional pain syndrome (CRPS) type II (formerly, major causalgia) is primarily distinguished from CRPS type I (reflex sympathetic dystrophy) by which of the following:

A. The presence of nerve injury.
B. Abnormal sudomotor activity.
C. Hyperalgesia beyond the territory of a single peripheral nerve.
D. The presence of edema.
E. Abnormal vasomotor activity.

ANSWERS AND DISCUSSION

■ ANSWERS AND DISCUSSION FOR CHAPTER 69

Answer 69-1: D

Discussion 69-1

A. Of all vascular injuries, 80% occur in the extremities.
B. The majority result from penetrating trauma. Blunt mechanism is responsible for only 10% of the cases.
C. Long-bone fracture, secondary to blunt trauma, is *not* a frequent cause of lower extremity vascular injury.
D. Most vascular injuries do occur in the lower extremities (correct answer).
E. Most lower extremity vascular injuries are still the result of penetrating trauma (gunshot wounds 70%–80%; stab wounds 10%–15%).

Answer 69-2: C

Discussion 69-2

A. Most peripheral arterial injuries present with signs of acute ischemia or expanding hematoma, not active bleeding. Only a minority will present with external bleeding.
B. In the chest, most penetrating injuries manifest as cavitary bleeding (hemothorax) and are diagnosed clinically by the presence of persistent bleeding after initial chest tube placement. *Blunt* aortic injuries present with a widened mediastinum.
C. The outcome after major abdominal arterial injuries is dependent on the presence of retroperitoneal tamponade (stems the bleeding) and anatomic location (the more proximal injuries carry the worst prognosis).
D. Ninety-five percent of all blunt thoracic aortic ruptures occur *distal to* the origin of the left subclavian artery in the proximity of the ligamentum arteriosum.
E. External bleeding from extremity arterial injury is usually easily controlled in the emergency department by applying external compression. Tourniquets may be difficult to apply in proximal wounds and can contribute to ischemia.

Answer 69-3: E

Discussion 69-3

A. False. Patients with a partial arterial transection, false aneurysm, or intimal flap injuries may have palpable pulses distal to the injury.
B. Common complications of penetrating injuries are pseudoaneurysms, AV fistulas, and thrombosis. AV fistulas (and pseudoaneurysms) are usually not discovered *soon* after injury and frequently go undiagnosed or untreated until later.
C. Arterial injuries presenting with significant external arterial bleeding are likely to be partial transections. Complete transections usually present with signs of acute ischemia rather than external bleeding, because of the retraction and constriction of the proximal and distal ends of the injured artery.
D. A penetrating wound in proximity to major axial vessels is no longer a mandatory indication for an angiogram.

In the absence of hard signs, like a distal pulse deficit or major external bleeding, or a decreased (<1.0) ankle-brachial index (ABI) or wrist brachial index, these patients are best served by serial pulse examinations over a 24-hour observation period.

E. Classically, signs and symptoms of arterial injury are divided into *hard* (absence of distal pulses, active external hemorrhage, signs of acute ischemia, pulsatile hematoma, and bruit or thrill) and *soft* (diminished distal pulses, injury in the proximity of a major vessel, neurologic deficit, and hemodynamic compromise). The former indicate the presence of a significant arterial injury, and prompt exploration is indicated. The latter *may or may not* be associated with a major arterial injury so they allow time for observation, resuscitation as needed, and further investigation (e.g., an ABI, a duplex scan, or some other study). Hemodynamic compromise or hypotension may be attributable to other causes and could even be responsible for diminished pulses.

■ ANSWERS AND DISCUSSION FOR CHAPTER 70

Answer 70-1: D

Discussion 70-1

A. Although acute ligation of the internal carotid artery may be tolerated if the patient has good colaterals including a complete circle of Willis, reports with good-quality arteriographic studies have demonstrated that the circle is intact in less than 50% of patients.
B. Prosthetic grafts may be used in uncontaminated wounds; however, autogenous tissue is preferable.
C. Even under protection of systemic heparinization, distal thromboembolism can occur. Acute ligation of this artery may be attended by a significant stroke.
D. Although it is true that the presence of brisk back bleeding from the internal carotid artery generally indicates rich collateral circulation, direct end-to-end anastomosis should still be performed if it is feasible. If the artery cannot be reapproximated without tension, an interposition graft of saphenous vein is recommended. Any form of reconstruction should be followed by a completion arteriogram or duplex ultrasound to detect any technical defects.
E. Extracranial to intracranial bypass is too complex a procedure to perform in this trauma setting, and it does not supply anywhere near as much flow as a carotid reconstruction. Acute ligation of the internal carotid artery may be a consideration if direct internal carotid artery reconstruction is technically impossible.

Answer 70-2: E

Discussion 70-2

A and B. In the past it was believed that repair was contraindicated in patients who experienced carotid artery trauma and were admitted with hemiparesis and/or alterations in consciousness because of the danger of converting a bland infarct into a hemorrhagic infarct. However, recent studies have indicated that this is an unlikely event, and although cerebral infarcts can develop micro-hemorrhages at the time of reperfusion, most are not converted to major hemorrhagic infarcts.

C. It has been shown that in most patients with carotid artery trauma, recovery of neurologic function is more likely if the artery is expeditiously repaired regardless of the pre-repair neurologic function.

D. There is the possibility of delayed complications, such as false aneurysm or AV fistula, if any penetrating trauma such as a stab wound to the internal carotid artery is not repaired. Patency can often be restored by local thrombectomy, after which repair should be performed.

E. Most experienced trauma and vascular surgeons now recommend repair of penetrating carotid artery injuries in most patients, if it is technically feasible, and especially if there is continued patency of the artery. Choosing ligation because of brisk back bleeding, assumed to indicate excellent collateral circulation, ignores the possibility of stroke from propagation/embolization of distal thrombus.

Answer 70-3: C

Discussion 70-3

A and E. Blunt trauma to the carotid artery can be difficult to diagnose because less than half of such injured patients at initial evaluation will have either symptoms or signs that suggest significant carotid injury. If the injury is severe, the patient usually develops symptoms within 24 hours, but in many patients, months or even years may pass before symptoms and signs related to the arterial injury become manifest.

B. External signs of injury to the superficial structures of the neck are present in only a minority of patients with a blunt carotid injury.

C. An evaluation for carotid injury should be undertaken in patients who have sustained a blunt injury to the head and neck and develop an unexplained Horner's syndrome or relate lateralizing symptoms consistent with a transient ischemic attack (correct answer).

D. The diagnosis is especially difficult in patients who have sustained cervical hyperextension injuries in which the artery is stretched forcibly over the transverse process of C2 and the body of C1 (not at C3). The stretch injury inflicts multiple medial and intimal tears that predispose to dissection and possible delayed thromboembolism.

■ ANSWERS AND DISCUSSION FOR CHAPTER 71

Answer 71-1: C

Discussion 71-1

A. Chest radiography is the most commonly used radiologic screening study for the patient who has sustained significant deceleration injury. A widened superior mediastinum is one of the most common findings in a patient with blunt disruption of the descending thoracic aorta, but it is also the most nonspecific.

B. Loss of the aortic knob contour, or in particular, a double shadow of the aortic knob, is one of the more specific findings on chest radiography for blunt disruption of the descending thoracic aorta.

C. An increased cardiac:thoracic ratio (heart:thorax width on AP projection) is *not* a finding specifically related to disruption of the descending thoracic area.

D and E. Depression of the left main stem bronchus greater than 140 degrees and deviation of the nasogastric tube are additional chest radiography findings associated with blunt disruption of the descending thoracic aorta.

Answer 71-2: D

Discussion 71-2

A. Patients with *penetrating* injuries to the thoracic aorta usually present with exsanguinating hemorrhage or tamponade and are usually explored empirically for these reasons. Patients with penetrating injuries to the thoracic aorta who are hemodynamically stable when they present to the hospital are uncommon. Aortography is used selectively. Other imaging methods, such as a CT scan, may be used because aortic injury is only suspected in a stable patient by presumed trajectory.

B. Because of the large dye column, small pseudo-aneurysms, as might be present in a stable patient, are often difficult to detect and localize by aortography.

C. In this setting, aortography can be easily and rapidly obtained using the Seldinger technique through femoral artery access.

D. If a diagnostic aortogram is ordered in a stable patient, views tangential to the proposed trajectory of the bullet should be obtained to detect small pseudoaneurysms (correct answer).

E. Because most victims of penetrating chest trauma and possible injury to the thoracic aorta are young healthy males empirically receiving copious amounts of intravenous fluids, contrast nephrotoxicity is not a major concern.

Answer 71-3: D

Discussion 71-3

A. Proximal control of the mid-distal left subclavian artery injury often requires a high (third interspace) left anterolateral thoracotomy combined with a supraclavicular incision. It is inappropriate for this injury.

B. Bilateral anterolateral thoracotomies are rarely performed now and would not be used here because proximal control of a right subclavian artery injury is best achieved by option D.

C. A right "book" thoracotomy *might* give enough exposure but is seldom used because of its significant morbidity.

D. The ascending aorta, innominate artery, aortic arch, and left common carotid artery are midline structures and most readily managed through median sternotomy with a cervical extension.

E. A left posterolateral thoracotomy can be useful in that it provides ready access to the descending thoracic aorta and the proximal left subclavian artery, lying just under the pleural surface of the mediastinum, but it is *not* appropriate here.

ANSWERS AND DISCUSSION FOR CHAPTER 72

Answer 72-1: E

Discussion 72-1

A. Retroperitoneal hematomas caused by blunt trauma rarely require exploration.

B. Exploration of a zone III (pelvic) hematoma caused by pelvic fractures may cause severe bleeding that might be difficult to control; however, they should be explored if there is an absent femoral pulse.

C. Routine exploration of zone II (perinephric) hematomas may result in the unnecessary loss of a kidney. Exploration is indicated if they are expanding or pulsatile, but remote proximal and distal control should first be obtained.

D. Exploration of stable midline hematomas is unnecessary, and exploring higher, retrohepatic hematomas is extremely dangerous and should not be attempted.

E. As an overall guiding rule, only expanding, pulsatile, or leaking retroperitoneal hematomas need to be explored. One exception is a pelvic hematoma associated with an absent ipsilateral femoral pulse (see B). The other is a hematoma at the root of the mesentery in the presence of ischemic (dusky) bowel, seeking possible superior mesenteric artery injury.

Answer 72-2: D

Discussion 72-2

A. The celiac artery originates from the anterior wall of the abdominal aorta, immediately below the aortic hiatus, at the T_{12} to L_1 level (not at L_2).

B. The rich collateral network of the celiac artery permits ligation without significant sequelae of upper abdominal (stomach, liver, spleen) ischemia because of the rich collateral circulation.

C. Same explanation as B.

D. Same explanation as B, and is the correct answer because it covers both lack of liver ischemia and splenic infarct.

E. The main celiac trunk or axis is only 1 to 1.5 cm long and gives its three major branches (tripod of Halles) at the upper border of the pancreas. Because of its high anatomic position and the extensive fibrous, nerve, and lymphatic tissues surrounding it, surgical dissection is difficult.

Answer 72-3: E

Discussion 72-3

A. The common iliac artery divides into the external and internal iliac arteries over the sacroiliac joint. The ureter crosses higher than the external iliac artery over the bifurcation of the artery.

B. The common iliac veins join at the L_5 level, but *below* the level of the aortic bifurcation and underneath the right common iliac artery, to form the inferior vena cava.

C. Stable hematomas of the pelvis caused by *penetrating* (as opposed to blunt) trauma should always be explored to determine whether a common, internal, or external iliac artery injury exists.

D. Ligation of the common or external iliac arteries should not be performed, even in unstable patients. Ligation is poorly tolerated by most patients, for it is associated with a high incidence of limb loss and subsequent attempts to revascularize the leg (even by femorofemoral bypass) may still result in reperfusion injury. E is a better solution.

E. In the hemodynamically critically ill patient, "damage control" with the placement of a temporary intraluminal shunt, and reconstruction of the iliac artery injury when stability is restored, is appropriate.

ANSWERS AND DISCUSSION FOR CHAPTER 73

Answer 73-1: D

Discussion 73-1

A. Observation in this clinical setting is only appropriate when the patient has both a normal pulse examination distal to the injury and the ABI or wrist (for upper extremity injuries) brachial index is greater than or equal to one. This patient has abnormal physical examination results and an abnormal ABI; therefore, observation is not indicated.

B. Immediate exploration in the OR is a possibility; however, this treatment plan is used more frequently for patients with profound ischemia, significant past or ongoing hemorrhage, or hemodynamic instability.

C. Duplex sonography does possess the sensitivity and specificity to diagnose a vascular injury. Unfortunately, the lack of 24-hour prompt availability of the equipment and experienced operators has limited its application in the trauma setting. An ABI or wrist-brachial index is easier and available. Significant decreases indicate an arterial injury, except in older patients who may have preexisting peripheral arterial disease. The next preoperative test is anatomic localization of that injury before exploration and repair (see D).

D. Although this patient is hemodynamically stable with Doppler signals present in the pedal vessels, a vascular injury is not excluded. With an ABI less than 1.0, the probability of a vascular injury is high; therefore an arteriogram of the lower extremity is indicated to confirm acute injury and localize it.

E. Local exploration in an attempt to remove the bullet is dangerous and inappropriate, TV and movie Westerns to the contrary.

Answer 73-2: B

Discussion 73-2

This injury is categorized as a minimal arterial trauma. Associated features include the following:

- Low-velocity injury
- Minimal arterial wall disruption (<5 mm) for intimal defects and pseudoaneurysms
- Adherent or downstream protrusion of intimal flaps
- Normal distal circulation
- No active hemorrhage

Therefore:

A. Operative intervention involving resection and vein bypass grafting would be an overly aggressive approach at this point in the patient's course and should be reserved for injuries that become more significant over time.

B. When treated nonoperatively, resolution, improvement, or stabilization of such "minimal" injury can be anticipated in more than 85% of cases. Follow-up of patients with "minimal" vascular injuries up to 10 years confirmed the safety of this treatment plan. Therefore, the most appropriate answer is for close observation for change in vascular status and discharge within 24 hours if there is no deterioration. There should be periodic outpatient follow-up over the next 6 months.

C. Same answer as in A (not indicated), but in addition, although a PTFE graft is readily available and might give short- to mid-term patency, this patient is 22 years old, and autogenous bypass is preferred for relatively small peripheral arteries.

D. There is no role for immediate endovascular management with this particular injury. A good outcome for bare or covered stents in this diameter peripheral artery has not been shown.

E. Anticoagulation is *not* required in the conservative treatment of a "minimal vascular injury."

Answer 73-3: B

Discussion 73-3

A. Although combined injuries are uncommon, the duration of ischemia is critical to the outcome. Therefore, in most cases the arterial repair should be performed first to restore circulation to the limb, before the orthopedic stabilization is addressed. However, in this case the massive musculoskeletal trauma has rendered a limb so unstable that external fixation must be placed before the vascular procedure.

B. With an unstable limb resulting from this type of fracture, selective use of intraluminal shunts followed by rapid installation of an external fixator will minimize limb ischemia and allow for a subsequent unhurried meticulous vascular repair. Nevertheless, this should be followed by fasciotomy (correct answer).

C. In this scenario, the patient has an intact motor and sensory examination; therefore, primary amputation is not indicated. Primary amputation is reserved for patients with massive orthopedic, soft tissue, and nerve injuries in whom salvage of a functional painless limb is not achievable, or in hemodynamically unstable patients (such as those with other serious injuries) in whom embarking on a complex vascular repair might jeopardize survival.

D. Traction is not appropriate management of this particular orthopedic injury.

E. This approach is not appropriate for this type of orthopedic injury. It would not likely achieve proper position and stabilization, and in the process it would endanger the arterial repair.

Answer 73-4: C

Discussion 73-4

A. This patient presents with a recurrent femoral artery pseudoaneurysm with signs of probable bacterial infection. Although direct thrombin injection has a success rate of more than 90% for the treatment of iatrogenic arterial false aneurysms, caution should be used in this setting because of the presence of an infection. Repeating

the treatment that produced this complication is inappropriate.

B. With a presumed bacterial infection and the location of the false aneurysm being the common femoral artery, endovascular stenting is contraindicated.

C. The most appropriate treatment would be for open surgical repair or reconstruction if need be. This would also include debridement of all necrotic or infected tissue, and copious irrigation of the wound with antibiotic solutions. In the presence of any infection or when large residual tissue defects persist, muscle coverage with either sartorius or rectus abdominis flaps over the repaired vessel should be used. The approach has been shown to produce good results in most cases; it gives better coverage and is more expedient and less time consuming and expensive than E.

D. Because of the skin necrosis, any form of compressive therapy, even ultrasound-guided compression, is contraindicated.

E. One *might* succeed with this approach, if lucky enough to not experience rupture and massive hemorrhage from the open wound. Also, the cost of continued hospitalization would be prohibitive and the late repair difficult through scar tissue.

■ ANSWERS AND DISCUSSION FOR CHAPTER 74

Answer 74-1: C

Discussion 74-1

Although the decision to perform a prophylactic lower leg fasciotomy is somewhat subjective, there are numerous clinical factors that increase the probability of developing a postoperative compartment syndrome. Such factors include a delay of more than 6 hours from the time of vascular injury, concomitant skeletal and soft tissue injuries (B), combined arterial and venous trauma (particularly if the venous injury is treated by ligation, A), site of vascular injury (more common in the popliteal area), mechanism of injury (more common in blunt trauma), and patients requiring large amounts of resuscitative blood products and fluids (E). If numerous positive predictive variables are present, strong consideration should be given for a prophylactic fasciotomy. Reperfusion of an ischemic extremity is one of the key elements to the development of a compartment syndrome, and the degree of ischemia (D) can be described as a positive predictor. However, the method of arterial repair has no bearing on compartment syndrome; therefore, the correct answer is C.

Answer 74-2: C

Discussion 74-2

Traditionally, absolute measures of compartmental pressure were used to guide therapy, and pressures greater than 40 to 45 mm Hg at any point, or sustained above 30 mm Hg for more than 3 to 4 hours, mandated fasciotomy. However, it was noted that compartment syndrome occasionally occurs at lower tissue pressures in hypotensive patients and fails to develop despite markedly abnormal tissue pressures in individuals who were well perfused. A more sensitive and specific predictive measure is the *arterial perfusion pressure,* the gradient between diastolic arterial pressure and the interstitial pressure. Fasciotomy is recommended at a measured compartment pressure 20 to 30 mm Hg less than systemic diastolic blood pressure or 30 mm Hg less than mean blood pressure. Continued observation or indiscriminate use of narcotics for the treatment of a developing compartment syndrome is inappropriate; therefore, C is the correct answer. A, B, D, and E are inappropriate, although popliteal patency might have helped in retrospect.

Answer 74-3: B
Discussion 74-3

Skeletal muscle viability is assessed by color, presence of arterial bleeding, and contraction to galvanic (electrocautery) stimulation. Muscle that does not contract is not viable and should be debrided. Exposed muscle should be reassessed every 1 to 2 days until complete wound closure or coverage is obtained. Debridement of nonviable muscle is critical to prevent infection that often compromises the eventual outcome when present. In the lower extremity, loss of one or two muscle compartments can be tolerated. With a comprehensive physical therapy program, ambulation is frequently regained. Unfortunately, the loss of more than two muscle compartments in the leg generally warrants amputation, but not at this point (D and E).

This patient's postoperative course has been complicated by muscle necrosis. Although closure of the fasciotomy site is the goal, closure at the time of muscle debridement is not recommended (A). Further muscle resection may be required. Likewise, placing a free flap in the defect after the muscle resection would not be recommended (C). Therefore, the correct answer is B.

■ ANSWERS AND DISCUSSION FOR CHAPTER 75

Answer 75-1: D
Discussion 75-1

A. Patients with stage I disease are generally treated conservatively, which may include non-narcotic drug therapy (phenytoin, amitriptyline, carbamazepine, combined with a nonsteroidal anti-inflammatory agent, and physical therapy with or without a transcutaneous electrical nerve stimulation [TENS] unit). A sympathetic block may be used in patients who have severe pain or are unable to undergo physical therapy. In stage I, a sympathetic block may last much longer than the duration of the local anesthetic agent used, even for weeks, allowing physical therapy to be pursued fully. Even with such remarkable lasting relief, sympathectomy should be withheld until stage II.
B. Patients who are allowed to progress to stage III do *not* respond to any therapy, including surgical sympathectomy.
C. Patients with stage II disease can continue to be treated with physical therapy, TENS, and steroid therapy, as long as relief is obtained. In those who fail medical treatment, a beneficial result from sympathectomy cannot be guaranteed in all, but response to sympathetic block will select those who will benefit (see D).

D. With failed medical therapy in stage II, as in C, confirmatory block should be performed before proceeding with sympathectomy. The response should be dramatic, with the patient reporting 75% to 100% relief, and the relief should last as long as the local anesthetic used. These are the patients in whom the greatest benefit can be predicted with confidence. Sham (saline) blocks are unnecessary; one only needs to have two blocks with two agents of significantly different durations (e.g., Xylocaine and Marcaine) and have the patient's reported duration of relief be consistent with this.
E. Sympathectomy has a nonspecific pain relief effect and hopeful patients may say they felt good relief from a trial block, even if the improvement is only modest (e.g., 25%–50%). Patients with causalgia-like pain, especially patients in whom the symptoms and signs are not totally convincing for causalgia, such as those in stage III, cannot be assured of significant and lasting benefit from sympathectomy. Poor patient selection, for example, the performance of such "hopeful" sympathectomies in those without a dramatic response to sympathetic block, has led to doubts as to its degree of benefit and durability in some reports.

Answer 75-2: C
Discussion 75-2

The diagnosis of causalgia is quite certain when the clinical presentation is classic and includes superficial burning pain in the distribution of a single somatic sensory nerve, hyperesthesia, and vasomotor abnormalities. In CRPS type I, formerly called minor causalgia or mimocausalgia, one or more of these three clinical features may be minimal or even absent, and yet the response to sympathetic block may still be good and lasting. A positive bone scan (A), and (B) radiologic evidence of osteoporosis in the affected part, are helpful, but (C) a strongly positive response to sympathetic blockade provides the best evidence for causalgia. In fact, the ultimate relief obtained by surgical sympathectomy can be best predicted from the response to sympathetic block. Thermometry (D) has been used to gauge sympathetic activity, and thus proof of adequate sympathetic block and (B) a sweat test can be used in a similar manner, but neither can be extended to diagnose causalgia with any certainty.

Answer 75-3: A
Discussion 75-3

A key diagnostic criterion for CRPS type II is that it is a pain syndrome that results specifically from a nerve injury (A). Classically, causalgia was first reported in war injuries, as a pain syndrome associated with *partial* nerve injury, as opposed to complete transection. In civilian cases, the nerve injury may be minor or obscure, but the pain follows the distribution of a nerve. However, (C) hyperalgesia *beyond* the distribution of a somatic nerve is seen in reflex sympathetic dystrophy (type I). In the latter, spontaneous allodynia or pain occurs that is not necessarily limited to the region of the injured nerve. Otherwise, both CRPS I and II can be similar in other aspects, with (E) abnormal vasomotor activity, and at some stages (B) abnormal sweating and even (D) edema.

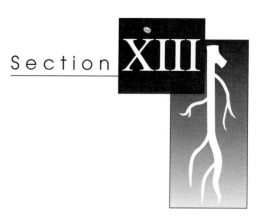

MANAGEMENT OF CHRONIC ISCHEMIA OF THE LOWER EXTREMITIES

STUDY QUESTIONS

■ QUESTIONS FOR CHAPTER 77

Question 77-1

An 80-year-old woman with end-stage chronic obstructive pulmonary disease presents with a small ulcer on the left great toe for 2 weeks and an ABI of 0.2. In counseling, regarding her risk of amputation, the following is correct:

A. Amputation is imminent without a revascularization procedure.
B. There is no risk of limb loss.
C. Limb loss is a possibility, but she might heal with conservative therapy.
D. She is likely to die in the next 6 months, so limb loss is irrelevant.
E. None of the above.

Question 77-2

Which endpoint is most appropriate in trials to evaluate the efficacy of pharmacotherapy in claudication?

A. Absolute claudication distance during treadmill exercise.
B. Initial claudication distance during treadmill exercise.
C. The change in ABI.
D. The number of blocks patients report being able to walk over the same course.
E. None of the above.

Question 77-3

In population studies, survival in patients with critical limb ischemia (CLI) correlates best with:

A. ABI.
B. Extent of pedal necrosis.
C. Male sex.
D. Presence of aortoiliac disease.
E. Smoking.

■ QUESTIONS FOR CHAPTER 78

Question 78-1

In evaluating a patient who presents with the recent onset of claudication but is otherwise in apparently good health, each of the following tests can be justified, *except*:

A. Carotid artery duplex imaging.
B. Stress electrocardiogram.
C. Segmental arterial pressure measurement.
D. Renal artery duplex imaging.
E. A standardized treadmill exercise study, documenting walking distances before the onset of pain and the need to stop.

Question 78-2

The initial hematologic evaluation of the patient with recent onset claudication should include all of the following *except*:

A. Screening for a hypercoagulable state.
B. Complete blood count including white blood cells and platelets.
C. Fasting blood glucose.
D. Fasting lipid profile.
E. Serum creatinine level.

Question 78-3

Which of the following is true regarding imaging studies used for the assessment of the patient with lower extremity arterial occlusive disease?

A. Obtaining an ABI value greater than 1.0 reliably excludes the presence of hemodynamically arterial occlusive disease.
B. Duplex imaging provides adequate preoperative imaging for planning distal arterial reconstruction surgery in patients with calcified vessels but is not essential for post-treatment surveillance.
C. Gadolinium-enhanced magnetic resonance imaging is a useful study for planning distal vascular reconstruction because it is able to identify patent distal tibial and pedal vessels.
D. Digital subtraction angiography is limited as an imaging modality because visualization of distal arteries is obscured by arterial wall calcium.
E. All patients presenting with the new onset of claudication symptoms should have a baseline arteriogram performed whether or not intervention is planned.

■ QUESTIONS FOR CHAPTER 79

Question 79-1

An end-to-side proximal anastomosis for an aortobifemoral (ABF) bypass graft for aortoiliac occlusive disease:

A. Has better late patency compared with grafts with an end-to-end proximal anastomosis in most published series.
B. Provides inferior early hemodynamic improvement than an end-to-end graft.
C. Has a lower incidence of embolic complications than end-to-end grafts.
D. Is associated with an increased incidence of postoperative impotence compared with an end-to-end anastomosis.
E. Is preferred for patients with severe bilateral external iliac occlusive disease.

Question 79-2

In a patient with combined aortoiliac and femoropopliteal occlusive disease, as demonstrated by preoperative arteriography, which of the following would be the best indicator of the need for a simultaneous distal bypass at the time of ABF grafting?

A. A severe profunda femoris origin stenosis.
B. A preoperative ABI of only 0.3.
C. Total occlusion of the entire length of the SFA.
D. A gangrenous toe.
E. An increase of ABI of only 0.2, measured in the OR after aortofemoral graft placement.

Question 79-3

Thrombosis of one limb of an ABF graft 3 years after implantation:

A. Is best treated by a femorofemoral bypass graft.
B. Usually indicates the need for a distal bypass graft for successful correction.
C. Is most often caused by recurrent or progressive aortic disease at the proximal anastomosis.
D. Is best treated by insertion of a new ABF graft.
E. Can usually be managed by graft limb thrombectomy and profundoplasty.

■ QUESTIONS FOR CHAPTER 80

Question 80-1

Which of the following is a true statement regarding femorofemoral bypass?

A. Medium- and long-term patency are comparable to aortofemoral bypass.
B. In the absence of significant occlusive disease in the aorta or donor iliac arterial systems, a femorofemoral graft will not produce a symptomatic "steal" from the donor leg.
C. Externally supported prosthetic femorofemoral bypass grafts are associated with better medium- and long-term patency than nonsupported grafts.
D. Hemodynamic performance of femorofemoral bypass is comparable to that of aortofemoral bypass.
E. Basing a femorofemoral bypass on a "donor" iliac artery treated with balloon angioplasty is associated with a sig-

nificantly poorer patency than an iliac artery without such previous intervention.

Question 80-2

Which of the following statements is true regarding axillofemoral bypass performed for chronic arterial occlusive disease?

A. Providing some redundancy of the axillary end of the axillofemoral component can help reduce the risk of "axillary pullout" after axillofemoral bypass.
B. Each advance in prosthetic graft technology over the last 40 years (i.e., improved graft material, external support) has been associated with increases in long-term patency.
C. Patency in patients with chronic critical ischemia is comparable to that in claudicants.
D. Patency is worse when there is occlusion of the SFA "outflow."
E. The axillofemoral component of an axillobifemoral bypass graft should be a minimum of 10 mm in diameter.

Question 80-3

Which of the following statements is true?

A. Obturator bypass should be performed with autologous graft material.
B. Patency of thoracofemoral bypass is inferior to that of aortofemoral bypass.
C. The axillobifemoral configuration provides better patency than the axillounifemoral bypass.
D. Femorofemoral bypass has superior patency to balloon angioplasty for treating discrete common iliac artery stenosis and should be the primary treatment.
E. "Extra-anatomic" bypass procedures should be reserved for patients not suitable for direct "anatomic" (e.g., aortofemoral or femoropopliteal) bypasses.

■ QUESTIONS FOR CHAPTER 81

Question 81-1

A 69-year-old man has rest pain with an ABI of 0.35 and a toe pressure of 30 mm Hg. Arteriography demonstrates an ipsilateral 75% distal common femoral artery stenosis involving the origin of the deep femoral artery and a flush SFA occlusion. Which one of the following factors suggests most strongly that isolated femoral endarterectomy and profundoplasty will be sufficient to relieve the patient's symptoms without requiring concomitant or staged distal infrainguinal reconstruction?

A. The patient has forefoot gangrene involving three toes.
B. The patient has diabetes mellitus.
C. The popliteal artery reconstitutes through profunda collaterals with a profunda-popliteal collateral index (PPCI) of 0.18.
D. The ipsilateral popliteal artery and trifurcation do not visualize, but the distal peroneal artery reconstitutes on late views and fills the dorsalis pedis through collaterals at the ankle level.
E. Remote failure of a previous above-knee femoropopliteal PTFE bypass.

Question 81-2

Which of the following most adversely affects the long-term patency of an infrainguinal bypass?

A. Use of an ipsilateral 4-mm reversed GSV as a conduit in the above-knee popliteal position.
B. Use of distal origin sites for the bypass, such as the deep femoral or popliteal arteries.
C. Use of contralateral GSV for a below-knee femoropopliteal bypass in a patient whose ipsilateral vein was previously harvested for coronary reconstruction.
D. Use of 6-mm PTFE for above-knee femoropopliteal bypass.
E. The presence of diabetes mellitus.

Question 81-3

Which of the following statements regarding infrainguinal bypass graft stenosis and surveillance is true?

A. Inflow and outflow lesions are more commonly identified causes of failing infrainguinal vein grafts in the first 3 postoperative years than intrinsic vein graft stenoses.
B. History, pulse palpation, and Doppler-derived ABIs are as sensitive as duplex surveillance in the detection of graft-threatening lesions after autogenous vein bypass.
C. Graft surveillance after PTFE infrainguinal bypass has been demonstrated to improve graft patency and reduce major limb amputation.
D. The majority of vein graft lesions are diffuse or long (>5 cm in length) and require interposition grafts to correct.
E. Repair (angioplasty or open revision) is indicated for focal graft stenoses identified by duplex surveillance and characterized by peak systolic velocity (PSV) >300 cm/sec and/or velocity ratio (VR) >4.0.

■ **QUESTIONS FOR CHAPTER 82**

Question 82-1

Profundoplasty as a lone revascularization is considered an alternative to distal bypass in which of the following:

A. Extensive forefoot gangrene.
B. Diabetic neuropathy.
C. Rest pain with minimal tissue loss.
D. Mild claudication.
E. Advanced foot sepsis.

Question 82-2

Which of the following preoperative factors are *not* useful in predicting a favorable outcome after an isolated profundoplasty?

A. Presence of a severe stenosis of the profunda origin.
B. A patent distal profunda with abundant collaterals in the thigh.
C. Good inflow to the femoral level.
D. Diabetes.
E. Patent popliteal and tibial arteries.

Question 82-3

You are evaluating a patient in the emergency department with an acutely ischemic right leg. He had undergone an ABF bypass for claudication 8 years ago, and recently he noted recurrence of mild symptoms with exertion. His foot was cool and pale, but his motor and sensory functions are intact, and the right femoral pulse is absent. All pulses are present in the left leg. An arteriogram confirms occlusion of the right limb of the ABF, occlusion of the SFA, and patency of the distal profunda. Which of the following is indicated?

A. CT to rule out graft infection.
B. Vein mapping in preparation for thrombectomy and concommittant distal bypass to improve outflow of ABF.
C. Thrombectomy or thrombolysis of the ABF followed by profundoplasty.
D. Intra-arterial papaverine at the time of the arteriogram to see if distal profunda dilates.
E. Protect the foot, keep it warm and dependent, and advise the patient to accept the mild symptoms.

■ **QUESTIONS FOR CHAPTER 83**

Question 83-1

Thrombosis of a PTFE above-knee femoral popliteal bypass 12 hours after surgery is *least* likely the result of:

A. Poor choice of inflow site.
B. Insufficient runoff.
C. Compression or kinking of the graft.
D. Inherent thrombogenicity of the graft.
E. Decrease in cardiac output with hypotension.

Question 83-2

A 68-year-old man had a femoral tibial saphenous vein bypass graft performed 9 months ago for ischemic rest pain. His graft has been examined with Doppler ultrasound at 3-month intervals, but this time it detects a focal flow disturbance with a velocity ratio of 3.0 at a localized site in the mid-part of the vein graft. He is asymptomatic but admits he has not been walking much. His rest pain has not returned, and peripheral pulses are readily palpable. Which of the following represents the most appropriate management of this patient?

A. Continue duplex surveillance and perform another duplex scan in 6 months.
B. Obtain an arteriogram if the ABI is more than 0.15 below postoperative baseline.
C. Initiate subcutaneous low molecular weight heparin therapy and obtain another duplex scan in 3 months.
D. Initiate subcutaneous low molecular weight heparin therapy and schedule the patient for elective reoperation with a new vein graft.
E. Obtain an arteriogram and plan to treat a confirmed localized vein graft stenosis with percutaneous transluminal angioplasty (PTA).

Question 83-3

In regard to intimal hyperplasia that develops in a femoral popliteal vein bypass graft, which of the following is *not* true?

A. It may involve the vein bypass in a diffuse manner.
B. Intimal hyperplasia is an important cause of graft failure in the early and middle follow-up periods.
C. It is most likely to be localized to one of the anastomoses than appear in the body of the graft.
D. The distal anastomosis is affected much more commonly than the proximal anastomosis.
E. When a significant stenosis is identified, graft revision is justified.

■ QUESTIONS FOR CHAPTER 84

Question 84-1

A completion arteriogram after a proximal external iliac artery balloon angioplasty shows a significant dissection. The foot looks good. The patient is not having pain. What is the most appropriate next step in management?

A. Repeat the balloon angioplasty to a slightly higher pressure for a longer period of time. If that does not work, consider using a larger balloon.
B. Place a stent in the proximal external iliac artery.
C. Place a stent from the origin of the external iliac artery to the origin of the common femoral artery.
D. Place the patient on heparin overnight, and send the patient home with clopidogrel.
E. Measure pressure across the arterial segment in question, and repeat the balloon angioplasty if there is a gradient of 10 mm Hg or more.

Question 84-2

A patient with multilevel occlusive disease presents with gangrene of the foot. There is a moderate iliac artery stenosis and diffuse femoropopliteal occlusion with reconstitution of the posterior tibial artery. What is the best approach to management?

A. Simultaneous iliac artery balloon angioplasty and femoral to posterior tibial bypass.
B. Leg amputation.
C. Femoral-femoral bypass with femoral-posterior tibial bypass if this inflow procedure is not adequate.
D. Immediate iliac artery balloon angioplasty followed by femoral-posterior tibial bypass in a few days.
E. Iliac artery stent-graft and femoral-posterior tibial bypass.

Question 84-3

Which of the following lesion scenarios is the *least* favorable for endovascular treatment?

A. A focal posterior tibial artery lesion in a diabetic patient with heel gangrene and end-stage cardiomyopathy.
B. Diffuse stenosis of the infrarenal aorta in a patient with severe claudication.
C. A focal SFA stenosis in a smoker with mild claudication.
D. Critical iliac artery stenosis and a 20-cm SFA occlusion in a patient with rest pain.
E. Stenosis of the aortic bifurcation in a patient with severe claudication.

■ QUESTIONS FOR CHAPTER 85

Question 85-1

Lumbar sympathectomy is *least* indicated in:

A. Hyperhidrosis.
B. Buerger's disease.
C. Causalgia.
D. Diabetic neuropathy.
E. Rest pain from peripheral atherosclerotic disease (PAD), which is not amenable to bypass.

Question 85-2

Lumbar sympathectomy in diabetic patients *may* produce a favorable response in all of the following except those with:

A. An ABI of ≥ 0.3.
B. Peripheral neuropathy.
C. Shallow ischemic ulcers.
D. Ischemic rest pain.
E. None of the above.

Question 85-3

When a lumbar sympathectomy is performed, it is important to know that the sympathetic innervation of the foot and lower leg is primarily conveyed through:

A. L1-L3.
B. L2-L4.
C. L2-L3.
D. L4-L5.
E. L5-S1.

■ QUESTIONS FOR CHAPTER 86

Question 86-1

Which of the following is true regarding the popliteal artery entrapment syndrome?

A. Patients most commonly present in the late teens or early twenties.
B. Popliteal artery aneurysm may be the presenting feature.
C. Once occlusion of the artery has occurred, treatment by thrombectomy and vein patch is adequate.
D. The popliteal artery usually lies deep and medial to the origin of the medial head of the gastrocnemius muscle.
E. The condition is seldom encountered in female patients.

Question 86-2

Which of the following is true regarding adventitial cystic disease?

A. The radial artery is the second most common site affected.
B. Treatment by angioplasty and stent placement will restore long-term patency.
C. The theory of repetitive micro-trauma has the most evidence to support this explanation for the formation of the cysts.
D. The cyst has a characteristic ultrasound appearance and can be confidently diagnosed on duplex Doppler.
E. Angiography is essential in making the diagnosis.

Question 86-3

In the young adult who presents with exercise induced claudication, which of the following is true?

A. Adventitial cystic disease of the popliteal artery is the most likely cause.
B. Angiography may appear totally normal in the resting position.
C. The symptoms usually have a slow progressive onset.
D. Normal ankle pressures at rest will exclude a vascular cause for the symptoms.
E. The popliteal artery may course lateral to the origin of the lateral head of gastrocnemius muscle.

■ QUESTIONS FOR CHAPTER 87

Question 87-1

With regard to the lower extremity microcirculation in diabetes mellitus, which of the following statements is correct?

A. Microalbuminuria correlates with abnormal capillary permeability.
B. A thickened capillary basement membrane increases resistance in the microcirculation.
C. There is arteriolar occlusion caused by periodic acid-Schiff–positive material.
D. Diffusion of oxygen is impaired.
E. Skin blood flow is diminished because of anatomic neuropathy.

Question 87-2

Compared with an injury in a nondiabetic person, injury to the skin in the diabetic foot is best characterized by which of the following?

A. Accentuated release of histamine from mast cells.
B. Diminished release of neuropeptides from fine motor nerves.
C. Diminished neuroinflammatory response.
D. Increased "wheal and flare" response.
E. Accentuated macrophage migration.

Question 87-3

Which of the following contributes to ulceration in the diabetic foot?

A. Increased sweat gland function with macerated skin.
B. Talipes equinovarus.
C. Loss of lumbrical muscle function.
D. Fixed dorsiflexion of the foot.
E. Oteomyelitis, creating a sinus tract through the skin.

■ QUESTIONS FOR CHAPTER 88

Questions 88-1

Declining erectile function and frequency are primarily related to:

A. Aortic occlusive disease.
B. Psychogenic causes.
C. Neurologic diseases.
D. Lack of a suitable partner.
E. Failure of smooth muscle relaxation.

Question 88-2

Female sexual dysfunction (FSD):

A. Is virtually nonexistent as abundant arterial collaterals supply the genital area.
B. Often responds to sildenafil citrate.
C. Is a common complaint.
D. Is associated with hyperthyroidism.
E. Is associated with diabetes and cardiovascular disease.

Question 88-3

A diagnostic approach to ED should:

A. Be based on a systematic screening sequence.
B. Use penile injection to assess blood flow.
C. Include neurologic screening.
D. Use selective arteriography.
E. Depend on response to initial pharmacotherapy.

ANSWERS AND DISCUSSION

■ ANSWERS AND DISCUSSION FOR CHAPTER 77

Answer 77-1: C

Discussion 77-1

The control groups in several pharmaceutical trials of CLI have demonstrated that near-term limb loss in patients with nonhealing ulcers is less than 50% and actual ulcer healing is 40%. In addition, improving her PaO_2 and eliminating anemia will help. Therefore, a period of conservative therapy for an octogenarian female with severe chronic obstructive pulmonary disease and a small nonhealing toe ulcer caused by CLI is justified before subjecting her to the risk and morbidities of revascularization.

Answer 77-2: A

Discussion 77-2

The most reproducible measurement in claudication pharmaceutical trials is (A) the absolute claudication distance, the point at which the patient cannot go further because of pain and demands the treadmill be stopped. This is measured using a standard treadmill exercise and is considered the standard for claudication trial efficacy. Some debate exists regarding the use of fixed versus graded treadmill testing. Graded treadmill testing has the advantage of differentiating the severely limited claudicant—the patient population who theoretically may realize the most benefit from claudication pharmacologic therapy. The initial point of claudication (B) is more variable, and patient reports of distance walked before stopped by claudication (D) are unreliable, even if the same course is followed. (C) The ABI may not change despite a walking distance benefit from pharmacotherapy and is useful only in revascularizations.

Answer 77-3: A

Discussion 77-3

Although serum albumin and C reactive protein will likely become additional CLI mortality markers in the future; currently the parameter that best correlates with mortality in population studies remains (A) the ABI. ABI correlates better than (B) pedal neurosis, (C) gender, (D) aortoiliac disease, or (E) smoking. These data are important, because patients with CLI who undergo surgical revascularization have significant morbidity. Reflecting this, several studies have demonstrated that a significant minority of patients with CLI die before healing incisions and pedal lesions after revascularization. Therefore, because of the abbreviated life expectancy in CLI, much of the care must be considered palliative, and predictors of near-term mortality are important in determining the choice between amputation and bypass in high-risk patients.

■ ANSWERS AND DISCUSSION FOR CHAPTER 78

Answer 78-1: D

Discussion 78-1

A. Patients with lower extremity ischemia also have an increased incidence of carotid artery stenosis. Several studies have documented that as many as 28% of patients with leg ischemia have hemodynamically significant carotid artery stenoses and more than 10% have critical stenoses (i.e., >75%). Therefore, comprehensive assessment of the claudicant warrants evaluation of the cervical carotid arteries by duplex imaging.

B. There is a significant association between a reduced ABI and coronary artery disease. The presence of coronary artery disease may be silent in more than 25% of claudicants because of their exercise restrictions. Because of this, an assessment of coronary artery disease is justified. A stress electrocardiogram, whether by treadmill or by pharmacologic means of simulating the stress of exercise, is useful in identifying the presence of coronary artery disease.

C. The measurement of segmental arterial pressures with calculation of the ABI and thigh-brachial index is the best initial study for assessing occlusive disease the lower extremity in the claudicant.

D. Claudicants with significant risk factors for atherosclerosis may have multifocal involvement. However, in the absence of severe difficult to control hypertension, with diastolic pressures greater than 115 mm Hg or an abnormal serum creatinine, renal duplex imaging is unlikely to identify renal artery stenoses significant enough to benefit from treatment, other than control of risk factors. Therefore, this test would *not* be indicated in the initial evaluation of the majority of claudicants.

E. Treadmill testing in the vascular laboratory permits the quantification of the ambulatory distance and both the initial onset of pain and maximum walking distance before being forced to stop walking. Those distances provide a valid baseline for future comparisons after treatment, whether by an exercise program or a vascular intervention. This study also is of benefit in uncovering subclinical stenoses that become flow limiting with exercise.

Answer 78-2: A

Discussion 78-2

A. Testing for the presence of a hypercoagulable state should be undertaken *only if* there is significant clinical suspicion based on prior thrombotic events or there is a strong familial history of hypercoagulable states. The development of symptoms of claudication is most often the result of progression of the atherosclerotic process rather than spontaneous thrombosis.

B. A complete blood count is a cost-effective method for identifying the presence of many blood-related problems, including abnormally high or low red cell or platelet counts (e.g., leukemia, anemia, thrombocytosis) that might require specific treatment, in addition to the symptom-directed treatment of claudication.

C. Diabetes is a significant risk factor for arterial occlusive disease. Patients may present with symptoms of claudication without prior documentation of diabetes. A fasting blood glucose level is a cost-effective screening test for this metabolic disorder.

D. A fasting lipid profile, including total cholesterol, high-density lipoprotein, low-density lipoprotein, and triglyceride concentration, is an important screening test for patients with the new onset of symptoms of claudication. There is an increasing body of evidence that suggests that careful control of lipid levels can reduce the risk of associated cerebral, coronary, and peripheral arterial occlusive disease.

E. A serum creatinine level is a useful and readily available test that can indicate the presence of renal disease. Risk factors for arterial occlusive disease, such as hypertension and diabetes, also adversely affect renal function. Chronic renal insufficiency and renal failure also have prognostic value in the assessment of risks and benefits of treatment.

Answer 78-3: C

Discussion 78-3

A. The ABI is an excellent and cost-effective method for assessing the presence of peripheral arterial disease in patients. However, an excessively high index (>normal, >1.0) or an index higher than the actual pressure may be found with the presence of arterial wall calcification, as in many patients with long-standing diabetes. Therefore, a higher than normal or expected ABI should be corroborated, that is, compared with pulse-volume recordings, Doppler velocity waveform analysis, or toe pressures, to determine its veracity.

B. Although duplex imaging technology continues to improve, this modality is limited by the presence of arterial wall calcification, especially in tibial vessels, as commonly encountered in diabetic patients. Thus, it has not yet become a universally reliable tool for planning distal arterial reconstruction. It is of benefit as part of a surveillance program and is able to detect restenosis at angioplasty sites, failing vein grafts, and anastomotic strictures.

C. Gadolinium-enhanced magnetic resonance imaging is very helpful in the evaluation of the arterial tree of the lower extremity, especially for examining distal tibial and pedal vessels. With delayed imaging and multiple data sets, magnetic resonance imaging can visualize small distal vessels without the excessive contrast load often required by conventional or digital subtraction angiography.

D. Although heavily calcified vessels distort ultrasound-based imaging studies and can be problematic for other studies, such as CT angiography, calcium does not distort the images obtained by conventional contrast angiography.

E. Advanced imaging studies are needed only if intervention is planned. In the absence of the need for intervention, a patient can be adequately treated on the basis of noninvasive tests (e.g., segmental arterial pressures and plethysmography). Treadmill testing is of value in documenting the effectiveness of conservative management over time, that is, an exercise program or pharmacotherapy.

■ ANSWERS AND DISCUSSION FOR CHAPTER 79

Answer 79-1: E

Discussion 79-1

A. No definitive comparative data are available because of differences in runoff and other factors affecting patency, and concurrent comparisons have not been done in case-matched series. Nevertheless, a number of major series have reported better late patency for grafts with an end-to-end proximal anastomosis, and, although other series have shown equivalent patencies, *none* has reported superior late patency for end-to-side grafts.

B. As determined by postoperative noninvasive studies, there is no difference in the degree of early hemodynamic improvement between the two types of proximal anastomosis.

C. End-to-side grafts may be at higher risk of distal embolic complications because of potential risk of flushing aortic debris after release of the aortic clamp, which can travel to the legs through preserved flow through the aortoiliac segment in the end-to-side configuration.

D. The incidence of impotence is potentially *less* with end-to-side proximal anastomosis because of maintenance of antegrade perfusion to the internal iliac arteries. This is difficult to prove because preoperative and postoperative sexual dysfunction are not well documented in reported series, but certainly the incidence of postoperative impotence is not greater with end-to-side proximal anastomosis than after end-to-end proximal anastomosis.

E. An end-to-side proximal aortic anastomosis has clear advantages if the aorta itself is not too severely diseased in patients with severe *bilateral external iliac occlusive disease*. In these circumstances, end-to-end grafts will not provide adequate retrograde iliac artery flow to maintain pelvic perfusion, increasing the likelihood of postoperative impotence and the possibility of persistent hip and buttock claudication, colon ischemia, or even spinal cord ischemia, related to a relatively acute pelvic devascularization.

Answer 79-2: D

Discussion 79-2

The decision of whether a distal bypass should be performed at the same time as an inflow reconstruction for a patient with multilevel disease is frequently encountered. Although satisfactory clinical improvement can usually be achieved with an ABF graft alone, certain patients are best managed by simultaneous inflow and outflow grafting. Although no single criterion exists for predicting successful outcome, some conclusions can be made.

A. A proximal profunda stenosis can be corrected by profundoplasty at the time of proximal grafting and should enhance the hemodynamic benefit of an inflow procedure and thus is *not* an indication for adding a distal bypass. On the other hand, a small or diseased *distal* profunda femoris would suggest the need for improving outflow by adding a distal bypass.

B. The preoperative ABI does indicate the severity of overall perfusion impairment, but it does not localize the segment with the greatest hemodynamic importance. Logically, the worse the proximal disease being bypassed, the greater the hemodynamic benefit of proximal bypass alone. Correction of severe inflow disease alone might well achieve significant improvement in postoperative ABI and give excellent clinical relief of ischemia. Thus a preoperative ABI as low as 0.30 does not, per se, dictate the need for distal bypass. Similarly, other noninvasive predictors have not reliably indicated which patients definitely will require distal bypass for an adequate result.

C. Even a totally occluded SFA may well be compensated by profunda-popliteal-tibial collaterals, so this alone is not an indication for adding a distal bypass.

D. The most reliable guide to considering adding a distal bypass is tissue necrosis of the foot (i.e., deep ulceration or gangrene), because healing such lesions or debridement/amputation requires a significantly greater improvement in distal perfusion than supporting intact tissue. Thus, although severe claudication or even rest pain will usually be adequately relieved by bypass of hemodynamically significant inflow disease alone, a gangrenous toe or deep ulceration/necrosis in the foot demands as total a revascularization as possible.

E. Intraoperative predictors, such as an ABI at completion of the proximal bypass, are limited by vasoconstriction of distal vessels for hours. It is well recognized that profunda revascularization often takes hours to days to fully improve distal perfusion.

Answer 79-3: E

Discussion 79-3

Occlusion of a graft limb is one of the most common late graft-related complications of aortofemoral grafting for occlusive disease. In the majority of cases, it is caused by obstruction of graft limb outflow by recurrent or new occlusive disease or intimal hyperplasia occurring at or just beyond the distal anastomosis. Most often, these patients have an occluded SFA, and the development of obstruction to profunda outflow results in graft limb thrombosis. Progression of proximal aortic disease (C) is relatively unusual and rarely is a cause of occlusion of *one* graft limb. If present, proximal disease usually causes failure of the entire graft. Unilateral graft limb thrombosis can usually be successfully managed by (E) graft thrombectomy *and* correction of the graft limb outflow problem, usually by some form of profundoplasty. *If* the profunda is small or diffusely diseased, a distal bypass (B) may be required to provide adequate runoff, but this is not usually the case. *If* graft limb thrombosis is chronic, thrombectomy may not be successful, in which case (A) a femorofemoral bypass can be a useful alternative, but only if the contralateral graft limb and its outflow are normal. Placement of an entirely new aortofemoral graft (D) is an extensive redo procedure with significantly greater risks. It should be considered only for failure of the entire graft be-

cause of some intrinsic problem (e.g., a generalized graft infection or fabric degeneration).

■ ANSWERS AND DISCUSSION FOR CHAPTER 80

Answer 80-1: B

Discussion 80-1

A. Although there are no randomized trials, case-control studies with efforts at matching patients have shown poorer patency for femorofemoral bypass.

B. A small decline in resting pressure may be detected in the donor limb of some cases, but symptomatic "steal" has not been a significant problem in the absence of proximal occlusive disease in the donor iliac artery system.

C. The concept of external support has "face validity," but there is no convincing evidence that an externally supported prosthesis provides any improvement in patency in this application, and it may complicate intervention should the bypass thrombose.

D. Femorofemoral bypass has been demonstrated to have residual hemodynamic abnormalities, especially with exercise testing, whereas aortofemoral bypass is associated with hemodynamic normalization.

E. The majority of published studies have concluded that balloon angioplasty of the donor iliac limb is associated with hemodynamic and patency performance indistinguishable from that in patients who did not require donor iliac angioplasty.

Answer 80-2: A

Discussion 80-2

A. Placing the axillary artery to graft anastomosis as medial (close to the clavicle) as possible and leaving some redundancy of graft in the axilla are both important to reduce the risk of anastomotic disruption when stressed by upper extremity abduction, the so-called axillary pullout syndrome.

B. There is no convincing evidence that graft material or its support have impacted or improved patency.

C. Published experience mostly indicates that axillofemoral patency is superior in claudicants compared with that in patients with chronic critical ischemia.

D. Published experience is not uniform, but the majority of studies have reported equivalent patency in patients with and without SFA patency.

E. There is no evidence to support this; in fact, theory would suggest that the risk of thrombosis may actually increase when axillofemoral graft diameters exceed 8 mm (i.e., graft diameters greater than outflow diameters should result in a reduction in graft flow velocity).

Answer 80-3: E

Discussion 80-3

A. Satisfactory patencies may also be achieved with prosthetic grafts. However, autologous grafts are preferred in the presence of infection.

B. Collected experience indicates that thoracofemoral bypass provides patency comparable to aortofemoral bypass.

C. Despite previous literature bias favoring axillobifemoral grafts, more recent comparisons suggest that the patency rates of axillounifemoral and axillobifemoral grafts are not significantly different.

D. Balloon angioplasty is the more appropriate primary treatment for discrete common iliac artery stenosis; it is less invasive and with as good or better long-term patency than femorofemoral bypass.

E. Although some have advocated "extra-anatomic" procedures as preferred primary treatment for most patients with lower extremity arterial occlusive disease, available evidence indicates that they are either less effective (patency and clinical improvement) or provide no risk reduction when compared with their direct "anatomic" counterparts (aortofemoral bypass and femoropopliteal bypass).

■ ANSWERS AND DISCUSSION FOR CHAPTER 81

Answer 81-1: C

Discussion 81-1

A. The presence of gangrene increases the likelihood that distal bypass will also be required to maximize foot perfusion in a patient who will need to heal either multiple toe amputations or a transmetatarsal amputation.

B. Patients with diabetes mellitus require higher forefoot and toe pressures to heal than nondiabetic patients. They are also much more likely to have atherosclerotic disease involving the distal profunda femoris artery and the tibial and pedal arteries. These factors diminish the potential that profundoplasty alone will suffice.

C. The arteriographic visualization of good collaterals between the deep femoral artery and the popliteal artery is a favorable sign. The PPCI is an objective predictor of response to profundoplasty. A PPCI exceeding 0.5 (indicating a significant gradient across the knee) has been consistently associated with failure of isolated profundoplasty, although a PPCI less than 0.20 predicts resolution of ischemic rest pain and healing of ischemic lesions in more than 90% of patients.

D. This anatomic situation (popliteal occlusion and severe tibial-pedal occlusive disease) would result in a high PPCI, and a lack of response to isolated profundoplasty could be expected.

E. The mere presence of a previously failed PTFE graft does not mean that the patient will not respond to profundoplasty. In fact, correction of hemodynamically significant distal common femoral and profunda disease is frequently useful in salvaging limbs in selected patients with occluded femoropopliteal grafts or when an infected PTFE graft must be removed.

Answer 81-2: D

Discussion 81-2

A. Ipsilateral GSV is the preferred conduit for all infrainguinal reconstructions if long-term patency is the primary goal of the procedure. Level I evidence supports the use of vein even in the above-knee position (5-year patency at least 15%–20% superior to PTFE).

B. Distal origin sites do not compromise long-term patency as long as there are no hemodynamically significant lesions proximal to the selected site of origin.

C. Results using contralateral GSV are equivalent to ipsilateral GSV except patency rates are lower in patients undergoing redo bypass (not the case in this instance in which the vein had been used for coronary bypass).

D. The 5-year patency of above-knee PTFE femoropopliteal bypass is only 50% to 60% in prospective randomized trials (vs. 68%–76% for vein). Although there are some arguments to considering above-knee PTFE bypass in selected patients, long-term patency is not one of them.

E. Diabetes does not adversely impact graft patency, although it is associated with an increased risk of delayed wound healing and major limb amputation.

Answer 81-3: E

Discussion 81-3

A. Of all failed or failing infrainguinal autogenous vein grafts in the first 3 to 5 years after implantation, 60% to 65% are caused by intrinsic vein graft lesions, 80% of which are focal and correctable.

B. Duplex surveillance is much more sensitive and accurate in the detection of graft stenosis than history, physical, and ABI measurements.

C. Surveillance of PTFE grafts has not proven to be clinically useful.

D. Eighty percent of vein graft lesions are focal and correctable by a variety of techniques including percutaneous transluminal angioplasty, open-patch angioplasty, excision and reanastomosis, and translocation. Long-segment lesions or diffuse graft narrowing account for less than 5% to 8% of intrinsic graft lesions.

E. The duplex criteria listed are indicative of severe graft stenosis and portend a high risk of subsequent graft occlusion. Repair is almost always indicated.

■ ANSWERS AND DISCUSSION FOR CHAPTER 82

Answer 82-1: C

Discussion 82-1

The indications for isolated profundoplasty are less clear and most dependent on the individual surgeon's judgment. Distal perfusion is improved but not to as great an extent as with distal bypass. Few patients with disabling claudication (D) should be considered for isolated profundoplasty as they will likely continue to have symptoms because of the remaining superficial femoral occlusion, although perhaps to a lesser extent. Patients with rest pain and ulceration with minimal tissue necrosis (C) are good candidates for profundoplasty, particularly when other possibilities for revascularization are not good, which include absence of saphenous vein or those patients who would not tolerate a more extensive procedure because of comorbidities. Those with (A) extensive forefoot gangrene, (E) advanced foot sepsis are unlikely to benefit, and, in general, those with diabetic neuropathy (B) do less well.

Answer 82-2: D

Discussion 82-2

The preoperative factors that help predict success of an isolated profundoplasty include (C) good inflow to the common femoral artery, (A) the presence of a significant proximal profunda lesion, and (B) a good distal profunda with good collaterals to (E) patent popliteal or tibial arteries. When most of these factors are not present, then reconsideration of a distal bypass should be entertained. (D) Diabetes is *not* a risk factor which correlates with favorable outcome.

Answer 82-3: C

Discussion 82-3

The most frequent cause for late failure of an ABF bypass is intimal hyperplasia at the distal anastomosis resulting in graft limb thrombosis. (C) Thrombectomy or thrombolysis of the graft is rarely sufficient alone, because the outflow stenosis must be corrected. When the superficial femoral is occluded and there is a significant proximal profunda stenosis, profundoplasty is indicated to maximize outflow and maintain graft patency. It had remained patent for a long time, and isolated profundoplasty is a low-risk procedure. (A) Graft infection is an unlikely cause. (B) Distal bypass should not be needed. (D) This use of papaverine is passé. (E) This advice is inappropriate when a simple procedure like (C) will relieve symptoms.

■ ANSWERS AND DISCUSSION FOR CHAPTER 83

Answer 83-1: C

Discussion 83-1

All are possible causes of bypass graft failure. Generally, *early* graft thrombosis is attributable to errors in technique or judgment. These can include a poorly constructed anastomosis or (A) poor choice of inflow or outflow sites. In addition, early graft thrombosis may occur for no apparent reason in technically adequate bypasses, as confirmed by completion arteriography. This might show an unsuspected compression or kinking of the bypass, but although there is a real risk of this in vein bypasses, it would be *very unlikely* for an above-knee femoral-popliteal bypass, particularly because tunneling devices are now so commonly used. Therefore, C is the correct answer. Unrecognized coagulopathy can cause early bypass graft, as soon as the heparin wears off, and although it is a rare cause, it bears investigation if no other cause is found. Owing to (D) the inherent thrombogenicity of a prosthetic graft, it can thrombose early in a low-flow setting. (E) A transient decrease in cardiac output with hypotension can contribute to this. Prosthetic grafts characteristically require a minimum threshold velocity for continued patency, but this becomes less of a factor with time after operation or insufficient runoff. (B) Poor runoff is often blamed and can be a factor in more distal bypasses, particularly in diabetic patients or redo bypasses, but poor

runoff is rarely a factor in *above-knee femoral-popliteal prosthetic* bypasses, which are more often done in claudicants with single-level disease.

Answer 83-2: E

Discussion 83-2

If the patient had any recurrence of ischemic symptoms or the surgeon detects either a diminution in peripheral pulses examination or other manifestations of ischemia, an explanation must be sought by further investigations. These duplex findings are a reliable indicator of a vein graft stenosis of a severity likely to result in graft thrombosis. Treating a failing graft requires a less complex procedure and is associated with better patency than treating a thrombosed graft. Therefore (A) continued monitoring of the graft at the standard intervals is inappropriate. (B) Monitoring the resting ABI, commonly done before duplex scanning, is less sensitive than the duplex scan and is unnecessary because a graft stenosis has already been identified. (C) Heparin therapy and repeating the duplex scan at an earlier interval might be appropriate earlier in the postoperative period *if* the duplex scan finding suggested a much lesser degree of stenosis, but even then an arteriogram should be obtained. (D) The heparin is appropriate to help prevent immediate graft thrombosis, but localized vein graft stenoses at this time interval postoperatively respond often enough to PTA (especially with the new cutting balloons) that it (E) is preferable in this patient to seeking a long length of autogenous vein and subjecting the patient to another long distal bypass. The later the graft stenosis develops, the greater the likelihood of successful salvage of the graft. Abandoning a potentially salvageable vein graft is not appropriate. Thus, in this patient, answer E is the most appropriate management.

Answer 83-3: C

Discussion 83-3

Intimal hyperplasia is an important cause of infrainguinal bypass graft failure. It may develop with prosthetic, modified biologic or vein grafts and in different locations.

A. It can involve any portion of a vein graft in a focal or *diffuse manner* and develop at either the proximal or distal anastomosis or somewhere in the mid-graft.
B. When significant intimal hyperplasia does occur, it usually produces infrainguinal graft failure between 2 and 18 months after operation. It is the most common cause of vein graft failure during the first 2 years, once beyond the immediate postoperative period, when technical inadequacy and low flow states are more likely causes of graft thrombosis.
C. In prosthetic grafts, intimal hyperplasia is more commonly localized to an anastomosis than be in the mid-graft, but this statement does not apply to *vein grafts*, so C is not true and is the correct answer.
D. However, anastomotic narrowing as the result of intimal hyperplasia can also occur in vein grafts with a greater predilection for the distal versus the proximal anastomosis.
E. A significant stenosis warrants repair to prevent graft thrombosis even if the patient is asymptomatic, particularly because autogenous conduits are a valuable and lim-

ited resource and, on the basis of patency rates and the complexity of a secondary procedure, treating a "failing" (stenosed) graft is far preferable to treating a "failed" (thrombosed) graft.

ANSWERS AND DISCUSSION FOR CHAPTER 84

Answer 84-1: B

Discussion 84-1

A. Answer A is incorrect; though it would be a reasonable approach to residual stenosis after iliac PTA.

B. When a significant dissection occurs as a result of iliac PTA, the best treatment is to place a stent at the location where the balloon angioplasty was performed. This is one of the most solid indications for stent placement in any vascular bed.

C. Answer C is incorrect because the stent is not required for the entire length of the external iliac artery. In addition, it is usually best, whenever possible, to avoid placing a stent that approaches the proximal common femoral artery because this is an arterial segment with a high degree of flexibility required.

D. Answer D is incorrect because this would be inadequate treatment for a significant dissection, which is unlikely to resolve under anticoagulant therapy.

E. Answer E is incorrect. This is a proper approach to *residual* stenosis. One may measure pressure across a dissection, but the pressure gradient across the dissection does not predict its behavior. One treats a dissection to prevent occlusion resulting from extension of the dissection.

Answer 84-2: A

Discussion 84-2

A. Simultaneous iliac artery balloon angioplasty and infrainguinal bypass have been shown to produce reasonably good results without the delay and complications of performing separate staged procedures to achieve leg revascularization.

B. Primary leg amputation is definitely *not* indicated with a readily salvageable limb.

C. The inflow iliac artery stenosis is moderate and treating it with a femoral-posterior tibial bypass is unlikely to improve flow to the foot and will only delay the performance of the leg bypass that is required for limb salvage.

D. The inflow iliac artery stenosis is moderate and treating it before leg bypass is unlikely to improve flow to the foot and will only delay the performance of the leg bypass that is required for limb salvage.

E. These could be performed, but *primary* stenting is not indicated for this lesion. Secondary stenting would be indicated if balloon angioplasty failed to produce a good hemodynamic result.

Answer 84-3: C

Discussion 84-3

A. The patient described in A would be at high risk for surgery, and PTA of the tibial artery lesion may be enough to heal the foot lesion.

B. The situations described in B and E are similar, and both may be treated with balloon angioplasty and selective stent placement.

C. The patient described in C should be managed medically, not with endovascular intervention. Even though the lesion is focal, making it favorable for PTA, the patient's symptoms are mild and the patient continues to smoke.

D. The patient described in D would probably be adequately treated with iliac artery balloon angioplasty alone because the iliac is critical and the patient has presented with rest pain but without tissue loss.

E. See B.

ANSWERS AND DISCUSSION FOR CHAPTER 85

Answer 85-1: D

Discussion 85-1

A. Hyperhidrosis is the most common indication for dorsal sympathectomy, but it is occasionally an indication for lumbar sympathectomy. Desiccating powders, often containing formaldehyde, are more commonly used for sweating feet.

B. Buerger's disease involving the feet with pain and ulceration has been frequently treated in the past by lumbar sympathectomy with some benefit in terms of initial relief, but lasting improvement requires smoking cessation.

C. Causalgia can be a valid indication for sympathectomy in the lower and upper extremities.

D. Diabetic neuropathy in its early "neuritic" phase can present with pain in the feet, often burning in character. Eventually the "burned out" phase supervenes with sensory (and some) motor deficit. This is *never* an indication for sympathectomy; in fact, studies have shown that in the later phases there is also an "autosympathectomy."

E. Rest pain from PAD that is not amenable to bypass is a debatable indication, but lumbar sympathectomy has been shown in some series to benefit up to 40% of selected cases with rest pain and shallow ulcers. Selection is made on the basis of unequivocal strong positive response to sympathetic block. However, with current distal bypass techniques, very few patients with critical ischemia from PAD are not amenable to bypass.

Answer 85-2: B

Discussion 85-2

Selected patients with critical ischemia, even diabetic patients, can benefit from lumbar sympathectomy.

A. Bergan and Yao showed benefit for patients with an ABI greater than 3.0, presumably because the circulatory improvement with sympathectomy is mild and would benefit only those close to the upper margin of critical ischemia (an ABI of 0.30 represents an ankle pressure close to 40 mm Hg).

B. A diabetic patient with peripheral neuropathy has deficits of the sensory and motor nerves, but this neuropathy also involves the sympathetic fibers, such that these patients already have what has been termed an "autosympathectomy." Therefore, *sympathectomy would have no effect or no benefit in such patients.*

C. Shallow ulcers can heal after sympathectomy. Deep ulcers with underlying tissues (tendons, joints, bone) exposed will not benefit.
D. Ischemic rest pain may respond to sympathectomy, particularly if fairly recent or the ABI is marginal (in the upper range for this category, e.g., 0.30 or higher).
E. Because B is correct, E is wrong.

Answer 85-3: C
Discussion 85-3

The preganglionic sympathetic fibers going to the lower extremity mostly exit and synapse with postganglionic fibers at the L2 and L3 levels, so an L2-L3 sympathectomy is adequate and C is the correct answer. Variations in the sympathetic chain have been documented in earlier anatomic dissections. For example, L1 is missing on one side or the other in most cases, so that the additional removal of L1 (A) on one side could impair sexual function. (B) The additional removal of L4, which is accessible, is harmless but really adds nothing. It is often done by those who are unsure of the levels being removed and want to make sure of an adequate sympathectomy. Unfortunately, a lumbar vein often crosses the sympathetic ganglion chain between L3 and L4, and when under stretch may be mistaken for a crossover fiber and divided, with annoying bleeding. (D) L5 and (E) S1 are not really accessible through the usual retroperitoneal exposure, but because they play no role in relaying sympathetic fibers to the extremities, they are of no importance in lumbar sympathectomy.

■ ANSWERS AND DISCUSSION FOR CHAPTER 86

Answer 86-1: B
Discussion 86-1

(A) Patients most commonly present in the fourth and fifth decade. (B) Aneurysms not uncommonly develop near the point of entrapment. (C) When occlusion of the popliteal artery occurs, the wall of the artery has degenerated to the point in which preservation of a portion of the wall leads to early failure of the reconstruction. (D) The popliteal artery only lies deep and medial to the origin of the medial head of the gastrocnemius muscle in type I entrapment, a relatively uncommon variant. (E) Although originally described mainly in men, this observation was probably biased by the military nature of the early-described series; more recent reports indicate a substantial proportion of women are affected.

Answer 86-2: D
Discussion 86-2

(A) The external iliac/femoral artery is the second most commonly affected site. (B) Stents do not fare well in the popliteal artery because of the degree of flexion that occurs in this artery, particularly in the young and active patient. Unless evacuated, the cyst wall will probably continue to secrete fluid, and this results in restenosis of the artery. (C) The

scientific evidence supporting the cell inclusion and embryologic derivation theory suggests that this mechanism is the most likely explanation for the formation of adventitial cystic disease. (D and E) The *diagnosis* can usually be made by ultrasound, but angiography is valuable in planning therapy.

Answer 86-3: B
Discussion 86-3

(A) Popliteal artery entrapment is far more common than adventitial cystic disease as a cause of claudication in the younger patient. (B) Angiography may be normal at rest and only demonstrate the abnormality in the plantar-flexed stress position. (C) Surprisingly, the symptoms are often of sudden onset, frequently precipitated by extreme effort such as running a marathon. (D) Ankle pressures may be normal at rest in both popliteal vascular entrapment and adventitial cystic disease if occlusion of the artery has not yet taken place. (E) In view of the embryologic development of the popliteal artery, it will never course *lateral* to the origin of the lateral head of the gastrocnemius muscle.

■ ANSWERS AND DISCUSSION FOR CHAPTER 87

Answer 87-1: A
Discussion 87-1

A. With long-standing diabetes, the capillary basement membrane becomes thickened with increased permeability to albumin. This capillary leak of albumin correlates with the presence of microalbuminuria, which is in turn a predictor of all of the complications of diabetes.
B. The thickened capillary basement membrane does *not* compromise the lumen of the capillary.
C. There is *no* confirmatory evidence of any occlusive lesion in the microcirculation, following some very early reports, poorly controlled, to the contrary.
D. The basement membrane abnormalities do *not* interfere with diffusion of oxygen.
E. Autonomic neuropathy results in sympathectomy and vasodilatation of the skin microcirculation.

Answer 87-2: C
Discussion 87-2

The neuroinflammatory response is mediated by the axon reflex in nociceptive, fine "C" fibers of the sensory nerves. (C) *This entire neuroinflammatory response is blunted early in the course of diabetic neuropathy.* (B) There is an *increased* release of packets of neuropeptides from these fibers in response to injury. The other listed responses are characteristic of a *normal* neuroinflammatory response and are thus diminished, not increased/accentuated, in diabetics. These include (A) the release of histamine, triggered by substance P, which causes mast cells to degranulate, which in turn produces (D) the wheal and flare response to skin injury, and the release of other cytokines, including tumor necrosis factor-;ga, which (E) stimulates macrophages to migrate to the site of injury. Thus, in diabetic patients, each of these three "normal" responses is decreased/diminished, not increased/accentuated.

Answer 87-3: C

Discussion 87-3

A. Autonomic neuropathy causes loss of sweat (eccrine) and oil (apocrine) gland function, not an increase.
B. Talipes is a congenital deformity not associated with diabetes.
C. Neuropathy of long fine motor fibers and consequent loss of lumbrical muscle function results in a "claw deformity" of the foot, which creates pressure points susceptible to ulceration.
D. Foot drop, rather than dorsiflexion is a consequence of motor neuropathy.
E. Osteomyelitis occurs secondary to ulceration, not as the initiating cause.

■ ANSWERS AND DISCUSSION FOR CHAPTER 88

Answer 88-1: E

Discussion 88-1

Aortic disease (A) accounts for only a small proportion of patients with ED, and although B, C, and D may all contribute to impotence, the main mechanism of most ED is E: failure of relaxation of cavernosal smooth muscle.

Answer 88-2: E

Discussion 88-2

(E) Women with diabetes and cardiovascular disease frequently have sexual dysfunction. Collaterals cannot compensate for interruption of the primary arterial supply. (B) Sildenafil citrate has not been effective in many cases and is not recommended for use in women. (C) Women tend to complain less of FSD and failure of lubrication and arousal may not be detected. (D) Hyperthyroidism may actually contribute to enhanced sexuality.

Answer 88-3: E

Discussion 88-3

(A) Although screening systems were previously used for the diagnostic evaluation of ED, the most accepted current approach is more limited and goal directed to detect the response to initial pharmacotherapy. In the absence of contraindications, phosphodiesterase type-5 inhibition (E) and modification of risk factors are used first. The other alternatives (B–D) are used with failure of response to pharmacotherapy but are now uncommonly invoked.

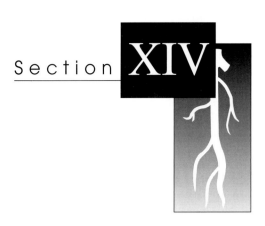
NEUROVASCULAR CONDITIONS INVOLVING THE UPPER EXTREMITY

STUDY QUESTIONS

■ QUESTIONS FOR CHAPTER 90

Question 90-1

The largest number of anatomic variations within the upper extremity arterial blood supply is seen within which of the following arterial segments:

A. Subclavian artery.
B. Superficial volar arch.
C. Deep volar arch.
D. Axillary/brachial/radial/ulnar arteries.
E. Innominate artery.

Question 90-2

A patient with a cool, moist, blue hand that is exquisitely painful to touch most of the time most likely has which of the following? Note: The patient has *not* had hemodialysis access, catheter access, or any other upper extremity invasive procedures previously.

A. Primary Raynaud's disease.
B. Scleroderma.
C. Reflex sympathetic dystrophy.
D. Secondary Raynaud's phenomenon.
E. Arterial embolism.

Question 90-3

The diagnosis of primary Raynaud's disease is suggested by:

A. Uniform color changes in response to cold in all digits.
B. Recovery of fingertip temperature within 10 minutes after immersion in ice water.
C. Trophic changes, ulcers, or severe pain.
D. Reactive hyperemia.
E. Use of vibrating tools by male worker.

Question 90-4

A peaked contour pulse on digital plethysmography, is associated with:

A. Proximal subclavian artery obstruction.
B. Digital artery occlusion.
C. Arteriovenous fistula.

D. Vasospastic disease (primary Raynaud's).
E. Thoracic outlet syndrome.

Question 90-5

When patients are evaluated for unilateral upper extremity vascular symptoms, arteriography should be performed:

A. From the second portion of the subclavian artery to the digital vessels.
B. With the arm in the neutral position only.
C. With and without vasodilatation.
D. By direct brachial artery puncture.
E. With visualization of all the arch vessels and their origins.

■ QUESTIONS FOR CHAPTER 91

Question 91-1

A 67-year-old man presents with a left-sided transient ischemic attack. High-grade stenosis is identified at the right carotid bifurcation on magnetic resonance angiography. The patient is also noted to have an aberrant origin of the right subclavian artery. Other anatomic abnormalities should be expected *except* for:

A. A "nonrecurrent" recurrent laryngeal nerve.
B. A right-sided thoracic duct.
C. A congenital cardiac abnormality.
D. A right vertebral artery that does not take origin from the subclavian artery.
E. Any of the above (i.e., none are associated with an aberrant right subclavian origin).

Question 91-2

Nonatherosclerotic diseases that have a known affinity to affect the proximal great vessels include all but:

A. Takayasu's arteritis.
B. Radiation arteritis.
C. Giant cell arteritis.
D. Syphilitic aneurysms.
E. All of the above.

Question 91-3

A 77-year-old man presents with recurrent angina during light upper body workouts 5 years after successful coronary artery bypass surgery. A stress thallium study indicates anterior wall ischemia. On physical examination, his left arm pressure is 30 mm Hg lower than the right. The best procedure to remedy his problem is:

A. Redo coronary artery bypass surgery using vein or radial artery graft.
B. Coronary angioplasty with drug-eluting stents.
C. Subclavian to carotid transposition.
D. Carotid to subclavian bypass.
E. Subclavian to subclavian bypass.

■ QUESTIONS FOR CHAPTER 92

Question 92-1

A 35-year-old female artist presents with a cold index finger and splinter hemorrhages. Arteriography reveals what appears to be fibromuscular dysplasia of the proximal brachial artery with distal emboli. What is the most appropriate treatment for this patient?

A. Thrombolytic therapy and long-term anticoagulation with warfarin.
B. Anticoagulation with warfarin to maintain an international normalized ratio between 2.0 and 3.0.
C. Arterial resection and vein graft interposition.
D. Dorsal sympathectomy.
E. Digital artery sympathectomy.

Question 92-2

Upper extremity nerve anatomy and function is important in diagnosing and treating upper extremity neurovascular conditions. The median nerve:

A. Is lateral to the brachial artery.
B. Is medial to the brachial artery.
C. Enervates the lumbrical muscles of the hand.
D. Is the sensory supply to the palmar and dorsal aspects of the thumb and index fingers.
E. Produces a claw-hand when injured.

Question 92-3

A 69-year-old man has paresthesia and some difficulty grasping with his left hand after a brachial puncture for cardiac catheterization. The left brachial pulse is intact. The arm pressure is normal. What is the next step in the patient's management?

A. Bilateral upper extremity blood pressure measurement.
B. Splinting of the elbow and close observation.
C. Duplex ultrasound to rule out pseudoaneurysm.
D. Arteriography to detect distal embolization.
E. Operative decompression of the median nerve.

■ QUESTIONS FOR CHAPTER 93

Question 93-1

Vasospasm of the fingers occurs:

A. With cooling of the distal fingertip and warming of the proximal portion of the finger.

B. With cooling of the proximal finger and warming of the distal fingertip.
C. With sympathetic nerve blockade.
D. With systemic hypertension; diastolic pressure greater than 90 mm Hg.
E. Primarily in young men.

Question 93-2

In patients with Raynaud's disease and underlying digital artery abnormalities, the most common associated disorder is:

A. Scleroderma.
B. Mixed connective tissue disease.
C. Atherosclerosis.
D. Hypersensitive angitis.
E. Buerger's disease.

Question 93-3

A 25-year-old woman presents with unilateral Raynaud's syndrome. What is the most appropriate next step in the diagnosis?

A. Complete blood count, including sedimentation rate.
B. Antinuclear antibody test.
C. X-ray film of the hand.
D. Complete upper extremity arteriogram, including the arch and peripheral vessels.
E. Cold recovery time.

■ QUESTIONS FOR CHAPTER 94

Question 94-1

A 29-year-old female secretary was involved in a rear-end automobile collision 6 months ago. Cervical spine x-ray films at the time were negative. She now presents with numbness and tingling in the fourth and fifth digits and cervical pain, which worsen when she is using her arms above her head. What is/are the appropriate next step(s) in the diagnostic evaluation?

A. Electromyography and nerve conduction velocity.
B. Cervical spine x-ray film.
C. Noninvasive vascular laboratory studies.
D. Magnetic resonance imaging of the cervical spine.
E. All of the above.

Question 94-2

As a cause of symptoms:

A. Neurogenic thoracic outlet compression is less common than venous thoracic outlet compression.
B. Arterial thoracic outlet compression is more common than neurogenic thoracic outlet.
C. Venous compression (Paget-Schroetter syndrome) is less common than cervical rib arterial compression.
D. Neurogenic thoracic outlet compression is more common than arterial or venous thoracic outlet compression, combined.
E. Trauma is less likely to produce neurogenic thoracic outlet compression than skeletal abnormalities.

Question 94-3

In a supraclavicular incision to deal with various types of thoracic outlet compression, the phrenic nerve must be visualized and protected from injury. The phrenic nerve passes:

A. Posterior to the anterior scalene muscle.
B. In the belly of the middle scalene muscle.
C. From lateral to medial on the anterior surface of the anterior scalene muscle.
D. From medial to lateral over the anterior scalene.
E. Anterior to the subclavian vein.

■ QUESTIONS FOR CHAPTER 95

Question 95-1

What is the most frequent cause of *arterial* compression in the thoracic outlet?

A. Lung cancer.
B. Healed clavicle fracture.
C. Complete cervical rib.
D. Hypertrophied anterior scalene muscle.
E. Hypertrophied middle scalene muscle.

Question 95-2

What sign or symptom most suggests a diagnosis of arterial thoracic outlet syndrome?

A. Bilateral cold intolerance and digital ulcers.
B. Atrial fibrillation.
C. History of radiation therapy for lymphoma.
D. Strong family history of abdominal aortic aneurysm (AAA).
E. Right arm exertional cramping.

Question 95-3

What structure is *not* commonly identified during a *supraclavicular* exposure for resection of a cervical rib?

A. Vagus nerve.
B. Phrenic nerve.
C. Anterior scalene muscle.
D. Subclavian artery.
E. Platysma.

■ QUESTIONS FOR CHAPTER 96

Question 96-1

A 25-year-old male weight lifter presents with right upper extremity swelling and slight bluish discoloration. The most likely underlying cause of his condition is:

A. Cervical rib.
B. Anomalies of the first rib.
C. Middle scalene hypertrophy.
D. Costoclavicular compression.
E. Hypertrophy of the pectoralis minor muscle.

Question 96-2

What is the next step in the above patient's management?

A. Venous duplex.
B. Venogram.

C. Chest x-ray film.
D. Chest computed tomography (CT) scan.
E. Magnetic resonance venography of the upper extremity.

Question 96-3

Catheter-related subclavian vein thrombosis is:

A. Rarely associated with pulmonary emboli.
B. Best treated with catheter removal alone.
C. Associated with long-term disabilities of the upper extremity.
D. A marker of a hypercoagulable condition.
E. Treated with anticoagulation and ace wrapping of the upper extremity.

■ QUESTIONS FOR CHAPTER 97

Question 97-1

Sympathectomy has accepted benefits in selected cases for all of the following *except:*

A. Hyperhidrosis.
B. Prolonged QT syndrome.
C. Angina.
D. Complex regional pain syndrome.
E. Cold-induced vasospasm.

Question 97-2

Which of the following is incorrect? Sympathectomy:

A. Reduces sweating.
B. Causes impotence.
C. Reduces the vasomotor response to cold.
D. Relieves anginal pain.
E. Causes postoperative neuralgia.

Question 97-3

The most common complication of bilateral thoracoscopic sympathectomy is:

A. Horner's syndrome.
B. Compensatory hyperhidrosis.
C. Intercostal neuralgia.
D. Injury to vagus nerve.
E. Injury to the phrenic nerve.

■ QUESTIONS FOR CHAPTER 98

Question 98-1

A 34-year-old auto mechanic presents with a 1-day history of numbness, tingling, pain, and discoloration of the tips of his fingers in his right hand. All of the following are true about hypothenar hammer syndrome (HHS) except (i.e., choose the false answer):

A. It involves the ulnar artery.
B. It is most commonly the result of repetitive localized trauma.
C. It may result in an arterial aneurysm.
D. The lesion is located in the forearm.
E. The cause may be fibromuscular dysplasia.

Question 98-2

A 22-year-old amateur baseball player comes to your office because of numbness in his right index and middle fingers after a successful 14-inning no hitter. Among baseball pitchers, the artery most likely to be injured from repetitive motion is the:

A. Axillary.
B. Brachial.
C. Anterior humeral circumflex.
D. Posterior humeral circumflex.
E. Suprascapular.

Question 98-3

A 23-year-old baseball player presents with cyanosis of his right index finger. Understanding the underlying condition requires knowledge of the anatomy of the quadrilateral space and the potential effects of repeated throwing (see question 98-2). In that regard, the quadrilateral space is composed of all of the following *except:*

A. Clavicle.
B. Teres minor.
C. Teres major.
D. Humerus.
E. Triceps.

ANSWERS AND DISCUSSION

■ ANSWERS AND DISCUSSION FOR CHAPTER 90

Answer 90-1: D

Discussion 90-1

A. The right subclavian artery will occasionally arise directly from the aortic arch or thoracic aorta (aberrant subclavian). The left subclavian can be joined by the left carotid at its origin. These are very important variants to be aware of but not the most numerous.
B. The superficial volar arch has nine variations grouped according to whether the arch is complete or incomplete.
C. The deep volar arch also groups its six variations based or whether the arch is complete or incomplete.
D. In the arteries of the upper arm and forearm, that is, distal to the subclavian artery down to the wrist, there are 12 major arterial variations of the upper limb, with multiple minor variations, *by far the greatest number.* One of the most confusing factors in dealing with occlusions is a high takeoff of the ulnar artery from the axillary.
E. The innominate or brachiocephalic artery, nominally the common stem of the right carotid and subclavian, can be absent if one or both of these two arteries originate separately from the aortic arch (the latter is rare; an aberrant subclavian is more common), and can include the origin of the left carotid (bovine arch, relatively common), but these different variations are still few in number, compared with some of the other segments included as possible answers.

Answer 90-2: C

Discussion 90-2

(C) Reflex sympathetic dystrophy or causalgia, in its dystrophic stage, may be mistaken for Raynaud's disease. However, individuals with Raynaud's disease, both (A) primary and (D) secondary, rarely exhibit hyperesthesia and the pain is not usually severe or continuous. Furthermore, in Raynaud's disease the hand is not typically moist (a reflection of increased sympathetic activity). Patients with (B) scleroderma can develop secondary Raynaud's phenomenon. These patients are more likely to have digital ulcerations/necrosis, and severe pain is associated with these lesions.

(E) Arterial emboli may produce pallor initially but then can progress to cyanosis, but the hypersensitivity is absent; in fact, hyposensitivity (and muscle weakness) should be sought.

Answer 90-3: D

Discussion 90-3

(D) Patients with primary Raynaud's disease classically develop reactive hyperemia on rewarming of the digits, after the cold-induced vasospasm ends. (C) Trophic changes, ulcers, and severe pain are typically seen in patients with *secondary* Raynaud's phenomenon and almost never seen in patients with primary Raynaud's disease. (B) A vasospastic response of digital arteries to cold is normal. In patients with primary Raynaud's disease this response is abnormal in that

it occurs earlier, with relatively milder cold exposure, and persists longer. In the cold-water immersion test, a healthy patient's fingers should recover within 10 minutes. Patients with primary Raynaud's disease often have a recovery delayed well beyond this normal cutoff point, for example, the fingers do not recover for 20 minutes or more. (A) Although one might expect a diffuse and even vasospastic response in primary Raynaud's disease, in contrast with certain fingers being much worse in secondary Raynaud's disease, this is not a reliable differentiation. Patients with primary Raynaud's disease often have an uneven digital response to cold exposure and rewarming. (E) Primary Raynaud's disease is more common in females, and secondary Raynaud's phenomena are seen in some workers using vibrating tools.

Answer 90-4: D

Discussion 90-4

A. Pulse volume recording of a patient with a proximal subclavian artery demonstrates diminished amplitude.
B. Digital artery occlusion, similarly, is found to have diminished amplitude at the level of the finger but preserved waveforms proximally.
C. An arteriovenous fistula will be associated with a rapid fall-off of the waveform.
D. The peaked pulse contour is classic for vasospasm and Raynaud's disease. It should be noted that this finding is not specific for this condition, in that it can also be seen in some patients with collagen vascular diseases involving the digital arteries (e.g., disseminated lupus and scleroderma), but these were not options among the answers.
E. In thoracic outlet syndrome the waveform is normal with the arm in the neutral position and diminished with abduction and external rotation.

Answer 90-5: C

Discussion 90-5

A. Complete visualization of the arterial tree from the aortic arch to the digital vessels is mandatory. The proximal subclavian artery is a common location for atherosclerosis with distal embolic potential. Introducing the catheter in too far, beyond the origin of the subclavian artery, may therefore miss a potential cause for upper-extremity ischemia.
B. Although upper-extremity arteriography yields important information with the arm in the neutral position, additional information can be gained from placing the arm in the abducted, external rotated position. Thoracic outlet arterial compression may be discovered even though the arteriogram in the neutral position is negative.
C. It is important to perform the distal part of the arteriogram with and without vasodilatation. Vasospasm is common with catheterization of distal arteries. The test may be interpreted incorrectly, apparently demonstrating distal digital obstruction, without the use of an intra-arterial vasodilator.

D. Direct brachial puncture for arteriography of the upper extremity is not appropriate for the same reason "A" was not true. Complete visualization of the subclavian from the arch to the digits is important.

E. For unilateral symptoms it is important to visualize the entire proximal subclavian artery, and although this might visualize some of the arch vessels (innominate and right carotid), unless lesions are seen with this, it is unnecessary to evaluate the entire arch and its branch arteries. Occasionally, depending on the findings, visualizing the *contralateral* arm vessels will be indicated, for example, if digital artery occlusive disease is found on the ipsilateral arm without an apparent proximal cause, the finding of similar lesions on the opposite arm would suggest diffuse disease, whereas its absence would refocus investigation on the cause in the ipsilateral lesions.

■ **ANSWERS AND DISCUSSION FOR CHAPTER 91**

Answer 91-1: C
Discussion 91-1

Although congenital cardiac abnormalities certainly can occur, they would not be expected, whereas (A) a "nonrecurrent" recurrent laryngeal nerve, (B) a right-sided thoracic duct, and (D) a vertebral artery that takes origin from the arch of the aorta, although not necessarily present, should be anticipated if neck surgery is anticipated.

Answer 91-2: C
Discussion 91-2

(A) Takayasu's arteritis is particularly known to affect the proximal great vessels as well as the descending aorta and its proximal branches. (B) Radiation arteritis involves the great vessels when they have been included in the field of irradiation. Radiation to the mediastinum, particularly for disorders of the thymus, was somewhat common in the past and is still done today. (D) Syphilitic aneurysms, although rare today, do effect the proximal great vessels. Only (C) giant cell arteritis, primarily involves more peripheral arteries, for example, the subclavian beyond the clavicle and the more distal arteries to the head, typically the temporal artery but also intracranial vessels.

Answer 91-3: D
Discussion 91-3

The patient's symptoms stem, in all likelihood, from a coronary subclavian steal related to a subclavian stenosis or occlusion proximal to an internal mammary artery (IMA)-coronary artery reconstruction. The safest effective procedure for this would be (D) a carotid to subclavian bypass because this could be performed without interrupting circulation through the left IMA bypass (or right IMA, if there is one) during the time of revascularization. (C) A subclavian to carotid transposition would give excellent patency for bypassing a proximal subclavian occlusion but would require clamping the subclavian proximal to the IMA reconstruction. (B) Coronary angioplasty, regardless of the type of stent used, would not address the problem. (A) Redo coronary

artery bypass surgery, replacing the LIMA with another graft through a redo sternotomy and mediastinal dissection, would be much more than necessary for this patient. (E) A subclavian-subclavian bypass might relieve symptoms but has the same objections as C, plus its patency rate is inferior. Depending on the approach, it would either cross the sternotomy or, if performed through bilateral neck exposures, double the risk of local complications.

■ **ANSWERS AND DISCUSSION FOR CHAPTER 92**

Answer 92-1: C
Discussion 92-1

A. Thrombolytic therapy and long-term warfarin anticoagulation may not inhibit arterial emboli from a disrupted intimal surface, although the former may help clear up the distal emboli, even this is not a certainty (see C, below).

B. Long-term anticoagulation alone does not treat the digital emboli, although it may inhibit further embolization.

C. The proper treatment for a proximal embolizing source in the brachial artery is resection and replacement with a vein interposition graft. The superficial location of the artery makes it ideal for resection and repair. It will also provide a pathologic diagnosis. Although balloon angioplasty has been used in other locations for embolizing arterial lesions, it has not been described in the brachial artery. Preoperative thrombolytic therapy may be considered for the treatment of the peripheral emboli; however, such distal lesions do not respond well to intra-arterial thrombolytic therapy.

D. Dorsal sympathectomy (D) is not indicated. Dorsal sympathectomy would only provide vasodilatation of the hand and would provide no protection against future embolization.

E. Digital sympathectomy in the hand is of little benefit because local vasodilatation is only short-lived and, again, does not prohibit future distal embolization.

Answer 92-2: B
Discussion 92-2

The median nerve is medial to the brachial artery (A, B) and provides sensory enervation to only the palmar aspects of the thumb and index fingers, with small portions of the dorsal aspects of the tips (D). The ulnar nerve innervates the lumbrical muscles (C). An injury to the median nerve results in difficulties with apposition of the thumb and ring finger, not a claw-hand (E).

Answer 92-3: E
Discussion 92-3

A. Bilateral blood pressure measurements are useful in detecting proximal occlusive lesions (e.g., a chronic subclavian stenosis). A difference in blood pressures between the two extremities of greater than 15 mm is significant. However, because this injury is distal to the brachial artery, an arm pressure measurement is of no use.

B. Splinting of the forearm and continued observation in this setting could soon result in permanent median nerve injury.

C. A duplex ultrasound scan of the artery may be entirely normal because bleeding has occurred in the neurovascular bundle.

D. Arteriography is of no value in detecting median nerve compression.

E. Operative decompression of the median nerve by evacuating the hematoma within the nerve sheath and controlling bleeding from the puncture site, if it has not already stopped (the usual case), is urgently needed to avoid a permanent median nerve deficit. Because the median nerve is within the neurovascular bundle, even a small amount of bleeding will result in nerve compression. Time is of the essence; operative decompression of the median nerve is needed urgently to prevent long-term sequelae.

■ ANSWERS AND DISCUSSION FOR CHAPTER 93

Answer 93-1: B

Discussion 93-1

Vasospasm of the fingers is a local event that occurs by *cooling at the base of the finger.* The opposite (A) is not true. Sympathetic blockade or interruption produces a warm, dry skin surface. Sympathetic stimulation produces a cooled, vasoconstricted hand. (D) Systemic hypotension, not hypertension, is associated with vasospasm. (E) Raynaud's disease is particularly common in young females with low resting blood pressures.

Answer 93-2: A

Discussion 93-2

(A) Scleroderma is found in 20% of patients with Raynaud's syndrome. Conversely, more than 90% of patients with scleroderma will have Raynaud's syndrome. Raynaud's syndrome is less common in patients with (B) mixed connective tissue disease (5%), (C) atherosclerosis (8%), (D) hypersensitive angitis (4%), and (E) Buerger's disease (4%).

Answer 93-3: D

Discussion 93-3

Unilateral Raynaud's disease is a marker for underlying arterial occlusive disease. Bilateral symptoms are associated with a systemic connective tissue disease, which would be diagnosed by (A) complete blood count and (B) antinuclear antibody test, or (C) a hand x-ray film. Arteriography (D) is mandatory in this patient because an underlying structural abnormality is most likely. Underlying abnormalities may represent thoracic outlet compression. Cold recovery time (E) is only appropriate in patients suspected of having primary Raynaud's syndrome with normal digital arteries. Cold recovery time is generally not performed unless there is a normal arterial blood flow study of the upper extremity.

■ ANSWERS AND DISCUSSION FOR CHAPTER 94

Answer 94-1: E

Discussion 94-1

The diagnosis of neurogenic thoracic outlet is made *by exclusion,* excluding all other possible causes of the patient's upper extremity neurologic symptoms. Clinical diagnosis in experienced hands may make this diagnosis almost certain, but certainty is important for effective treatment, physiotherapy, or a possible intervention.

A. Electromyography will rule out peripheral nerve entrapment (cubital or carpal tunnel syndromes). Occasionally, the test result may be positive in true neurogenic thoracic outlet. In these instances, there is motor latency in the median nerve distribution and ulnar sensory abnormalities.

B. A cervical spine x-ray film should be either repeated or the cervical spine x-ray film from the outside institution should be obtained to rule out the presence or absence of cervical ribs or cervical spine pathology.

C. Noninvasive vascular laboratory studies are helpful and should be performed with the arm in provocative positions. Demonstrated compression of the artery implies potential compression of the nerve. The artery and the nerve are closely related anatomically.

D. Magnetic resonance imaging of the cervical spine is needed to rule out any cervical disk disease, syrinx, or other spinal cord abnormalities.

Answer 94-2: D

Discussion 94-2

(D) Neurogenic thoracic outlet is far more common than venous or arterial thoracic outlet, in that order. Approximately 95% of all cases of *symptomatic* thoracic outlet compression are classified as neurogenic, 4% as venous, and 1% as arterial. Thus, A, B, and C are incorrect, and D is correct. (E) Trauma plays a significant role in precipitating symptomatic *neurogenic* thoracic outlet compression, in anatomically susceptible patients, but skeletal abnormalities do not. The latter do play a major role in thoracic outlet *arterial* compression.

Answer 94-3: C

Discussion 94-3

The phrenic nerve passes over the anterior surface of the anterior scalene muscle from lateral to medial. Thus, C is correct and the other answers are wrong. The nerve then passes between the subclavian artery and vein into the thoracic cavity. Temporary phrenic nerve paralysis occurs in approximately 10% of patients undergoing thoracic outlet decompression using the supraclavicular approach or anterior scalenectomy.

■ ANSWERS AND DISCUSSION FOR CHAPTER 95

Answer 95-1: C

Discussion 95-1

A. Lung cancer may present with neurologic symptoms from invasion, but rarely causes arterial compression.

B. A clavicle malunion or callus may compress the artery, but is less common than a cervical rib and clavicular abnormalities, and often causes compression of the vein, which is located more anterior than the artery.
C. This is the correct answer. Most patients with thoracic outlet syndrome have a bony abnormality, and a complete cervical rib is the most common abnormality.
D. Scalene muscles can hypertrophy in throwing athletes and lead to arterial compression, but is less common than cervical ribs.
E. Scalene muscles can hypertrophy in throwing athletes and lead to arterial compression, but again is less common than cervical ribs.

Answer 95-2: E

Discussion 95-2

A. Bilateral symptoms are more common with systemic disorders such as vasculitis, diabetes, and calciphylaxis. Arterial thoracic outlet syndrome is most often unilateral.
B. A dysrhythmia is more consistent with cardiac embolism.
C. Radiation therapy can cause a localized vascular injury with stenosis or embolism that is *not* associated with compression in the thoracic outlet.
D. Aortic aneurysm is not associated with arterial thoracic outlet compression. The latter patients tend to be younger and free of atherosclerotic risk factors.
E. This is the correct answer. Patients with arterial thoracic outlet syndrome often have *unilateral* ischemic symptoms without the usual medical history suggestive of primary arterial pathology.

Answer 95-3: A

Discussion 95-3

A. This is the correct answer. The vagus nerve courses medial to the standard exposure of a cervical rib, outside of the usual operative field.
B. The phrenic nerve lies anterior to the anterior scalene muscle and requires careful attention to reduce risk of injury from direct trauma or retraction.
C. The anterior scalene muscle often needs to be divided to expose the cervical rib. Removal of the anterior scalene muscle helps decompression.
D. The subclavian artery lies anterior to the cervical rib and needs to be retracted to excise the cervical rib.
E. The platysma is divided and subplatysmal flaps are elevated early in the dissection during the supraclavicular approach.

■ ANSWERS AND DISCUSSION FOR CHAPTER 96

Answer 96-1: D

Discussion 96-1

A. Similar to anomalies of the first rib, cervical ribs are also uncommon. Again, the incidence is well less than 1% in many series. Cervical ribs are more commonly associated with arterial injuries.
B. Anomalies of the first rib are extremely uncommon. In screening chest radiography studies, it is between 0.46%

and 1.5%. Although anomalous first rib may produce compression of the subclavian vein by narrowing the costoclavicular space, its likelihood is uncommon.
C. The middle scalene muscle is posterior to the artery and the brachial plexus. Hypertrophy of this muscle is uncommon, and if it were to occur, it would most likely compress the nerve or artery.
D. The subclavian vein passes through the costoclavicular space. Compression of the costoclavicular space occurs by hypertrophy of the subclavius muscle or overuse of the upper extremity as occurs in weight lifters, tennis players, and kick boxers.
E. Hypertrophy of the pectoralis minor muscle would not cause occlusion of the subclavian axillary vein. Hypertrophy of the pectoralis minor muscle does produce arterial occlusion with the arm abducted and externally rotated in professional athletes. Effort vein thrombosis most commonly occurs in the costoclavicular space and not in the subpectoral region.

Answer 96-2: B

Discussion 96-2

A. The venous duplex is a useful screening tool and is noninvasive. However, it is sometimes difficult to perform in muscular patients and has a sensitivity of 94% and a specificity of 96%. Clear visualization of the subclavian vein under the clavicle is difficult, and often the only indication of vein patency is respiratory variation.
B. Venogram is the diagnostic study of choice. The venogram is useful not only in the diagnosis of the condition but also for transcatheter thrombolysis should thrombosis be found.
C. The chest x-ray film may be useful, but it is not diagnostic. The chest x-ray film will rule out any bony anomalies and Pancoast tumors.
D. Chest CT, similar to chest radiography, is useful in identifying bony abnormalities and pulmonary malignancies.
E. Magnetic resonance venography can be performed in the upper extremity but does not provide the clear detail or the therapeutic potential of a venogram.

Answer 96-3: E

Discussion 96-3

A. Pulmonary emboli do occur with upper extremity venous thrombosis. Incidence ranges between 3% and 16% when specifically sought.
B. Because of the possibility of clot propagation and pulmonary emboli, catheter removal alone is not adequate and the patient must be anticoagulated.
C. Unlike patients with effort vein thrombosis or primary subclavian vein thrombosis, long-term disability rarely occurs after subclavian vein thrombosis secondary to catheterization. Few symptoms occur because important collaterals are preserved by the discrete nature of the clotting process.
D. Catheter-related subclavian vein thrombosis is not a marker of a hypercoagulable condition. The most likely cause is secondary to venous trauma in the presence of a foreign body. *Primary* upper extremity venous thrombosis, however, can be a marker of a hypercoagulable condition.

E. Patients with catheter-related subclavian vein thrombosis are best treated with anticoagulation and ace wrapping of the upper extremity. The catheter may be left in place if the patient requires this site for venous access. In general, however, the catheter is removed and replaced in other locations.

■ ANSWERS AND DISCUSSION FOR CHAPTER 97

Answer 97-1: C

Discussion 97-1

A. Hyperhidrosis remains the best indication given its favorable long-term results and high patient satisfaction rates.
B. The treatment of prolonged QT syndrome with sympathectomy is a limited but acceptable alternative for certain patients who are refractory to pharmacologic treatment.
C. The use of sympathectomy for the treatment of angina can be effective in alleviating the symptoms of angina, *but* it does not treat the underlying coronary artery disease; as a result, it does nothing to reduce the risk of death from myocardial infarction, and thus should not be used for this indication.
D. Complex regional pain syndrome, which includes variants formerly called causalgia and reflex sympathetic dystrophy, is a valid indication for sympathectomy, if it has progressed beyond stage I, when it is potentially treatable by medication and physiotherapy and may spontaneously resolve. A dramatic response to sympathetic block, lasting the duration of the anesthetic agent used, is the best approach to patient selection.
E. Sympathectomy is effective in reducing the exaggerated vasomotor response to cold exposure and can be used in severely symptomatic patients who have not received relief from, or cannot tolerate, calcium blockers or other drugs and in whom cold avoidance (moving or changing jobs) is not practical. However, in time, some restoration of sympathetic tone is common, leaving patients improved but not asymptomatic. This outcome was not acceptable in the past with open sympathectomy but is less objectionable when it can be performed endoscopically.

Answer 97-2: B

Discussion 97-2

A. Sympathectomy is well established as an effective treatment for essential hyperhidrosis, with overall success rates ranging from 93% to 100%.
B. Contrary to concerns of the past concerning bilateral lumbar sympathectomy, L2-3 ganglionic chain sympathectomy does not cause impotence, but by causing retrograde ejaculation, it can cause sterility in younger patients. Sympathectomy performed at the time of aorto-iliac surgery led to concerns over impotence, but the additional dissection of pre-aortic and pre-iliac fibers (unlike L2-L3 ganglionectomy), or the reconstructive procedure itself, may well have been responsible.

C. Sympathectomy reduces cold-induced vasospasm, but its application for primary Raynaud's disease is limited because of gradual return of intrinsic vasomotor tone.
D. Sympathectomy can relieve anginal pain but is not used for this because it does nothing for the underlying coronary disease that causes it and may remove a valuable warning symptom.
E. Sympathectomy is associated with postoperative neuralgia, in dermatomes adjacent to the level of ganglionectomy, in 25% to 45% of patients. It appears 1 week postoperatively and can last 4 to 6 weeks, but subsides spontaneously.

Answer 97-3: B

Discussion 97-3

A. The incidence of Horner's syndrome ranges from 0% to 40% but can be minimized by avoiding damage to the stellate ganglion.
B. Compensatory hyperhidrosis is by far the most common complication, with occurrence rates reported as high as 100%. It is most prominent in the dermatome distribution below the level of ganglionectomy. The mechanism of compensatory hyperhidrosis is complex and may involve factors including genetics, climate, and individual changes in the thermoregulatory process.
C. "Intercostal" neuralgia is also an important potential complication, reportedly occurring in up to one third of patients, and is usually transient.
D. Injury to the vagus nerve is rare when proper surgical technique and patient selection are performed.
E. Injury to the phrenic nerve, a complication seen with the open supraclavicular approach to dorsal sympathectomy, should not occur with the thoracoscopic technique.

■ ANSWERS AND DISCUSSION FOR CHAPTER 98

Answer 98-1: D

Discussion 98-1

A. HHS predominantly affects the ulnar artery because of its superficial location in the hypothenar eminence of the hand.
B. The cause of HHS is thought to be repetitive localized trauma to a focal area of the vessel. The most characteristic form of trauma is in the form of blunt trauma such as experienced at work by carpenters and mechanics.
C. One of the recognized long-term sequelae of HHS is localized aneurysm formation as the result of destruction of the media of the vessel wall. Others may develop segmental arterial occlusion because of intimal injury.
D. HHS is found only in the ulnar artery, in the wrist, not in the forearm.
E. Recent reports suggest that fibromuscular dysplasia may be an underlying factor in the development of HHS.

Answer 98-2: D

Discussion 98-2

Compression of (D) the posterior humeral circumflex artery within the quadrilateral space has been shown to occur with the arm in the "cocked" position (abduction and external rotation). Chronic compression and trauma to this artery among throwing athletes, particularly pitchers, can lead to aneurysmal dilation or occlusion. Aneurysms in this location are prone to distal embolization in the hand.

Answer 98-3: A

Discussion 98-3

"Quadrilateral space syndrome" is most frequently found among throwing athletes, particularly pitchers. The quadrilateral space is defined as the area bordered by (B) the teres minor superiorly, (D) the humeral shaft laterally, (C) the teres major inferiorly, and (E) the long head of the triceps muscle medially. The clavicle (A) is not involved. Found within this space are the posterior humeral circumflex artery and the axillary nerve. Chronic compression and trauma caused by excessive, repetitive abduction and external rotation of the arm can lead to the development of arterial occlusion or aneurysmal formation of the posterior circumflex artery. Small aneurysms in this space are prone to distal embolization. These can be diagnosed by angiography and may require surgical ligation for definitive treatment.

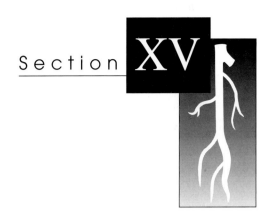

ARTERIAL ANEURYSMS

STUDY QUESTIONS

■ QUESTIONS FOR CHAPTER 99

Question 99-1

Arterial enlargement greater than 50% of normal diameter diffusely involving several adjacent arteries is termed:

A. Ectasia.
B. Aneurysm.
C. Arteriomegaly.
D. Aneurysmosis.
E. Multiple aneurysms.

Question 99-2

The most common cause for an AAA is:

A. Degeneration.
B. Dissection.
C. Infection.
D. Anastomotic disruption.
E. Connective tissue disorder.

Question 99-3

Most false aneurysms:

A. Contain only two layers of the normal arterial wall.
B. Are caused by infection.
C. Are iatrogenic.
D. Occur at arterial anastomoses.
E. Require surgical treatment.

■ QUESTIONS FOR CHAPTER 100

Question 100-1

Which of the following *correctly* applies? AAAs:

A. Can be reliably detected by a careful physical examination if the diameter is greater than 4 cm.
B. Can be treated effectively with beta-blockade to prevent expansion.
C. Are more likely to rupture in men than women at a given diameter.
D. Will require repair within 3 years in the majority of patients with initial diameters of 4.0 to 5.5 cm in a surveillance program using a diameter of greater than 5.5 cm or symptoms as indications for intervention.
E. Carry a related mortality (from elective repair or rupture) that cannot be reduced by ultrasound screening in men aged 65 to 75 years.

Question 100-2

Which of the following is *true*? Elective AAA repair:

A. Should be recommended to all patients with AAA diameter greater than 5.5 cm.
B. Is associated with an average operative mortality for open repair of approximately 5% in the United States.
C. Mortality in individual patients is influenced more by cardiac disease than pulmonary or renal disease.
D. Will result in a 5-year life expectancy equivalent to the general population.
E. Should not be performed without preoperative arteriography.

Question 100-3

Which of the following is *true*? Repair of AAAs:

A. With involvement of visceral and renal arteries is associated with no increased risk of morbidity and mortality compared with infrarenal AAA.
B. Followed by diarrhea in the first 48 hours is indicative of an early return of normal gastrointestinal function.
C. That are inflammatory is best performed through an anterior transperitoneal approach.
D. Should be aborted if an incidental colon cancer is detected at laparotomy.
E. Should be performed with perioperative beta-blockade in almost all patients.

■ QUESTIONS FOR CHAPTER 101

Question 101-1

A 60-year-old woman with several myocardial infarctions in her history presents with an infrarenal AAA of 6 cm in diameter. The left common iliac artery is aneurysmal (3 cm in diameter). The right common iliac artery has a diameter of 1.8 cm. The preferred option for endovascular treatment is the following:

A. Aorto-aortic straight tube graft repair.
B. Aorto-uniiliac endograft repair to the left external iliac artery with coil embolization of the left hypogastric artery, occluder-cuff blocking of the right common iliac artery, and femorofemoral bypass.
C. Aorto-biiliac repair with extension of the left iliac limb to the external iliac artery. In addition, a coil occlusion of the left hypogastric artery will be performed.

D. Aorto-biiliac endografting to both common iliac arteries, using a 36-mm wide left iliac limb (bell-bottom stent-graft iliac limb configuration).
E. Conventional surgical aneurysm repair.

Question 101-2

A 73-year-old man was treated 3 years ago by implantation of an aorto-biiliac modular endograft for an infrarenal AAA. The diameter of the aneurysm at the first postoperative CT examination was 62 mm. Follow-up CT scans have been performed at 6, 12, 18, and 24 months. A gradual increase to a diameter of 70 mm was noted. No evidence of endoleakage has been observed at any of the CT scans or at arteriography, despite the use of multiple projections and contrast injections at different levels proximal, within, and distal from the reconstruction. Intra-aneurysmal pressure measurement by direct translumbar puncture was performed, and a pulsatile pressure wave (130 mm Hg systolic, 100 mm Hg mean pressure) was recorded. The patient was in good medical condition. The next step in the management of this patient with *endotension* of the aneurysm should involve:

A. Conversion to open surgical repair of the expanding aneurysm.
B. Continuation of a wait-and-see policy.
C. Laparoscopic clipping of lumbar arteries and the inferior mesenteric artery.
D. Translumbar puncture of the aneurysm, aneurysmography, and coil embolization of any lumbar artery that communicates with the aneurysm sac.
E. A "banding" procedure (ligature around the infrarenal neck).

Question 101-3

A 50-year-old man was treated by endograft repair for a 6.2-cm large aneurysm 6 months previously. Spiral CT examination demonstrated a type II endoleak from a lumbar artery. The aneurysm diameter has remained unchanged since the procedure. What would you propose for further management in this patient?

A. Laparoscopic clipping of the lumbar artery.
B. Intra-aneurysmal pressure measurements by direct translumbar puncture of the sac.
C. Selective catheterization of the lumbar artery through a hypogastric artery and coil embolization.
D. Continuation of surveillance by CT examination at 6-month intervals.
E. Conversion to open surgical repair of the aneurysm.

■ **QUESTIONS FOR CHAPTER 102**

Question 102-1

During repair of a ruptured AAA (RAAA), which of the following statements are *true*?

A. The use of the retroperitoneal exposure has been shown to have adverse effects on outcome.
B. Red cell salvage can reduce the need for banked coagulation products.
C. Inadvertent arterial or venous injuries do not significantly increase mortality.

D. Abdominal closure without significant tension is possible in the majority of cases.
E. Hypothermia is not associated with any adverse clinical events.

Question 102-2

A successful open RAAA repair has been performed and the patient is currently 48 hours postoperative and remains in the intensive care unit. Which of the following statements regarding the prognosis for survival is true?

A. Although infrequent, the development of colon ischemia is a highly lethal complication.
B. Renal dysfunction requiring dialysis is not associated with a statistically significantly worse prognosis.
C. Myocardial infarction is rare in this patient population; however, it does negatively affect prognosis.
D. Respiratory dysfunction is common; however, it is easily supported by modern day ventilators and does not have an overall negative effect on short- and long-term prognoses.
E. Multiple organ dysfunction after RAAA is a relatively uncommon cause of death.

Question 102-3

The intervention that is most likely to reduce the *overall* mortality secondary to RAAA is:

A. Endovascular AAA repair.
B. Anti-inflammatory drugs, which help prevent the development of organ dysfunction after RAAA.
C. Better training of first responders (emergency department physicians and nurses) to improve early recognition of patients with RAAA.
D. Widespread screening programs that identify asymptomatic aneurysms.
E. Better prediction of AAA rupture risk using new technology.

■ **QUESTIONS FOR CHAPTER 103**

Question 103-1

The use of adjunct distal aortic perfusion and cerebrospinal fluid (CSF) drainage has reduced the incidence of immediate neurologic deficit after thoracoabdominal aortic repair to:

A. 2.4%.
B. 6.8%.
C. 10%.
D. 29%.
E. 1.2%.

Question 103-2

Which of the following describes the extent V thoracoabdominal aortic aneurysm (TAAA)?

A. The aneurysm begins distal to the left subclavian artery and ends above the renal arteries.
B. The aneurysm begins distal to the left subclavian artery and ends below the renal arteries.
C. The aneurysm begins from the sixth intercostal space and ends below the renal arteries.

D. The aneurysm begins from the sixth intercostal space and ends above the renal arteries.

E. The aneurysm begins from the twelfth intercostal space and ends below the renal arteries.

Question 103-3

A 68-year-old man underwent repair of TAAA, extent II. The patient awoke neurologically intact. On postoperative day 2, the patient developed delayed paraplegia. The patient's *mean* arterial blood pressure was 50 mm Hg and hemoglobin level was 7.0 g/dL. His CSF drain was blocked. What should be undertaken to reverse the delayed neurologic deficit?

A. Immediately take measures to increase the patient's blood pressure aiming for a mean arterial pressure of 90 mm Hg or greater, to improve spinal cord perfusion.

B. Transfuse packed red blood cells to improve oxygen-carrying capacity.

C. Immediately reinstitute free CSF drainage by either readjusting the existing CSF catheter or inserting a new one.

D. A, B, and C.

E. Delayed neurologic deficit cannot be reversed by any of the above measures.

■ QUESTIONS FOR CHAPTER 104

Question 104-1

Mortality associated with acute proximal (Stanford type A, DeBakey type I) aortic dissection:

A. Is equivalent to distal (Stanford type B) dissections because of equal risk of aortic rupture.

B. Increases in patients with Marfan syndrome.

C. Is largely related to the central cardioaortic complications of aortic rupture, coronary artery compromise, and aortic valve disruption.

D. Is less than 5% when emergency ascending aortic repair is undertaken.

E. Is unrelated to the anatomic extent or complexity of the dissection process.

Question 104-2

Clinical features and diagnostic testing in acute aortic dissection indicate:

A. Clinical signs and symptoms are generally indistinguishable from acute coronary syndromes and pulmonary embolism.

B. Diagnostic attention should be focused on those patients with risk factor profiles typical for atherosclerotic cardiovascular disease.

C. Severe hypertension is nearly universal at presentation, as is a history of hypertension.

D. Plain chest radiography and surface echocardiography in combination provide effective diagnostic sensitivity and specificity.

E. Fine-cut, contrast-enhanced CT scanning is both an effective and the most commonly used diagnostic modality.

Question 104-3

Aortic branch compromise from acute dissection:

A. Is nearly always corrected by a definitive proximal aortic grafting procedure.

B. Always produces clinical sequelae requiring invasive intervention.

C. Is definitively diagnosed by contrast-enhanced CT scanning.

D. Has variant mechanisms and implications for therapy.

E. Always produces relevant clinical sequelae within minutes to hours of symptom onset.

■ QUESTIONS FOR CHAPTER 105

Question 105-1

Which of the following statements about femoral aneurysms is *true*?

A. The presence of a femoral aneurysm is an indication for surgical repair in the majority of cases.

B. The diameter must be at least 2.5 cm to qualify as a femoral artery aneurysm.

C. Femoral aneurysms may be associated with pain caused by nerve compression.

D. Because of its superficial location, femoral aneurysm can be reliably diagnosed by physical examination alone.

E. The best treatment of a femoral aneurysm is noninvasive endovascular treatment with a stent graft.

Question 105-2

Which of the following statements about popliteal aneurysms is *true*?

A. The presence of a popliteal aneurysm in association with aneurysms of the abdominal aorta is more common than the reverse, the presence of AAAs in association with the finding of a popliteal artery aneurysm.

B. Popliteal aneurysms are often caused by repetitive trauma by compression between the gastrocnemius muscle and the femur condyle.

C. Close to one third of the patients who have popliteal aneurysms present without symptoms.

D. Popliteal aneurysms are a common finding in patients with absent pedal pulses caused by silent distal embolization from the aneurysm.

E. Until popliteal aneurysms become more than 2 cm in diameter, the diameter is not relevant for the occurrence of symptoms.

Question 105-3

Which of the following statements about popliteal aneurysm treatment is *true*?

A. A popliteal aneurysm with a diameter of 3 cm can be followed safely. The risk of ischemia is low, and if this complication occurs, it can easily be treated with thrombolysis.

B. Popliteal aneurysms should be treated by proximal and distal ligation in combination with a bypass anastomosed end to side both proximally and distally.

C. In acute thrombosis producing ischemia with an incomplete neurologic deficit, angiography and catheter thrombolysis are preferred first as initial treatment to clear the outflow vessels.

D. A small popliteal aneurysm in combination with absent distal pulses is an indication for surgical repair.

E. In a patient with both a 6-cm asymptomatic aortic aneurysm and a popliteal aneurysm that also has an indication for treatment, the aortic aneurysm should be treated first because of the risk of rupture.

■ QUESTIONS FOR CHAPTER 106

Question 106-1

Proximal subclavian artery aneurysms are:

A. Usually syphilitic in origin.
B. Usually repaired through a supraclavicular incision.
C. Associated with aortoiliac and other peripheral aneurysms.
D. Best treated by an endograft.
E. Usually asymptomatic until rupture.

Question 106-2

Axillary-subclavian artery aneurysms associated with cervical ribs:

A. Are most commonly encountered in male athletes.
B. May be treated with long-term anticoagulant therapy if intraluminal thrombus is present.
C. Should be treated only if symptomatic.
D. Are best treated with aneurysm resection, removal of the cervical and possibly the first rib, and vein graft replacement.
E. Require clavicular resection for adequate operative exposure.

Question 106-3

Ulnar artery aneurysms:

A. Are usually congenital in origin.
B. Usually present as a pulsatile mass in the hypothenar area.
C. Often cause digital ischemia to the first three fingers.
D. Are best treated with a small-caliber vein graft using microvascular reconstructive techniques.
E. Do not respond well to lytic therapy.

■ QUESTIONS FOR CHAPTER 107

Question 107-1

Which is the correct *order of decreasing frequency* of the splanchnic artery aneurysms included in the answers?

A. Splenic artery, hepatic artery, celiac artery, superior mesenteric artery (SMA).
B. SMA, celiac artery, hepatic artery, splenic artery.
C. Hepatic artery, splenic artery, celiac artery, SMA.

D. Splenic artery, hepatic artery, SMA, celiac artery.
E. Celiac artery, splenic artery, SMA, hepatic artery.

Question 107-2

A 36-year-old grand multiparous woman presents to the emergency department with severe left upper quadrant pain and dizziness. On physical examination, she is found to have a blood pressure of 90/60 mm Hg that responds to 1 L of fluid. A hematocrit is drawn and is 31%. However, she feels much better after receiving intravenous (IV) fluid and is leaving the emergency department when she collapses. The likely diagnosis is:

A. Splenic artery aneurysm.
B. Hepatic artery aneurysm.
C. SMA aneurysm.
D. Ruptured AAA.
E. Gastroduodenal artery aneurysm.

Question 107-3

Categorically, the most common reported cause of *all* hepatic artery aneurysms is:

A. Mycosis.
B. Biliary sepsis.
C. Atherosclerosis.
D. Medial degeneration.
E. Traumatic pseudoaneurysms.

■ QUESTIONS FOR CHAPTER 108

Question 108-1

As originally described, *mycotic* aneurysms occur as a complication of which of the following?

A. Endocarditis.
B. Microbial arteritis arising from bacteremia.
C. Bacterial transformation of existing aneurysms.
D. Septic needle puncture of a normal artery.
E. Fungus infection of an existing aneurysm.

Question 108-2

Which of the following strategies is appropriate in the management of an infected aneurysm presenting as an emergency, with sepsis?

A. Avoid operation in septic patients; a better outcome will be obtained after extended treatment with antibiotics.
B. After control of hemorrhage, debride all infected or devitalized tissue.
C. At operation, only obtain aerobic cultures because open operations remove the opportunity to obtain valid anaerobic cultures. Anaerobic cultures can only be obtained under closed circumstances, for example, in a radiology suite by CT or ultrasound-guided needle aspiration.
D. Never reestablish direct arterial continuity during the first operation, because it will usually lead to later hemorrhage from an infected anastomosis.
E. The anastomosis should be wrapped in adipose tissue excised from the omentum.

Question 108-3

Which statement regarding the vascular surgical complication encountered by narcotic addicts "shooting" drugs obtained on the "street" is supported by clinical experience?

A. First-time users are the patients most likely to experience an infected false aneurysm of the femoral artery. Experienced users have learned how to avoid them.

B. Once the superficial veins of the upper and lower extremity are no longer available, most parenteral drug users switch to smoking "crack."

C. Blood cultures usually grow out a single dominant organism, predominantly a *Staphylococcus aureus*.

D. These patients require no special precautions against hepatitis and human immunodeficiency virus.

E. None of the above.

ANSWERS AND DISCUSSION

■ ANSWERS AND DISCUSSION FOR CHAPTER 99

Answer 99-1: C

Discussion 99-1

A. Ectasia is arterial dilation less than 50% of normal diameter.
B. Aneurysm is a localized arterial dilation more than 50% of normal diameter.
C. Arteriomegaly is diffuse arterial enlargement greater than 50% diameter, involving several different arterial segments, without focal discrete aneurysms.
D. Aneurysmosis is a term applied to patients with multiple discrete aneurysms.
E. Multiple aneurysms are discrete isolated aneurysms involving different arteries.

Answer 99-2: A

Discussion 99-2

A. Most AAAs result from a complex biologic process in which there is a degeneration of connective tissue within the aneurysm. They are usually associated with atherosclerotic changes in older patients, but represent a distinctly different process than occlusive atherosclerosis, and are better termed degenerative than atherosclerotic.
B. Dissection is the cause of many if not most thoracic aneurysms, but causes only a small percentage of AAAs. After an arterial dissection, the wall of false channel, consisting of only part of the normal mural components, is subject to dilation and aneurysm formation.
C. Infection is the most frequent cause of superior mesenteric aneurysms, but is a rare, albeit complicated cause of AAAs.
D. Anastomotic disruption causing a false aneurysm after arterial reconstruction most commonly occurs in the femoral artery after aortofemoral bypass, but much less commonly occurs at an abdominal aortic anastomosis.
E. Connective tissue disorders, most frequently Marfan syndrome, can cause AAAs, but this is an uncommon cause.

Answer 99-3: C

Discussion 99-3

A. Classically false, or pseudo-aneurysms are described as not containing all three layers of the arterial wall, to differentiate them from true aneurysms. Most false aneurysms, however, contain none of the normal arterial layers, but rather begin as a contained hematoma arising from a localized disruption in an artery and thus consist of organized surrounding connective tissue.
B. Although infection can result in local arterial disruption and a resulting false aneurysm, this is not a common cause.
C. Because of the steady proliferation of percutaneous catheter-based procedures, iatrogenic injury of the common femoral artery has become the most common cause of arterial pseudoaneurysm. Many of these resolve spontaneously, and many are now treated with compression or percutaneous thrombin injection to induce thrombosis of this contained hematoma.
D. Once the most common cause of false aneurysms, disruption of arterial (usually femoral) anastomoses has been substantially overtaken by iatrogenic catheter injury as the most common cause of false aneurysm.
E. Most false aneurysms result from femoral artery iatrogenic trauma and can be treated with ultrasound-guided thrombin injection. Surgical treatment is required for some, and for most of those involving bypass graft disruption, although endovascular treatment is now possible for some anastomotic aneurysms.

■ ANSWERS AND DISCUSSION FOR CHAPTER 100

Answer 100-1: D

Discussion 100-1

A. AAAs are detected by a careful physical examination in only 50% of AAAs 4 to 5 cm and only 75% of AAAs greater than 5 cm. Ultrasound and CT are reliable methods of detecting AAA.
B. Although animal studies suggested beta-blockade might reduce AAA expansion, this has not been observed in subsequent human trials.
C. AAAs are more likely to rupture in women than men at a given diameter. This is likely because of the relatively smaller diameter of the normal aorta in women compared with men.
D. In both the United Kingdom and ADAM trials, more than half of the patients randomized to surveillance underwent repair of their AAA within 3 years of randomization. For those with AAA diameters 5.0 to 5.4 cm, more than three fourths eventually underwent repair.
E. Several randomized and nonrandomized trials have demonstrated approximately 50% reduction in AAA-related mortality with ultrasound screening in men aged more than 65 years.

Answer 100-2: B

Discussion 100-2

A. In addition to the rupture risk associated with an AAA greater than 5.5 cm, one must also consider the operative risk and life expectancy of the individual patient to determine whether prophylactic AAA repair is appropriate, rather than apply this threshold diameter to ALL patients.
B. Although centers with high volume and surgeons with high volume have lower mortality rates, the *average* mortality in the United States for elective AAA repair is approximately 5%.
C. Renal failure is associated with a threefold increased risk of death, whereas cardiac and pulmonary diseases are associated with an approximate twofold increased risk of death after AAA repair.
D. Life expectancy after AAA repair is lower than that of the general population, likely because of the increased prevalence of comorbid disease in this population.

E. Routine infrarenal AAA repair in patients without significant occlusive disease can safely be performed without preoperative arteriography. In centers with appropriate experience, CT angiography can provide adequate imaging to obviate arteriography even in patients with occlusive or aneurysmal disease of the iliac, renal, and visceral vessels.

Answer 100-3: E

Discussion 100-3

A. Suprarenal AAA and type IV thoracoabdominal aneurysms are associated with increased operative mortality and increased risk of renal failure. Most surgeons therefore use a higher diameter threshold to recommend open repair of these aneurysms.

B. Early diarrhea after AAA repair is suggestive of colon ischemia and should prompt investigation with sigmoidoscopy. This complication can be minimized by reimplantation of a patent inferior mesenteric artery that does not have pulsatile back bleeding after restoration of aortic flow to the lower extremities.

C. Inflammatory aneurysms are associated with a dense fibrosis that lies mostly anteriorly and frequently involves the duodenum. The posterolateral aorta is often spared facilitating repair approached from that direction (i.e., using the left retroperitoneal approach).

D. Nonobstructing, asymptomatic colon cancer, with no metastases, can be treated *after* recovery from the AAA repair. Obstructing colon cancer should in general be treated before AAA repair.

E. Several randomized trials have demonstrated a lower morbidity and mortality related to cardiac events with the routine use of perioperative beta-blockade. There are very few absolute contraindications to its use.

■ ANSWERS AND DISCUSSION FOR CHAPTER 101

Answer 101-1: C

Discussion 101-1

A. Straight tube endografts have largely been abandoned for the treatment of AAAs. The distal aortic cuff (adjacent to the bifurcation) is rarely of adequate length to provide durable sealing and fixation.

B. Aorto-uniiliac endografts may be used in case one of the iliac arteries is occluded and cannot be successfully treated by angioplasty. Another indication for use of aorto-uniiliac devices is emergency aneurysm repair, because expedient exclusion of the aneurysm can be obtained. There is no particular advantage of this device configuration in patients with common iliac aneurysm.

C. Aorto-biiliac endograft repair with iliac limb extension into the external iliac artery is currently the treatment of choice in case of an iliac aneurysm. Coil occlusion of the ipsilateral hypogastric artery is indicated to avoid a type II reperfusion endoleak. In the near future new devices consisting of an iliac endograft with a side branch into the hypogastric artery may come into use in cases with common iliac aneurysms.

D. Bell-bottomed stent grafts should be limited to mildly aneurysmal common iliac arteries (<30 mm).

E. The risk from open surgery in this cardiac-compromised patient may be prohibitive.

Answer 101-2: A

Discussion 101-2

A. Conversion to open surgery is considered the preferable treatment in patients with typical endotension, provided the medical condition of the patient is acceptable. Large-diameter aneurysms are considered to increase the risk of post-endovascular abdominal aneurysm repair rupture.

B. A wait-and-see policy is not justified in a patient with progressive expansion.

C. Laparoscopic clipping of lumbar arteries may be attempted when culprit lumbar arteries are visualized.

D. Translumbar puncture of the aneurysm and trans-sac coil embolization was demonstrated as an effective procedure. However, a visualized type II lumbar artery endoleak is a prerequisite for this procedure.

E. In a proven type I proximal endoleak, a banding procedure may be used to obtain a proximal seal. However, this procedure is not indicated in a typical case with endotension.

Answer 101-3: D

Discussion 101-3

A. Laparoscopic clipping of type II endoleaks was demonstrated to be an effective procedure. However, if the aneurysm is not expanding, observation and CT surveillance only are preferable.

B. Direct translumbar sac pressure measurement is helpful in determining the indication for further interventions in cases of endotension (with growth of the aneurysm). If there is no gradual expansion, measurement of the intrasac pressure will not determine clinical management.

C. Type II endoleaks only need treatment in case of aneurysm expansion.

D. Type II endoleaks without expansion are benign findings. However, surveillance at 6-month intervals is indicated because the possibility of late-onset expansion has not been ruled out at this time.

E. Conversion to open surgical repair is only indicated in cases in which no adequate endovascular treatment can be offered in cases with type II endoleak associated with aneurysm growth.

■ ANSWERS AND DISCUSSION FOR CHAPTER 102

Answer 102-1: D

Discussion 102-1

A. The retroperitoneal incision in a retrospective study has been shown to have some benefits (less hypotension) and reduced mortality. Thus, it does not have a *negative* effect on outcome.

B. Red cell salvage can reduce the need to red blood cells; however, coagulation products are removed, and thus using red cell salvage does not reduce replacement of coagulation products.

C. Inadvertent arterial and venous injuries contribute significantly to the mortality in this patient population. They are present in up to 68% of those who die of this condition.

D. The abdomen can be closed without undo tension in approximately 70% of patients. However, a temporary mesh can be useful in the 25% to 30% whose abdomens cannot be closed and is suggested to reduce the incidence of abdominal compartment syndrome, renal failure, and possibly the incidence of multiple organ dysfunction.

E. Hypothermia is associated with an increase the incidence of coagulopathy, wound infection, and cardiac events.

Answer 102-2: A

Discussion 102-2

A. Colon ischemia is infrequent (3%–13%); however, it is highly lethal (73%–100%). Thus, this statement is true.

B. Renal dysfunction is common; however, the development of dialysis-dependent renal failure has a much poorer prognosis, with a 76% to 89% mortality.

C. Myocardial infarction is not rare; it is a common complication and has a negative effect on early and late survival.

D. Respiratory dysfunction is common with an incidence of 26% to 47%. It does have a negative predictive effect on both early and late survival.

E. Multiple organ dysfunction is a common cause of death in patients with RAAA. Some recent articles suggest that this may be the most common cause of postoperative death.

Answer 102-3: D

Discussion 102-3

A. Endovascular AAA repair of RAAA is still in its infancy. It requires specially trained individuals, with access to a selection of devices and the team at the ready to facilitate implantation. This therapy has early promising results (lower mortality in selected cases); however, general access to the technology is limited to date. The mortality is still at least 20%.

B. The development of anti-inflammatory therapy has received a lot attention; however, no therapy has yet to be identified in humans that is promising enough to form the basis of a randomized clinical trial. Although this remains a possibility, such an approach is far from clinical practice at present.

C. Early recognition by first responders may be worthwhile; however, once an aneurysm has ruptured, the mortality is between 68% and 90%. So although this approach may be useful, it is unlikely to change the natural history of the disease and its overall mortality impact.

D. Randomized and nonrandomized trials have conclusively shown that screening for AAAs can reduce AAA-related mortality by 42% to 64%. Thus, screening, by identifying those with AAAs and candidates for elective repair, can reduce the incidence of RAAA and its impact on overall mortality more than any other single intervention at the present time.

E. Better prediction of rupture may help a proportion of the population with an AAA. However, the majority of patients who present with an RAAA were previously asymptomatic and unaware they had an aneurysm. Thus, better prediction of rupture will not help those in whom an AAA is not identified.

■ ANSWERS AND DISCUSSION FOR CHAPTER 103

Answer 103-1: A

Discussion 103-1

A. The use of adjunct distal aortic perfusion and CSF drainage has reduced the incidence of immediate neurologic deficit after thoracoabdominal aortic repair to 2.4%.

B. The incidence of immediate neurologic deficit after thoracoabdominal aortic repair *without adjunct* is 6.8%.

C. The current average reported *30-day mortality* for thoracoabdominal aortic repair is approximately 10%.

D. In the clamp-and-sew era, patients with extent II TAAA had the highest incidence of neurologic deficit at 29% (without adjuncts).

E. This is achievable only in selected low-risk subsets.

Answer 103-2: D

Discussion 103-2

A. Extent I TAAA begins distal to the left subclavian artery and ends above the renal arteries.

B. Extent II TAAA begins distal to the left subclavian artery and ends below the renal arteries. Extent II TAAA is the most extensive type and is still associated with the highest risk of neurologic deficit and death. With the current use of adjunct distal aortic perfusion and CSF drainage, the classification may be simplified as extent II versus non-II.

C. Extent III TAAA begins from the sixth intercostal space and ends below the renal arteries.

D. Extent V TAAA begins from the sixth intercostal space and ends above the renal arteries. The use of a classification system is helpful when it has clinical significance. With the addition of extent V (which used to be classified as either I or III) to Crawford's original classification, we have found that extent III TAAA incurred a higher risk of neurologic deficit.

E. Extent IV TAAA begins from the twelfth intercostal space and ends below the renal arteries, also known as total AAA.

Answer 103-3: D

Discussion 103-3

A. When a patient develops delayed neurologic deficit after thoracoabdominal aortic repair, it is frequently associated with hypotension. Increasing the patient's blood pressure, aiming for a mean arterial pressure of 90 mm Hg or greater, with infusion of blood products (packed red blood cells and fresh frozen plasma), fluid solutions (crystalloid and colloid), or vasopressors if necessary, can help reverse the delayed neurologic deficit. However, only increasing the blood pressure may not be sufficient.

B. Similarly, transfusion of packed red blood cells increases the oxygen-carrying capacity and helps reverse delayed neurologic deficit but may not be sufficient without additional measures.

C. Restoring free CSF drainage is an important step in reversing delayed neurologic deficit but by itself may not be sufficient. We have observed that all patients who developed delayed neurologic deficit but did not have CSF drainage failed to recover function.

D. Delayed neurologic deficit can occur as early as 2 hours and as late as 2 weeks after surgery in 2.7% of patients. We have found no single risk factor responsible for delayed neurologic deficit. However, using multivariable analysis, we identified acute dissection, extent II TAAA, and renal insufficiency as significant preoperative predictors for delayed-onset neurologic deficit. In addition, we have subsequently found that postoperative mean arterial pressure of less than 60 mm Hg and CSF drain complications were significant postoperative predictors in the development of delayed-onset neurologic deficit, independent of preoperative predictors. To optimize postoperative spinal cord perfusion in patients with delayed neurologic deficit, we drain CSF and keep the mean arterial pressure greater than 90 to 100 mm Hg, hemoglobin greater than 10 mg/dL, and cardiac index greater than 2.0 L/min.

E. Delayed neurologic deficit can be reversed. With our multifaceted approach, we have seen improvement in 57% of our patients who developed delayed neurologic deficit. Seventy-five percent of patients recovered function when the CSF drain was still in place at the onset of delayed neurologic deficit; 43% recovered neurologic function if the CSF drain had to be reinserted at the time of the delayed neurologic deficit.

■ ANSWERS AND DISCUSSION FOR CHAPTER 104

Answer 104-1: C
Discussion 104-1

A. Overall mortality for DeBakey type I dissections is increased compared with more distal (DeBakey type III) dissections related both to a much increased risk of early rupture and the necessity (in the majority of patients) for urgent ascending aortic graft replacement. In addition to rupture risk, central nervous system complications, particularly spontaneous and perioperative stroke, are generally seen only with type I dissections.

B. Patients with Marfan syndrome typically sustain acute type I dissection in the circumstance of aneurysmal dilatation of the aortic root. Accordingly, prophylactic repair of such root aneurysms is indicated in young people with Marfan syndrome. Despite unique potential technical issues related to aortic valve reconstruction, patients with Marfan syndrome tend to be younger and do well with surgical treatment in both acute and elective settings.

C. This fact constitutes the rationale for urgent ascending aortic graft replacement for most patients with acute type I dissections. Exceptions include those patients with profound neurologic deficits at presentation and those in whom some other (aside from the potential complications listed above) vascular complication (e.g., abdominal aortic obstructions or mesenteric vascular compromise) constitutes the immediate threat to life and therefore assumes treatment priority.

D. Operative mortality when urgent ascending aortic repair is performed for acute dissection generally runs in the 20% range, even in series reported from major centers.

E. Mortality increases as a function of the extent and complexity of the dissection. Independent of aortic rupture, the presence of additional aortic branch compromise, particularly that causing stroke and mesenteric vascular insufficiency, clearly increases overall mortality.

Answer 104-2: E
Discussion 104-2

A. Abrupt onset of severe chest and/or back pain is present in more than 90% of patients with acute dissection. Because this is described as "the worst ever" by some 90% of patients, a typical corollary is that the patient seeks medical attention shortly after symptom onset. Acute coronary syndromes have a much broader range of pain severity and acuity; acute pulmonary embolism may be painless.

B. Not true. Acute dissection, particularly proximal dissections frequently occur in patients less than 60 years of age. Degenerative aortic disease is not, per se, a risk factor for development of acute dissection, although a dissecting process can complicate a preexistent degenerative aneurysm

C. This often-quoted clinical sign is, in fact, not true. Less than 50% of patients presenting with acute dissection display severe hypertension. With respect to a history of treatment for hypertension, there is distinction between proximal (younger patients, ≈50% with history of hypertension) and distal dissections. The latter patients are on average 10 years older, and some 75% will relate a history of hypertension.

D. Although abnormal chest radiography findings occur commonly in acute dissection, these are nonspecific and almost never diagnostic. Technical limitations on aortic imaging limit the utility of transthoracic echocardiography. However, transesophageal echocardiography has high sensitivity and specificity, making it a useful diagnostic modality in the acute setting.

E. Because of its accuracy (specificity approaches 100%) and availability, contrast-enhanced CT scanning is the most widely applied initial diagnostic modality in acute dissection. The entire aorta should be imaged, both to define the extent of dissection and initiate evaluation and potential treatment of vascular complications related to the dissection. Defining whether the ascending aorta is involved can be a limitation, but this can be pursued with transesophageal echocardiography. Aortography is generally not needed in contemporary practice as a diagnostic modality, nor is it generally helpful before ascending aortic graft replacement. Its use is limited to those circumstances wherein an endovascular intervention is contemplated.

Answer 104-3: D

Discussion 104-3

A. The anatomic goals of "definitive" proximal aortic grafting, whether performed by open surgical or endovascular stent graft repair, are to repair/resect the entry tear (thereby eliminating the risk of rupture) and reconstruct the aortic wall layers. The latter, at least, in theory, eliminates false lumen flow and thus allows for reexpansion of the true lumen. Although this rationale would correct so-called dynamic obstruction (see B), in fact, persistent false lumen flow is noted in at least 50% of patients after proximal operation. In addition, vessels compromised with static obstruction (see B) would not be effectively treated with proximal operation.

B. Branch compromise may fluctuate in severity and spontaneously resolve as a function of the dynamic relationships of the true versus false lumen flow. Furthermore, effective medical therapy can favorably influence dynamic obstruction. Finally, obstruction of a subclavian origin or an incomplete iliac obstruction may be well tolerated and require no specific intervention in the acute setting.

C. Although contrast-enhanced CT scanning potentially affords an accurate three-dimensional image of the aortic topography, significant branch compromise may have to be inferred from, rather than demonstrated by, the CT images. In the most common (80%) mechanism of obstruction, vessels originating from a narrow, compressed (by a bulging false lumen) true lumen usually will not have total anatomic obstruction and the CT scan may be interpreted as "adequate perfusion." The key to diagnosis is the CT scan demonstration of a slit-like (even disappearing) true lumen.

D. As alluded to above, two principle mechanisms of branch compromise occur. In the more common (80%) scenario, a bulging pressured false lumen greatly narrows the true lumen, compromising vessels arising therefrom, even though the vessel origin itself is anatomically intact. This occurs when the dissection process itself encompasses at least two thirds of the aortic circumference. The therapeutic implication is that relief of true lumen compression with fenestration (open or endovascular) or entry tear site repair will accomplish revascularization. In a static obstruction, the dissecting process itself extends into the compromised vessel typically with more distal (i.e., beyond the aortic origin) obstruction. These more complex lesions require directed individual vessel revascularization procedures.

E. Because the absolute degree of branch compromise is often something less than 100%, and such compromise may fluctuate with blood pressure and/or medical therapy, morbid clinical sequelae in the acute phase of the disease may evolve over days or even weeks after symptom onset. For example, marginal mesenteric perfusion may be manifest only when oral food intake is initiated.

■ ANSWERS AND DISCUSSION FOR CHAPTER 105

Answer 105-1: C

Discussion 105-1

A. Incorrect. With small aneurysms, limb-threatening complications occur in less than 5% of the cases during follow-up without surgical repair. Specific indications are needed.

B. Incorrect. The normal diameter of the femoral artery ranges between 0.78 and 1.12 cm in men. An aneurysm is present if the diameter of an artery has increased more than 50%, in this case to approximately 1.5 cm.

C. Correct. Because of the narrow space under the inguinal ligament, a larger aneurysm of the femoral artery may produce compression of (branches of) the femoral nerve causing pain and/or weakness of the rectus femoris muscle.

D. Incorrect. A femoral aneurysm can be suspected by physical examination. Although seemingly simple and accurate, one third of all femoral aneurysms are missed by physical examination alone.

E. Incorrect. The best treatment is by surgical reconstruction. Endovascular treatment has almost no advantages and many disadvantages: hip flexion with groin compression may result in stent fracture or dislocation, and precise positioning, while maintaining adequate flow in the profunda artery, may be very difficult.

Answer 105-2: C

Discussion 105-2

A. Incorrect. The prevalence of popliteal aneurysms in patients with aortic aneurysms is approximately 3% to 10%, whereas the prevalence of aortic aneurysms in patients with popliteal aneurysms is more than 35%.

B. Incorrect. Although popliteal aneurysms may be caused by popliteal entrapment, this remains a rare cause for the development of an aneurysm.

C. Correct. A systematic review of the literature reveals that only 37.2% of popliteal aneurysms (range 5%–58%) were asymptomatic, limb ischemia was the presenting symptom in 55% (range 38%–90%), local compression was present in 6.5% (range 0%–23%), and rupture was present in 1.4% (range 0%–7%).

D. Incorrect. Most patients with absent pedal pulses have lower limb ischemia caused by femorodistal atherosclerotic disease. In patients with popliteal aneurysms, distal pulsations may be absent because of distal embolization; however, the opposite, i.e., finding a popliteal aneurysm as the cause of absent pedal pulses, is rare.

E. Incorrect. The occurrence of symptoms is clearly related to the size of the aneurysm. The median diameter of asymptomatic aneurysms is approximately 2 cm, and those associated with ischemia have a larger median diameter of approximately 3 cm. The risk of complications progressively increases with an increase in the diameter of the aneurysm.

Answer 105-3: D

Discussion 105-3

A. Incorrect. In low-risk patients, the treatment of a popliteal aneurysm should be considered if the aneurysm is greater than or equal to 2 cm. Watchful waiting is associated with the risk of (silent) distal embolization and acute, limb-threatening ischemia that cannot always successfully treated.

B. Incorrect. Although this approach is a good option for small aneurysms, it is not for large aneurysms because the aneurysm is left intact. The disadvantage of this technique is that compression caused by the aneurysm is not relieved, which is a problem with symptoms related to compression. In addition, the aneurysm may not thrombose if there is sufficient collateral circulation and thus may still expand causing compression and even resulting in rupture (much like type II endoleaks).

C. Incorrect. Although thrombolysis can be applied in acute thrombosis with ischemia, it takes a number of hours before the circulation is reestablished to the lower leg. During this delay, irreversible major tissue loss may occur. In these cases, direct surgical repair with intraoperative thrombolysis or thrombectomy of the tibial and pedal vessels, if necessary using an arteriotomy at the level of the ankle, is required because substantial distal embolization will have occurred.

D. Correct. Absent pedal pulses must be considered secondary to embolization, and thus the aneurysm can no longer be considered benign. Asymptomatic aneurysms can produce asymptomatic distal emboli, emphasizing the risk for progressive occlusion of the infrapopliteal arteries, with a high risk of complications. The risk of developing complications, including acute thrombosis and chronic thromboembolism, was 36% at 3 years for patients with normal pedal pulses.

E. Incorrect. In most cases the popliteal aneurysm should be treated first because acute thrombosis of the popliteal aneurysm may occur within 24 hours after the operation for an abdominal aneurysm, that is, aneurysm repair is a reported risk factor for acute thrombosis of a popliteal aneurysm.

■ ANSWERS AND DISCUSSION FOR CHAPTER 106

Answer 106-1: C

Discussion 106-1

A. Most subclavian aneurysms are degenerative or atherosclerotic in origin. Less common causes include fibromuscular dysplasia, cystic medial necrosis, congenital causes, and syphilis.

B. Proximal right subclavian artery aneurysms usually require limited sternotomy with extension into the supraclavicular fossa to gain adequate exposure and proximal control. In cases of proximal left subclavian aneurysms, a left thoracotomy combined with supraclavicular closure may be necessary.

C. From 30% to 50% of patients with degenerative subclavian artery aneurysms have aortoiliac and other peripheral aneurysms of similar type.

D. Although endovascular stent graft treatment of subclavian aneurysms has been reported, it is best reserved for unstable patients with multiple medical comorbidities. In addition to uncertain durability, a potential complication of stent graft placement in the proximal right subclavian artery includes stroke from embolic debris dislodged into the right common carotid artery. In addition, coverage of the vertebral artery on either side may lead to cerebral ischemia.

E. Presenting symptoms of subclavian aneurysms include chest, neck, and shoulder pain from expansion; upper extremity acute and chronic ischemic symptoms from thromboembolism; upper extremity pain and neurologic dysfunction from brachial plexus compression; hoarseness from compression of the right recurrent laryngeal nerve; respiratory insufficiency from tracheal compression; transient ischemic attacks and stroke from retrograde thromboembolism in the vertebral and right carotid circulation; and hemoptysis from erosion into the apex of the lungs.

Answer 106-2: D

Discussion 106-2

A. Cervical ribs are more common in women who appear more susceptible to arterial complications from associated axillary-subclavian aneurysms. The condition is not predominant in athletes.

B. If intraluminal thrombus is present, aneurysm resection and vein graft replacement along with removal of the cervical rib are necessary. Because the first manifestations in this setting may be limb-threatening ischemia, an aggressive surgical approach is warranted.

C. Asymptomatic subclavian aneurysms may harbor intraluminal thrombus that may subsequently embolize. Once again, an aggressive surgical approach is warranted because symptomatic thromboembolic events may lead to limb or digit loss.

D. In addition to cervical rib removal, complete resection of the axillary-subclavian artery aneurysm is necessary. In rare cases, vascular reconstruction can be accomplished by proximal and distal mobilization of the ends of the arteries and end-to-end anastomosis. Most cases, however, require a short interposition of vein graft. Although synthetic grafts have been used successfully, most patients are relatively young and a saphenous vein graft of adequate size would be the most optimal and durable conduit for reconstruction.

E. Supraclavicular and infraclavicular incisions are used to mobilize the distal subclavian and proximal axillary arteries. Resection of the clavicle is unnecessary. The cervical rib can be resected through the supraclavicular incision by accepted techniques.

Answer 106-3: D

Discussion 106-3

A. Ulnar artery aneurysms are most commonly seen in men younger than 50 years of age. The most accepted cause is trauma to the hypothenar area with compression of the artery against bony structures in the hand. More recently, histopathologic studies have suggested that some of these aneurysms may be related to fibromuscular dysplasia of the ulnar arteries.

B. Ulnar artery aneurysms usually present with symptomatic digital ischemia. These aneurysms are one of the most common causes of ischemia limited solely to the digits.

C. The fourth and fifth digits are most commonly involved with ischemia if it ensues. However, any digit or combination of digits may be involved with the exception of the thumb, which is invariably spared because of its radial artery blood supply.

D. Most experts recommend resection and microsurgical vascular reconstruction of the ulnar artery aneurysm because it eliminates the thromboembolic source, removes the painful aneurysmal mass that may cause ulnar nerve compression, adds the vasodilatory effects of local periarterial sympathectomy, and improves digital perfusion. Resection of the aneurysm and placement of a vein interposition graft is the optimal treatment for either a patent ulnar artery aneurysm with clinical or radiographic evidence of distal embolization or a thrombosed ulnar aneurysm that has resulted in profound digital ischemia.

E. Adjunctive preoperative thrombolytic therapy has been reported to yield excellent results. The benefit of thrombolytic therapy is restoration of patency to digital arteries, thus reducing adverse sequelae and improving distal runoff, theoretically enhancing patency of the reconstruction that would still be indicated.

■ ANSWERS AND DISCUSSION FOR CHAPTER 107

Answer 107-1: A
Discussion 107-1

Splenic artery aneurysms are the most common splanchnic artery aneurysms accounting for close to 60% of aneurysms in most series. They occur in a 4:1 female-to-male ratio. They are usually saccular and occur at vessel branchings. Hepatic artery aneurysms are the second most common splanchnic artery aneurysm of which 80% are extraparenchymal. As opposed to the splenic artery aneurysms, hepatic artery aneurysms occur twice as often in men. Celiac and SMA aneurysms are much less common, but in that order, so A is correct.

Answer 107-2: A
Discussion 107-2

The descriptors in the stem make this case almost classic for (A) splenic artery aneurysm. Splenic artery aneurysms occur in approximately 0.8% of the population in the United States. Most splenic aneurysms occur at branching points. The three main risk factors for developing a splenic artery aneurysm include: medial fibrodysplasia, portal-hypertension, and grand multiparity. In this particular patient, the patient initially presented with severe abdominal pain and was stabilized with IV fluid. The stabilization in the setting of a ruptured splenic artery aneurysm is likely secondary to the "double rupture" phenomena. These patients initially present with rupture into the lesser sac. When the blood is contained in the lesser sac, the

patient may be responsive to IV fluid. However, with time, blood escapes the lesser sac and flows freely into the peritoneal cavity with subsequent cardiovascular collapse. This is a surgical emergency, and operative therapy is needed to save the patient's life.

Answer 107-3: D
Discussion 107-3

A. Mycotic aneurysms of the hepatic artery, previously considered to be the most common type of hepatic artery aneurysm, now only cause approximately 10% of hepatic artery aneurysms, occurring most often as a complication after illicit intravenous drug use.

B. Even though in close proximity to the extrahepatic course of the hepatic artery, biliary sepsis is a very infrequent cause.

C. Some atherosclerotic changes are found in approximately 30% of hepatic artery aneurysms. However, these are considered secondary phenomena rather than a primary etiologic process.

D. Medial degeneration is the most common cause of hepatic artery aneurysms occurring in approximately 24% of these lesions. Medial defects appear to be acquired and are seemingly unrelated to other congenital abnormalities.

E. Pseudoaneurysms of the hepatic artery as a consequence of trauma are the second most common reason hepatic artery aneurysms form, occurring approximately 22% of the time. Conceivably, they may become recognized as the most common hepatic artery aneurysm in the future with early CT examinations being more frequent for trauma victims.

■ ANSWERS AND DISCUSSION FOR CHAPTER 108

Answer 108-1: A
Discussion 108-1

A. Sir William Osler, who coined the term *mycotic aneurysm,* recognized that mycotic aneurysms were an embolic complication arising distal to an infected cardiac valve or endocarditis. Infected debris is discharged from the upstream source and lodges in an artery (usually at a branch point) and initiates the arterial wall infection, which culminates in the mycotic aneurysm. It is a misnomer to refer to any other arterial infections as "mycotic."

B. Inoculation of a diseased artery with blood-borne microorganisms may give rise to a microbial arteritis.

C. Existing aneurysms may become secondarily colonized or even infected by blood-borne or contiguous infections. These are referred to as infected aneurysms.

D. Septic complications of needle punctures of arteries are referred to as posttraumatic and are not caused by endocarditis.

E. Although "mycotic" may suggest fungus, by traditional usage, the term *mycotic aneurysm* has a cardiac embolic source.

Answer 108-2: B

Discussion 108-2

A. Although administration of preoperative, intraoperative, and postoperative antibiotics is necessary, seldom would it be sufficient for a patient with an infected aneurysm presenting with sepsis. The source of sepsis must be controlled. Despite anecdotes suggesting cures from antibiotic administration alone, emergency presentation ordinarily requires prompt operation, and this is considered the safer, more conservative course.

B. Basic *surgical* principles apply and certainly include hemostasis and debridement of devitalized or infected tissue.

C. Tissue samples for aerobic, anaerobic, and fungal analysis are routine and easily obtained at the time of open operation. The results obtained direct the selection of postoperative antimicrobial therapy.

D. The decision for reestablishment of arterial continuity after arterial ligation and debridement depends on many factors, such as severity of limb or organ ischemia anticipated after ligation, ability to control sepsis with the initial operation, available conduit, and patient condition. Reestablishment of arterial continuity during an emergency operation for an infected aneurysm may be the best choice depending on circumstances.

E. Although an omental pedicle has been used to wrap in situ aortic reconstructions, and has been pulled down into groin wounds to cover femoral vessels, it is impractical to use elsewhere and has no special value if not in continuity.

Answer 108-3: E

Discussion 108-3

A. Most of the patients with infected false aneurysms resulting from illicit injections of "street" drugs are long-time users.

B. Many if not most who have exhausted all superficial veins are undaunted by the difficulties encountered with venous access. When superficial veins are exhausted, rather than switch to different drug abuse modes, they adopt a pattern of escalating recklessness in persisting with parenteral drug abuse, in which deep system veins in the groin or neck are targeted. The common femoral artery, carotid artery, and innominate artery are sites of infected arteries not infrequently encountered. These arteries are inadvertently entered/injured when attempts to access the adjacent veins are unsuccessful.

C. Most of these infections are polymicrobial.

D. Unfortunately, many of these patients have other infectious disease problems including polymicrobial infections and endocarditis, and are likely to be serology positive for hepatitis and human immunodeficiency virus.

E. Thus, none of the previous statements are true.

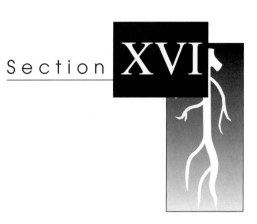

Section **XVI**

ARTERIOVENOUS FISTULAS, VASCULAR MALFORMATIONS, AND VASCULAR TUMORS

STUDY QUESTIONS

■ QUESTIONS FOR CHAPTER 110

Question 110-1

A 14-year-old boy has "always" had a birthmark on his left thigh. Prominent veins were noticed in early youth, but now there is a large network of distended tortuous veins over the thigh, and the patient says his leg tires easily and feels heavy after activities. Which of the following would be the single most useful *initial* diagnostic study?

A. An arteriogram.
B. An ascending venogram.
C. A computed tomography (CT) scan.
D. A magnetic resonance imaging (MRI).
E. Noninvasive testing including a duplex scan.

Question 110-2

A 14-year-old boy (similar patient as in question 110-1) has "always" had a birthmark on his left thigh. Prominent veins were noticed in early youth, but now there is a large network of distended tortuous veins over the thigh. A bruit and thrill can be detected over the mid-thigh.

Which of the following noninvasive study findings, compared with the contralateral leg, would *not* indicate significant congenital arteriovenous fistulas (AVFs) in the left thigh?

A. Pulse volume recording (plethysmographic) tracings increased at the thigh level, normal at the ankle level on the left, compared with the opposite leg.
B. Thigh brachial index higher and ankle brachial index lower than the opposite leg.
C. Thigh brachial index higher than and ankle brachial index equal to the opposite leg.
D. Greater peak to trough velocity swings in the left femoral artery velocity tracings.
E. Higher end-diastolic velocity in the left femoral artery.

Question 110-3

Which of the following would be of most practical help in studying a large arteriovenous (AV) malformation involving the left iliac arteries?

A. Comparison of thigh plethysmographic tracings.
B. Comparison of thigh pressure indices.
C. Comparison of velocity tracings from the femoral arteries.
D. MRI/magnetic resonance angiography (MRA).
E. Three-dimensional (3D) reconstruction computed tomographic arteriography (CTA) data.

Question 110-4

A 5-year-old boy is brought to you by his mother, who has noticed prominent veins appearing on his right thigh in the last year. The boy has no complaints and is very active. You observe a cluster of atypically located varicosities near what his mother identifies as a "birthmark." The legs are equal in length and girth, and no discoloration, local warmth, masses, or thrills are noted.

The *first* diagnostic test you should obtain in this setting is:

A. A venogram.
B. An arteriogram.
C. A duplex scan.
D. A CT scan.
E. An MRI.

Question 110-5

A 17-year-old girl presents with varicose veins (VVs) on both sides of the left thigh and calf that first appeared before puberty but have become more extensive. They are associated with a large birthmark and mild limb enlargement (the extremity is 2 cm diameter larger in girth than the right and is of a deeper hue). She says that the VVs are painful and unsightly, and she requests their removal.

Before you strip out her varicosities, you should:

A. Rule out deep venous hypoplasia/aplasia.
B. Determine the extent of venous reflux.
C. Rule out underlying AVFs.
D. Warn the patient that her varicosities might recur if stripped.
E. All of the above.

131

■ QUESTIONS FOR CHAPTER 111

Question 111-1

A 68-year-old man presents to the emergency department with abdominal and flank pain of 6 hours duration. The patient is diaphoretic with a blood pressure of 110/50 mm Hg and a pulse rate of 115 beats/min. The abdomen is tender, and there is a loud bruit in the periumbilical area. Both legs are edematous. A contrast-enhanced CT scan of the abdomen visualizes an 8.5-cm abdominal aortic aneurysm (AAA) and the inferior vena cava (IVC), but no retroperitoneal hematoma. The *most likely* diagnosis is:

A. Symptoms from a rapidly enlarging but not yet ruptured AAA.
B. Ruptured AAA with aortocaval fistula.
C. A large and expanding AAA compressing the IVC and producing leg edema.
D. An inflammatory AAA with involvement of adjacent lymphatics producing lymphedema of the legs.
E. An aorta-left renal vein fistula producing flank pain and some retrograde vena cava flow.

Question 111-2

In a patient with suspected aortocaval fistula, the ideal way to manage this problem in the operating room is:

A. Ligate the IVC above and below the fistula, after repairing the AAA.
B. Place an IVC filter intraoperatively after AAA repair.
C. Suture the caval defect from within the aneurysm sac, then repair the AAA.
D. Repair the AAA and the IVC separately under deep hypothermia and circulatory arrest.
E. Clamp the IVC above and below the fistula, open the AAA sac and repair it, and then dissect off the IVC and repair it separately to avoid narrowing it.

Question 111-3

A 44-year-old woman presents with vague abdominal pain. On examination, a loud abdominal bruit is heard in the right lower quadrant. The history is significant for a lumbar laminectomy 5 years before presentation. Of the following, the best *next* step is:

A. CT scan of the abdomen without contrast.
B. Iliofemoral venography.
C. Arteriography and open repair of an ilio-iliac fistula if one is found.
D. Arteriography and placement of a covered stent to occlude the traumatic ilio-iliac AVF if it is found.
E. Emergency abdominal exploration with quadruple ligation of the iliac artery and vein.

■ QUESTIONS FOR CHAPTER 112

Question 112-1

A 21-year-old man sustains a shotgun blast to the lower extremity. Dorsalis pedis and posterior tibialis pulses are palpable. The ankle-brachial index is 0.95 in the injured extremity.

What is the most appropriate diagnostic test for this patient?

A. No further diagnostic workup is necessary.
B. Duplex ultrasonography.
C. Digital subtraction arteriography
D. Computed tomographic arteriography (CTA).
E. Magnetic resonance angiography (MRA).

Question 112-2

A 65-year-old man is noted to have a continuous bruit in the groin after undergoing a cardiac catheterization 2 days prior. There is mild swelling of the leg. Dorsalis pedis and posterior tibialis pulses are palpable. The ankle-brachial index is 0.8. A duplex ultrasound of the groin reveals high systolic and diastolic flow in the common femoral artery and higher than normal velocity in the adjacent common femoral vein with variations in velocity that are synchronous with the cardiac, not the respiratory cycle.

What is the *most likely* diagnosis?

A. High grade narrowing of the common femoral artery, possibly secondary to dissection.
B. An AVF between the superficial femoral artery and an adjacent vein.
C. A to-and-fro ventricular septal defect modifying the pattern of extremity flow.
D. A pseudoaneurysm of the common femoral artery.
E. A deep venous thrombosis of the superficial femoral vein, increasing femoral artery flow but decreasing common femoral vein flow.

Question 112-3

A 52-year-old man presents with aching pain along the medial thigh. He has a history of a stab wound to the anterior thigh several years prior for which he never sought medical care. Prominent VVs are evident along the upper greater saphenous vein. Pulse examination reveals normal results. The ipsilateral ankle-brachial index is 0.85.

The most appropriate next step in the management of this patient is:

A. Vein stripping of the greater saphenous vein.
B. Operative exploration of the superficial femoral artery adjacent to the stab wound.
C. Prescription of full-length graded compression stockings.
D. Venous duplex scan.
E. Digital subtraction arteriography.

■ QUESTIONS FOR CHAPTER 113

Question 113-1

A 3-month-old infant presents with a 4-cm diameter red violaceous "birthmark" on the forehead near the hairline. It has enlarged from the small pea-sized lesion first noticed at 3 weeks of age. It is slightly uneven and slightly raised. There is a prominent draining vein toward the front of the ipsilateral ear. Duplex ultrasonography shows a pattern of high velocity and low resistance, with increased venous velocity. The most likely diagnosis is:

A. Venous malformation (VM).
B. AVM associated with a "port wine" stain.
C. Pyogenic granuloma.
D. Infantile hemangioma (IH).
E. Capillary malformation (CM).

Question 113-2

Both present as a vascular birthmark, but which of the following does *not* help distinguish between capillary malformation (CM) and infantile hemangioma?

A. Endothelial turnover rate.
B. Growth rate in early infancy.
C. Appearance at birth.
D. "Strawberry" color.
E. Flow characteristics.

Question 113-3

All of the following are used in managing infantile hemangiomas of the head and neck. Which should be used *most frequently*?

A. Observation.
B. Flashlamp pulsed-dye laser.
C. Surgical excision.
D. Cortisone injections.
E. Interferon or vincristine.

Question 113-4

A capillary malformation, presenting as a birthmark, can be a red flag for an underlying structural abnormality. Which of the following is *unlikely* to carry such a risk?

A. Midline occipital CM.
B. CM over the cervical or lumbosacral spine.
C. Facial CM with V_1-V_2 distribution.
D. Lateral buttocks CM.
E. CM with mandibular (V3) involvement alone.

■ QUESTIONS FOR CHAPTER 114

Question 114-1

A 22 year old has had increasing pelvic pain and intermittent lower gastrointestinal bleeding. MRI and MRA indicate a large pelvic AVM adjacent to the rectum. What is the most appropriate next step in management?

A. Surgical exploration and resection under deep hypothermia and cardiac arrest.
B. Observation to see whether symptoms resolve.
C. Arteriogram with embolization.
D. Surgical ligation of the main feeding vessels.
E. Percutaneous ultrasound-guided sclerotherapy.

Question 114-2

The main role of surgical intervention for arteriovenous malformations (AVMs) is:

A. Palliation of symptoms after initial transcatheter embolization.
B. Complete surgical resection of the lesion with ligation of all feeding vessels.

C. Ligation of main feeding vessels to reduce hemodynamic effects of the AVM.
D. Treatment of late recurrence of AVMs after prior embolization.
E. Resection of adjacent structures that may be affected by the AVM.

Question 114-3

A 30-year-old woman presents with an ulcerated, bleeding lesion on the tip of her left thumb. She states the thumb has been larger than her right thumb since she was a teenager, and is often tender. There is a prominent left radial pulse and an audible bruit over the base of the thumb. The thumb is warm and hyperemic. The most likely diagnosis is:

A. Venous malformation (VM).
B. Embolus to the digital artery of the thumb.
C. Arteriovenous malformation (AVM).
D. Venous thrombosis.
E. Raynaud's disease.

■ QUESTIONS FOR CHAPTER 115

Question 115-1

Which of the following agents is *not* used for the embolotherapy of high-flow vascular malformations?

A. Platinum nester coils.
B. n-butyl-2-cyanoacrylate.
C. OK432.
D. Ethanol.
E. Polyvinyl alcohol foam (PVA).

Question 115-2

Which of the following statements about the endovenous obliteration of venous malformations (VMs) is *not* true?

A. Direct puncture of the VM can be used to advantage.
B. Collapse, compression, or exsanguination of the VM makes sclerotherapy more effective.
C. Sclerotherapy of VMs uses only the same available agents used for sclerotherapy of VVs.
D. Sclerotherapy of VMs is mostly applied to extratruncal localized mass lesions.
E. The majority of VMs are managed conservatively, e.g., by compression therapy and intermittent elevation.

Question 115-3

Which of the following are *not* significant complications of the embolotherapy/sclerotherapy of vascular malformations?

A. Tissue necrosis and scarring.
B. Nerve injury.
C. Hemosiderosis.
D. Pulmonary embolism.
E. Intravascular thrombosis and consumptive coagulopathy.

■ QUESTIONS FOR CHAPTER 116

Question 116-1

A 59-year-old man presents with acute onset of multiple skin infarcts involving both feet. He denies any abdominal, back, or chest pain. He has neither tachycardia nor an irregular heart rhythm. His abdomen is soft and nontender, but his aorta feels somewhat prominent. He has palpable pulses in both lower extremities at all levels. Ultrasound of the abdominal aorta identifies a 4.1-cm infrarenal AAA, and this is confirmed by noncontrast abdominal CT that identifies no other abnormalities. Blood laboratory values are essentially normal.

What is the most appropriate *next* step in the patient's management?

A. Recommend long-term treatment with antiplatelet agents.
B. Evaluate the entire thoracic and abdominal aorta with arteriography.
C. Proceed with AAA repair.
D. Recommend long-term treatment with warfarin.
E. Evaluate the heart, entire thoracic, and abdominal aorta with noninvasive imaging (i.e., CT, MRI/MRA, and transesophageal echocardiography).

Question 116-2

A 62-year-old man presents with a 4-hour history of severe pain, numbness, and paralysis of the right lower extremity. He gives no history of claudication or heart palpitations, and he has a regular heart rhythm. His abdomen is soft and nontender, and his aortic width feels normal. He has normal left lower extremity pulses at all levels but absent pulses in the right lower extremity below the right femoral artery. His right lower extremity is pale, cool, and insensate from the knee distally, and there is diminished motor function of the foot and toes. Chest x-ray film, electrocardiogram, and blood laboratory study results are normal. Heparin has been administered.

Femoral embolectomy in this patient should:

A. Be followed by transthoracic echocardiography in the postoperative period.
B. Be followed by pathologic examination of the retrieved embolus, postoperative maintenance of anticoagulation,

and noninvasive evaluation of the heart and proximal arterial tree.
C. Be performed only if thrombolysis fails to dissolve the clot and relieve symptoms within 24 hours.
D. Be preceded by on-the-table open fasciotomies.
E. Be followed by long-term anticoagulation.

Question 116-3

In a "good-risk" 52-year-old woman, an isolated polypoid lesion identified in the distal descending thoracic aorta should be treated with:

A. A covered stent graft.
B. Long-term warfarin anticoagulation.
C. Localized aortic endarterectomy.
D. Localized aortic resection with interposition grafting.
E. Axillobifemoral bypass grafting with bilateral ligation of the external iliac arteries above the femoral anastomoses to prevent distal embolization.

Question 116-4

A 69-year-old man presents with acute onset of right lower extremity ischemia. The patient undergoes successful right femoral embolectomy with return of normal lower extremity function. Two days later, the pathologist reports that the embolectomy specimen tested positive for a sarcoma based on positive vascular endothelial antigenic stains to von Willebrand factor, CD31, CD34, and Ulex europaeus agglutinin-1 in association with an atypical spindle cell morphology. The *next* step in management of this patient should be:

A. Continue with therapeutic heparin and conversion to oral anticoagulants with subsequent discharge.
B. Continue with therapeutic heparin and initiate search for primary tumor and evidence of metastatic disease.
C. Provide referral to oncology for definitive treatment.
D. Return to the operating room for en bloc resection of the right femoral artery where the embolus was located and femoral artery reconstruction.
E. Provide referral to radiation therapy for definitive therapy.

ANSWERS AND DISCUSSION

■ ANSWERS AND DISCUSSION FOR CHAPTER 110

Answer 110-1: E
Discussion 110-1

A. If the patient has a large congenital AVF, an arteriogram through the opposite femoral artery might well be diagnostic but is *not necessary* unless intervention is indicated and imminent, so would *not* be indicated as an *initial* diagnostic study.
B. The described patient could also have either venous outflow obstruction or a venous anomaly, that is, a Klippel-Trenaunay syndrome. An ascending venogram might visualize venous truncal anomalies but usually will not properly define a proximal/iliac obstruction. In either situation, intervention is unlikely and an invasive test should be avoided if possible.
C. A CT scan is not likely to be definitively diagnostic and would require a large dye load.
D. An MRI would avoid a large dye load and visualize a vascular *mass lesion* in the thigh (e.g., AVM), and its multiplanar views could define its anatomic limits, and is very useful for this purpose, but it would not be an appropriate *initial* study.
E. Noninvasive testing would distinguish between a venous anomaly and AVFs, and give information about both. In the latter instance, comparing velocities with a duplex scanner of the ipsilateral versus the contralateral (normal) inflow artery would give a relative impression of the degree of AV shunt flow, and deeper probes might be used to actually visualize an AVM by demonstrating a vascular mass with characteristic turbulent flow with yellow flashes. Such testing in a nearby vascular laboratory would be quicker, noninvasive, and less expensive than the other options, give valuable information about both arterial and venous pathology, and thus provide an adequate basis for initial diagnosis and decision making and advising patient and parents regarding prognosis and the likely need for intervention eventually.

Answer 110-2: D
Discussion 110-2

Noninvasive testing produces characteristic findings in the presence of a significant extremity AVF. (A) Plethysmographic tracings are increased at the level of AVFs but may be either normal or, if there is a significant distal steel, decreased at the calf and ankle levels. Although large AVFs lower resistance and thus *mean* systolic pressure, they produce greater *pressure* swings at the level of the fistulas, and this produces an increase in the thigh pressure, which is a *systolic* measurement. B and C could both be found, depending on the size of the fistula and the degree of distal steel. The velocity tracings over the inflow artery will show increased *mean* velocity and a loss of the end-systolic reversal normally seen in the lower extremity at rest. In addition, the end-diastolic velocity is increased (E) and continuous throughout diastole, increasing the velocity tracings well above zero baseline, but these combine to *decrease* the peak to trough swings in the velocity tracings, so the findings described in D would *not* be found in the presence of a significant AVF.

Answer 110-3: D
Discussion 110-3

One of the weaknesses of noninvasive physiologic testing applied to AVFs is that their useful application is limited to lesions *in* the extremities. Thigh cuffs for plethysmographic tracings or pressure measurements are applied well below the groin and will not reflect any significant changes below fistulas at the iliac artery level. Femoral artery velocity tracings, being closer to the lesion, may demonstrate some changes downstream, but not significant enough for definitive diagnosis as a sole test, although with appropriately deep probes, a duplex scan could at least partially interrogate a pelvic AVM. Therefore answers A, B, and C are wrong. (D) MRI/MRA would be able to visualize the arterial and venous components of a pelvic AVM originating in the iliac arteries and would provide an estimate of its size, flow, and anatomic limits, using multiplanar views. One might think that 3D reconstruction of CTA data (E) would visualize this vascular mass, and it would show the blood vessels but, by subtracting all of the surrounding tissues, one would not get any perspective of its anatomic extent or flow, and it is more expensive than an MRI. It is for this reason (plus time and expense) it has not been found to be a practical study.

Answer 110-4: C
Discussion 110-4

The age and the location of the varicosities are against them because they are primary VVs caused by superficial venous (saphenofemoral) incompetence. They could reflect venous outflow obstruction, but the thigh/leg is not swollen or different in color compared with the other leg. The combination of prominent veins and a birthmark in the patient this young suggests underlying congenital AVFs. This possibility, as well as the other two diagnoses, can be best initially investigated with (C) a duplex scan. The duplex scan findings that would indicate an AVF are high velocities in the right femoral artery compared with the left, a high velocity pattern on the arterial tracing (high end-diastolic velocity elevating the tracing above the zero baseline and eliminating the end-systolic reversal normally seen in the arteries of limbs at rest), and, if the AVF flow is large, "arterialization" of the venous flow patterns when interrogating the femoral vein, and even the VVs.

A standard venogram (A) would not show the AVF, and a proximally injected arteriogram (B) might well be diagnostic and visualize the AVF, but in a child this age it would carry increased expense, discomfort, and risk of arterial catheter injury and would probably require general anesthesia. Most important, it is not needed to make a diagnosis and is only indicated at the time when therapeutic intervention is soon to be undertaken, unlikely in an asymptomatic 5 year old. A CT scan (D) would require contrast media and would not visualize an underlying AVM as well as an MRI. An MRI (E) would provide multiplanar views and avoid a contrast load (but use gadolinium). It can better delineate the anatomic extent of an AVM, but this advantage is best used in mass lesions, which is not the case here.

Answer 110-5: E

Discussion 110-5

This patient presents with a triad associated with the Klippel-Trenaunay syndrome (birthmark, varicosities, limb enlargement), a well-known venous anomaly, but this same triad can be associated with the so-called Parkes Weber syndrome, the latter having underlying AVFs. Obviously, (C) ruling out AVFs would be important before operating and stripping out her VVs. This may be simply done by comparing segmental limb pressures and segmental plethysmography and arterial velocity waveforms between the two lower extremities, and the latter can be studied by duplex scan at the same time it is being used to (B) evaluate the extent of the superficial reflux and the VVs. The AVFs in Klippel Trenaunay may be diffuse micro-AVFs, and their presence or absence may not be obvious from the above studies. In such case, a shunt quantification study using radionuclide-labeled albumen microspheres can be definitive. Some patients with Klippel-Trenaunay syndrome have abnormalities obstructing their deep veins (e.g., a hypoplastic or aplastic segment), and this needs to be ruled out before stripping the superficial veins and making things worse. (A) Again, duplex scan can be used to interrogate the deep and superficial veins. If there are no deep venous abnormalities, painful varicosities can be removed with cosmetic benefit and relief of symptoms, but there is a significant rate of recurrence (>30%), so the patient should be forewarned of this (D). Thus all of the above (E) should be done.

■ ANSWERS AND DISCUSSION FOR CHAPTER 111

Answer 111-1: B

Discussion 111-1

A. A rapidly enlarging AAA might produce discomfort and tenderness but not the other findings.
B. This is the most likely diagnosis. The clinical findings are compatible with it, and it explains the visualization of the AAA and the IVC at the same time. The rupture is into the IVC and does not produce any surrounding hemorrhage.
C. AAAs rarely if ever compress the IVC enough to produce leg edema. This could happen in the unlikely event of caval thrombosis but the cava visualizes as being patent.
D. Inflammatory AAAs may involve adjacent lymphatics with localized edema, but leg edema would not occur. Also, this edema has developed too quickly.
E. An aorta-left renal vein fistula can produce a bruit and left flank pain, and the left kidney might not visualize later with contrast studies, but the flow goes rapidly up the vena cava and would not result in visualization of the vena cava below the renal veins. It would not produce leg edema.

Answer 111-2: C

Discussion 111-2

A. It is unnecessary to ligate the IVC, but if it were to be done *after attempting* the AAA repair, caval bleeding into the sac would prevent the repair and might lead to exsanguinations.
B. An IVC filter *after the repair* is unnecessary (the risk of embolism of AAA sac thrombus is in the manipulation before the repair). The cava needs repair, not filtration, at this point.
C. This is the ideal technique. After aortic clamps are applied proximally and distally (which also reduces venous return through the IVC), the AAA sac is opened and the fistulous defect is oversewn from within, using compression by sponge clamps above and below the defect to reduce flow through it.
D. Hypothermia and circulatory arrest are unnecessary, as is separate repair of the IVC.
E. Dissecting the caval enough to clamp it above and below the fistula invites caval injury and massive hemorrhage, and separation of the caval to repair the defect is unnecessary. It will not be narrowed from oversewing the defect from within the aortic sac, and the latter approach is safer.

Answer 111-3: D

Discussion 111-3

The presumptive diagnosis is a traumatic ilio-iliac AVF related to a 5-year-old injury during discectomy. It must be small to have been asymptomatic for 5 years or have developed recently because previously injured tissues broke down (unlikely). The vague abdominal pain might be unrelated.

A. A CT scan without contrast would not make the diagnosis, but a gadolinium MRI (not listed) might well demonstrate the fistula.
B. An ascending femoroiliac venogram could show dilution of the iliac vein contrast from iliac artery inflow, but flow is also diluted near this point by blood flowing in from the opposite iliac vein.
C. An aortogram would show the fistula better than a venogram, but embarking on an open repair in this treacherous area behind the iliac artery as it crosses over the iliac vein for a small AVF poses significant technical problems in achieving vascular control, and is associated with significant risk.
D. With the access used for the arteriography, a well-placed covered iliac artery stent could be used to close this small fistula, preventing it from enlarging in the future. This would be *the preferred initial management*, and its success could be confirmed at that time with an additional contrast injection. At worst, inability to accurately place the stent and completely close the fistula would not interfere significantly with subsequent repair and may help in reducing fistula flow.
E. Quadruple ligation is an unnecessary penalty to pay for such a small fistula. Opening the artery and simply closing the small fistulous opening and then repairing the artery with a patch, prosthetic graft, or even using a crossover bypass, as deemed most appropriate, would be preferable.

■ ANSWERS AND DISCUSSION FOR CHAPTER 112

Answer 112-1: C

Discussion 112-1

A. The pulses and ABI within normal limits suggest there might not be an occlusive injury of a major axial artery, but false aneurysms and/or AVFs are possible, and may be located in branch vessels, and these should be excluded by further diagnostic studies. Patients sustaining such injuries are notoriously difficult to follow.

B. Duplex scanning might visualize a major occlusive arterial or venous injury if its likely location were known, but it would not pick up smaller branch lesions and would be difficult to perform through tissues injured by a shotgun blast.

C. Digital subtraction arteriography would be best, allowing one to visualize lesions of major and branch arteries, even nonocclusive lesions such as pseudoaneurysms and AVFs. Resuscitation can be ongoing in an angiogram suite.

D. CT with contrast would require the multiple slices fortuitously placed to capture all the potentially multiple lesions. Using 3D reconstruction of the CTA data would be expensive and time consuming and would require subtracting bone, muscle, and nerves to reconstruct the vessels, but subtracting associated anatomy would interfere with anatomic localization of the lesions demonstrated. It is a technical, involved study that is costly and takes time, and thus does not fit into this trauma setting.

E. MRA has the advantage over CTA of giving multiplanar views with surrounding anatomic structures visualized, but the radiating artifacts produced by the metal shotgun wound pellets on MRA would interfere with clear visualization. It shares other associated problems (e.g., isolation) with CTA, inasmuch as both are likely to be performed in a remote radiology unit.

Answer 112-2: B

Discussion 112-2

A. A high-grade stenosis of the common femoral artery, if just proximal to the point of duplex interrogation, might produce similar peak systolic and diastolic arterial velocity changes but not the venous velocity changes described.

B. All of the findings are compatible with an AVF, which is the correct answer. Usually the fistula is not with the common femoral vein but with the large medial tributary of the profunda femoris vein that crosses under the superficial femoral artery near its origin.

C. This cardiac lesion might affect flow in and near the heart but not flow in the common femoral vessels. Only tricuspid insufficiency is likely to have such remote flow effects, and these would be mainly in the venous system.

D. A pseudoaneurysm is the most common iatrogenic injury from groin access, but it would not produce these duplex findings.

E. Superficial femoral vein thrombosis would likely be visualized by the duplex scan, but being just below the point of duplex interrogation it would produce some indirect changes in common femoral flow, but with a compensatory increases in profunda femoris flow these would be difficult to detect and would not mimic those described. Also, this DVT would produce greater leg edema.

Answer 112-3: E

Discussion 112-3

A. These varicosities are not typical of primary saphenous varicosities, which would appear distally as well, and usually earlier there.

B. Exploration of the superficial artery should not be made without a lesion being diagnosed and anatomically localized.

C. This might relieve symptoms stemming from venous hypertension but not correct the underlying cause.

D. A venous duplex scan would not be definitive, and it would take a very experienced operator to spot the associated venous changes, perform an arterial scan, and localize the lesion.

E. The most likely lesion is an AVF somewhere along the course of the superficial femoral artery, but it must be visualized and exactly localized before undertaking repair. Digital subtraction arteriography can best do this.

■ ANSWERS AND DISCUSSION FOR CHAPTER 113

Answer 113-1: D

Discussion 113-1

A. VM at or near the skin surface (old term "cavernous hemangioma") can be this color, but VMs do not grow quickly or have a high-flow pattern.

B. This lesion could be mistaken for an AVM because of its high flow, characteristic of hemangioma's proliferative phase, but AVMs do not enlarge rapidly in infancy.

C. Pyogenic granuloma is an exophytic cutaneous vascular tumor that is commonly confused with hemangioma. It usually has a central facial location and rarely appears before 6 months of age, and when it grows rapidly, it becomes raised and pedunculated.

D. The correct answer is IH. Its appearance after 2 weeks of age and rapid growth during the first year are typical of the proliferative phase. It is very vascular with high-flow characteristics. Nevertheless, it will regress during childhood.

E. CM appears as a "birthmark" but does not expand rapidly; it grows commensurate with the child and remains macular.

Answer 113-2: D

Discussion 113-2

A. IHs have a rapid endothelial turnover; CMs do not.

B. IHs have a rapid growth rate during their early proliferative stage; CMs do not.

C. IHs may be represented by a nascent lesion at birth but are usually not clearly visible until after 2 weeks. CMs are full size at birth.

D. Both may have a reddish-pink color so this does not help. As the saying goes, "Not all hemangiomas look like strawberries" and "Not all strawberries are hemangiomas."

E. IHs, during their proliferative stage, have distinctly high-flow characteristics. CMs are slow-flow lesions.

Answer 113-3: A

Discussion 113-3

A. Most IHs are harmless small tumors. In general, these lesions should be allowed to undergo proliferation and involution under observation. Such lesions will leave normal or slightly blemished skin. Involution begins at approximately 1 year of age and continues until 5 to 7 years of age when the last traces of color typically disappear. Involution is complete in approximately 50% of children by 5 years of age and in 70% of children by 7 years of age. Gradual improvement is observed uniformly through age 12 years. Intervention, using some of the other listed options, is reserved for problematic lesions in which serious (e.g., ulceration, deformity, obstruction) or life-threatening (e.g., intrahepatic hemangiomas with congestive failure) complications occur, or the rapidly growing tumor infringes on orifices (mouth, nose, tongue) or other vital organs (e.g., the eyes).

B. Flashlamp pulsed-dye laser penetrates only 0.75 to 1.2 mm into the dermis; therefore only the superficial portion of the hemangioma is affected, resulting in moderate lightening of the color. However, these superficial hemangiomas are the very tumors that would be expected to regress in time, leaving nearly normal skin. Laser is not used for deep tumors. Overzealous use of the laser can result in ulceration, partial-thickness skin loss, hypopigmentation, and consequent scarring. On the other hand, there is no controversy about the useful role of pulsed-dye laser for telangiectasias that often persist in the involuting/involuted phases.

C. There are generally accepted indications for excision of IH during the proliferative phase. One example is a well-localized or pedunculated lesion, particularly one that is ulcerated or bleeds repeatedly. Common locations for early excision are the scalp and thorax. A problematic hemangioma of the upper eyelid that does not respond to pharmacologic therapy can be either excised or debulked. Staged or total excision of a large or protuberant involuting-phase hemangioma should be considered in the preschool period. Excision of hemangioma in early childhood is indicated (1) if it is obvious that resection is inevitable, (2) if the scar would be the same were excision postponed until the involuted phase, or (3) if the scar is easily hidden.

D. Injection of corticosteroid into the tumor should be considered but mainly for a small, well-localized cutaneous hemangioma and is typically used for lesions located on the nasal tip, cheek, lip, or eyelid. Intralesional corticosteroid can effectively stabilize an ulcerated hemangioma and facilitate subsequent healing. The goal is limited to minimize the volume of the deformity and diminish cutaneous sequelae.

E. Interferon or vincristine should be considered a second-line treatment after corticosteroid for serious or life-threatening hemangiomas. Indications for such chemotherapy include (1) failure of response to corticosteroid, (2) contraindications to prolonged systemic corticosteroid, (3) complications of corticosteroid, and (4) the rare instance of parental refusal to use corticosteroid.

Answer 113-4: E

Discussion 113-4

A. Midline occipital CM can overlie an encephalocele or ectopic meninges.

B. CM over the cervical or lumbosacral spine can be a clue to occult spinal dysraphism.

C. Sturge-Weber syndrome is composed of a facial CM associated in the V1–V2 distribution with ipsilateral ocular and leptomeningeal vascular anomalies.

D. A CM over the buttock can be association with underlying AVMs, as part of the Parkes Weber syndrome.

E. In contrast with C, a patient with a CM with mandibular (V3) involvement alone is at *no* risk for having ophthalmic or intracranial anomalies.

■ ANSWERS AND DISCUSSION FOR CHAPTER 114

Answer 114-1: C

Discussion 114-1

A. Surgical exploration often results in significant hemorrhage and damage to surrounding structures, particularly if not preceded by transcatheter embolization of the AVM. Some have been successfully resected in the past without this, using deep hypothermia and circulatory arrest, but this is no longer done with the advent of embolotherapy.

B. The AVM is symptomatic, and treatment is indicated. Once symptomatic, AVMs rarely abate for long. Without intervention there will be ongoing bleeding and pain.

C. Angiogram and embolization delivered to the nidus of the AVM will provide significant relief of symptoms and should result in decrease in size of the AVM. It may even make the AVM amenable to surgical resection. If relief of symptoms is achieved but the lesion remains difficult to resect, no other surgical treatment is indicated, but further embolization may be required during long-term follow-up.

D. Surgical ligation of feeding vessels does not allow resection of the AVM. It is usually incomplete, and commonly the AVM will revascularize through collaterals and continue to cause symptoms. Thus, even the goal of reducing the AVM's hemodynamic effects is not achieved. Furthermore, it may well make later attempts at transcatheter embolization impossible.

E. Percutaneous sclerotherapy with absolute ethanol is contraindicated for AVMs, which must be treated with catheter-guided injections. However, percutaneous injections may be useful in the sclerotherapy treatment of superficially placed VMs.

Answer 114-2: B

Discussion 114-2

A. Surgery should not be used for palliation after embolization. If there are residual symptoms, and the lesion does not appear on imaging studies to be completely resectable, then further embolization is indicated.

B. Complete surgical resection remains a valid goal, but it should only be attempted as definitive therapy. If the AVM appears to be localized and surgically resectable and is not invading important adjacent structures, particularly after preoperative transcatheter embolization has reduced its vascularity, resection is indicated.

C. Ligation of main feeding vessels alone does not eradicate the AVM, does not reduce its hemodynamic effects for long, and makes later transcatheter embolization difficult or impossible.

D. Treatment of late recurrence after prior embolization should be further embolization. This is common, and patients have improvement or resolution of symptoms in up to 80% of cases with repeat embolization as sole therapy.

E. Resection of adjacent structures is rarely necessary. If the AVM is invading adjacent structures, the primary treatment should be embolization to avoid extensive, debilitating, and risky extirpative surgery. Embolotherapy will often achieve relief of symptoms.

Answer 114-3: C
Discussion 114-3

A. VMs do not have associated bruits or prominent pulses from feeding arteries because of the lack of an arterial component.

B. Emboli result in distal ischemia, but swelling and ulceration are rare. Were this the diagnosis, the affected digit would be cool and pale.

C. Increased flow through feeding arteries can result in hypertrophy of the involved parts. Audible bruits are produced by turbulent flow through the AVFs. Ulceration may result from ischemia secondary to distal steal and is made worse by increased pressure in the subcutaneous tissues. These are common presentations of peripheral AVMs.

D. Venous thrombosis is not associated with bruits or prominent pulses, and rarely causes skin ulceration. A finger would be an unusual location for a spontaneous venous thrombosis.

E. Raynaud's disease (primary Raynaud's) is characterized by episodic spasm of digital arteries, usually in response to cold exposure. The resultant Raynaud's phenomena are seen as pale, cool, painful digits, which go through color changes as the spasm abates and reactive hyperemia follows. It is often precipitated by cool temperatures, and the symptoms are intermittent in nature. Bruits are not heard.

■ ANSWERS AND DISCUSSION FOR CHAPTER 115

Answer 115-1: C
Discussion 115-1

A. Nester coils are soft, long platinum fiber coils, which are excellent for packing an AV connection and are available in 0.035-inch and 0.018-inch diameters.

B. The adhesive polymer n-butyl-2-cyanoacrylate has been used for decades to treat AVMs. It results in permanent occlusion because it polymerizes to form a solid mass conforming to the shape of the embolized vessel, and because polymerization is an exothermic reaction that causes transmural vessel necrosis. Unfortunately, precise placement of this material is difficult, and arterial rather than nidal occlusion usually occurs. It is therefore no longer nearly as popular as it once was.

C. OK432 is a "superantigen" made by suspending killed Streptococcus A in a solution of penicillin. This agent has been shown to be very effective in treating macrocystic *lymphatic* malformations, *not* high-flow malformations. It is not commercially available in the United States.

D. Ethanol rapidly denatures proteins in the endothelial lining of vessels. Having a low viscosity, it passes readily through AV shunts making it suitable for embolization of AVMs but only in conjunction with supraselective catheterization of the nidus itself. The latter is important; it should never be injected into a proximal feeding artery. Dosage and technique are important in avoiding complications. Alcohol causes local neurolysis, and, if too much gets into the circulation, systemic effects can occur, including central nervous system depression, hypoglycemia, hypertension, hyperthermia, cardiac arrhythmias, pulmonary vasoconstriction and hypertension, and electromechanical dissociation.

E. PVA is used for preoperative embolization to reduce the size and vascularity of a localized AVM and make its resection easier. It is not good for *primary* embolotherapy. PVA particles greater than 250 μm are relatively safe, and, after the flow through the AVM is interrupted by these particles, more proximal occlusion of the feeding arterial trunks with Gelfoam pledgets is useful in preventing early recanalization.

Answer 115-2: C
Discussion 115-2

A. Most VM mass lesions are peripheral and have poor connection to the main venous channels, so direct puncture has been used as a practical means of access.

B. Emptying the VM reduces the dose of sclerosant required, brings it into better contact with the endothelium, and reduces the likelihood of tender thrombosed venous masses with pigmentation (much like VV sclerotherapy). However, this is more difficult to do with VMs than with VVs.

C. Sclerotherapy of VMs usually is performed with either ethanol or sodium tetradecyl, although polidocanol and ethanolamine have been reported to be effective as well. Ethanol is *not* used for VV sclerotherapy, and sodium tetradecyl is no longer commercially available and must be made up by a pharmacy by special request. VV sclerotherapy now uses the latter two plus other milder sclerotherapy agents, often with foam preparations.

D. Diffuse extra-truncal (peripheral) and truncular (axial deep vein) VMs are not very amenable to sclerotherapy, or their symptoms are either too mild or not responsive to sclerotherapy, which is therefore mainly applied to extratruncular mass lesions.

E. If one considers that the majority of VMs are *either* axial/truncular VMs (deep vein aplasia, hypoplasias, localized webs, or aneurysms, comprising 45% of the total) *or* extra-truncular (peripheral) VMs (which are either too diffuse or less symptomatic to qualify for sclerotherapy), only the minority of VMs are amenable to embolo-sclerotherapy, and symptomatic enough to justify it. Popliteal venous aneurysms require surgery and some deep vein *obstructive* lesions may also, but most are well collateralized by the time they present and, along with diffuse lesions, are managed conservatively for practical considerations.

Answer 115-3: C

Discussion 115-3

A. Damage to skin or more extensive tissues is the most common complication of liquid embolization or sclerotherapy of vascular malformations. Approximately 10% of patients having sclerotherapy of VM have some skin necrosis resulting in scarring.

B. Neurologic injury can result from three mechanisms. Extravasation of ethanol around a nerve trunk can result in a demyelinization and necrosis. Penetration of arteries supplying nerve trunks can result in ischemic necrosis. Severe swelling caused by intravascular sclerotherapy can cause compartment syndrome and subsequent nerve injury.

C. Pigmentation from hemosiderin deposits in the skin is seen frequently after sclerotherapy of VMs, but *hemosiderosis* does *not* result from this.

D. Massive pulmonary embolism is an infrequent but potentially fatal complication of embolization of malformations involving large conducting channels. Migration of microthrombi during sclerotherapy, particularly if there are multiple sessions, can also affect the pulmonary vascular reserve and result in cardiovascular collapse.

E. Endovascular treatment of large vascular malformations results in intravascular thrombosis and consumption of clotting factors.

■ ANSWERS AND DISCUSSION FOR CHAPTER 116

Answer 116-1: E

Discussion 116-1

Despite the fact that AAAs may be the source of embolic debris, (E) one needs to take advantage of the full spectrum of noninvasive imaging to exclude other potential sources in the proximal thoracic and abdominal aorta as well as in the heart. It must be remembered that primary aortic tumors may first present with embolization. (B) Full aortography, introducing catheters and using power injections, carries a risk of precipitating embolization and should not be performed until a more proximal lesion (than the AAA) has been excluded. Only then may a proximal aortogram, preferably from a brachial or axillary approach, be performed. Long-term treatment with (A) antiplatelet agents or (D) warfarin anticoagulants only has a role in managing patients with an intracardiac thrombus, an isolated large aortic mural

thrombus (in a high risk for surgery), or a diffusely shaggy aorta. After a thorough investigation has identified the apparent source of embolism it can be eliminated/controlled by direct surgery in reasonable-risk patients. The role of stent grafts for aortic embolic sources other than aneurysm has yet to be fully defined and requires demonstration of long-term durability, especially if placed in relatively young, fit patients.

Answer 116-2: B

Discussion 116-2

Embolectomy alone, although alleviating the patient's acute limb ischemia, ignores the source of the embolus and its potential for recurrent embolization. Although 90% of the distal emboli originate from the heart, other potential sources must be excluded. All arterial emboli retrieved at the time of surgery should be submitted for pathologic examination to exclude the rare possibility of a tumor embolus. Thus, B is the proper approach here. With evidence of severe motor and sensory deficits, thrombolysis (C) would be inappropriate because of the time required to restore circulation and salvage the leg. Also, an embolus that is newly arrived in the leg may nevertheless be old and organized, having developing over time at its site of origin, and thus may not lyse quickly. (D) Fasciotomies may well be required in this patient, but they can be performed as indicated *after* restoration of flow. They do not improve circulation unless muscle swelling inside tight fascial compartments has impaired it, and this does not happen until *after* revascularization. (E) Long-term anticoagulation has improved late outcomes after arterial embolism, by reducing recurrences, and thus is commonly indicated, but it is indicated *only if* the embolic source is not identified and/or controlled.

Answer 116-3: D

Discussion 116-3

A polypoid lesion in the aorta could be either a benign mural thrombus based on an ulcerative aortic plaque or a primary aortic tumor. Therefore, in a "good-risk" patient, (D) resection of the involved portion of the aorta with interposition grafting not only is diagnostic but also provides the best chance of obtaining free margins if the lesion proves to be malignant. This possibility, of it being an aortic tumor, is the reason for not blindly giving (B) long-term warfarin anticoagulant therapy (which is not without risk), for not performing (C) a localized endarterectomy, or for not using (A) a stent graft. The latter's lack of proven durability is another consideration in this relatively young, good-risk patient. (E) An axillofemoral bypass, tempting in older, high-risk patients, also ignores the possibility of an aortic tumor, but, even if the lesion was a thrombus developing on an aortic plaque, this procedure would not protect the kidneys or splanchnic viscera from embolism.

Answer 116-4: B

Discussion 116-4

A. Long-term anticoagulation has *not* been proven to be protective of further embolization.

B. Although the patient should be initially maintained on heparin postoperatively, an exhaustive diagnostic workup should be carried out to find the primary source of the tumor embolism. This should include a trans-esophageal echocardiography and CT of the chest, abdomen, and pelvis. Unfortunately, many of these patients have evidence of metastatic disease at the time of diagnosis with an average life expectancy of only 14 months. However, if no evidence of metastatic disease is identified, primary resection of the tumor should be performed and has the only chance of curing the patient.

C. The role of chemotherapy in improving long-term survival has not been established.

D. Resection of the artery where the embolism lodged is not indicated.

E. The role of radiation therapy in improving long-term survival remains unclear.

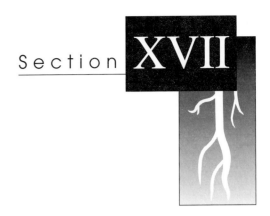

ARTERIOVENOUS
HEMODIALYSIS ACCESS

STUDY QUESTIONS

■ QUESTIONS FOR CHAPTER 117

Question 117-1

A 50-year-old man presents for his first hemodialysis access procedure. He has a history of hypertension but no previous extremity vascular procedures. Assuming that his physical examination supports it, his best primary access would be:

A. Radiocephalic straight forearm prosthetic arteriovenous (AV) shunt.
B. Radiocephalic autogenous AV fistula.
C. Brachiocephalic prosthetic loop shunt.
D. Forearm basilic vein transposition.
E. Brachiocephalic autogenous AV fistula.

Question 117-2

A 60-year-old woman is being evaluated for creation of a hemodialysis access. She has already failed a forearm autogenous access in her nondominant arm and is currently being dialyzed through a tunneled subclavian catheter on her dominant side. Aside from a physical examination, which test would most appropriately assure success and choose the best location of the future access?

A. Venous duplex scan.
B. Upper extremity arteriogram.
C. Platelet and coagulation studies.
D. Bilateral upper extremity venograms.
E. Heparin antibody titer.

Question 117-3

To be in compliance with the Dialysis Outcomes Quality Initiative (DOQI) guidelines, one should create which percentage of autogenous accesses among patients with dialysis-dependent renal failure?

A. 30%.
B. 40%.
C. 50%.
D. 60%.
E. 70%.

■ QUESTIONS FOR CHAPTER 118

Question 118-1

Venous transposition:

A. Is not recommended as a primary access by the DOQI guidelines.
B. Requires two separate anastomoses.
C. Can be accomplished in both the forearm and the upper arm.
D. Has a patency rate inferior to prosthetic in a similar position.
E. Is ill-advised in the diabetic patient.

Question 118-2

A 45-year-old female patient with diabetes presents for hemodialysis access creation. Although not yet on dialysis, she underwent a radiocephalic fistula several months previously in her nondominant arm, which failed at 6 weeks postoperatively. Assuming that her history and physical examination are favorable, the next most appropriate access would be:

A. A brachial-cephalic direct fistula in her dominant arm.
B. A radiocephalic straight prosthetic shunt in her nondominant forearm.
C. A brachiobasilic transposition in the nondominant arm.
D. A brachiobasilic straight prosthetic shunt in her nondominant arm.
E. A forearm basilic transposition in her nondominant arm.

Question 118-3

Six hours after the creation of a brachiobasilic transposed autogenous access fistula in his left arm, a 65-year-old patient returns to the emergency department with pain and numbness of the left hand. He had a previously failed radiocephalic straight prosthetic access in the same arm, and on examination, his hand is cool with poor capillary refill and its strength is weak relative to the right hand. His radial pulse is not palpable, and a strong thrill is felt over the access. To confirm your clinical diagnosis, the next step would be:

A. Compression of the fistula to observe if the radial pulse returns.
B. Duplex scan of the old prosthetic graft to detect thrombosis.

C. Exploration of the brachial artery with passage of Fogarty catheters distally.
D. Heparin anticoagulation, supportive care, and observation.
E. Digital subtraction arteriography of the affected limb.

■ QUESTIONS FOR CHAPTER 119

Question 119-1

The modality that has been unequivocally proven to have the best outcome in the treatment of a thrombosed hemodialysis access is:

A. Surgical thrombectomy with revision or patch angioplasty.
B. Systemic thrombolysis.
C. Percutaneous mechanical thrombectomy with percutaneous transluminal angioplasty (PTA) of underlying stenoses.
D. Percutaneous catheter-directed thrombolysis (CDT) with PTA of underlying stenoses.
E. None of the above has been proven superior over the others.

Question 119-2

A 57-year-old male patient is referred by his nephrologist who noted that his 2-year-old, left forearm brachiobasilic loop prosthetic access shunt had failed. On examination, there appears to be no evidence of infection and there is a strong radial pulse. In the operating room, the technique *most likely to succeed* in clearing the access of thrombus is:

A. Simple thrombectomy through a transverse graftotomy in the body of the graft.
B. Longitudinal graftotomy along the venous anastomotic hood with patch angioplasty or interposition bypass.
C. Longitudinal graftotomy along the arterial anastomotic hood with patch angioplasty or interposition bypass.
D. Transverse graftotomy across the venous anastomotic hood with patch angioplasty or interposition bypass.
E. Resect and redo an anastomosis after thrombectomy through each opening.

Question 119-3

Which of the following techniques can be combined in the open and endovascular treatment of thrombosed prosthetic AV shunts placed for angioaccess?

A. Balloon angioplasty of the arterial anastomosis, venous anastomosis, or outflow tract stenoses.
B. Angiographic imaging of the entire graft, arterial anastomosis, venous anastomosis, and venous outflow through angiographic sheaths inserted through the graftotomy.
C. Balloon catheter thrombectomy through a small transverse graft incision far removed from the venous and arterial anastomoses.
D. All of the above.
E. None of the above.

■ QUESTIONS FOR CHAPTER 120

Question 120-1

A 56 year old with end-stage renal disease has been undergoing hemodialysis three times each week for 2 years through an autogenous wrist (Brescia-Cimino) AV fistula. He is taking recombitant human erythropoietin. He has received the same dose of heparin at each session. Flow rates have been adequate. For the past 2 weeks the dialysis technicians have had to hold pressure for much longer than usual to gain hemostasis at his access puncture sites, and he presented to a local emergency department on one occasion for bleeding, which restarted at home after his dialysis session.

The most appropriate next step is:

A. Check protein C and S levels.
B. Administer vasopressin (deamino-D-arginine-vasopressin), 0.3 mg/kg one-half hour before the completion of each dialysis session.
C. Obtain a venous duplex to rule out venous outflow obstruction.
D. Initiate oral conjugated estrogens to aid in providing long-term procoagulant effect.
E. Increase the patient's dose of recombinant human erythropoietin.

Question 120-2

A 79-year-old diabetic woman is receiving hemodialysis through a right internal jugular dialysis catheter placed 6 weeks ago. She is noted to be somewhat lethargic before starting her dialysis session. Her blood glucose level is 269 mg/dL, and her temperature is 38.9°C (102.0°F).

Initial management could include all of the following, *except*:

A. Immediate computed tomography scan of the head and lumbar puncture to rule out bacterial meningitis.
B. Initiation of antibiotics active against both gram-negative and gram-positive organisms while awaiting culture results.
C. Obtainment of blood cultures through the dialysis catheter and a peripheral stick.
D. Administration of insulin.
E. Removal of catheter or exchange of catheter over a guidewire.

Question 120-3

A 62-year-old man had an autogenous brachiocephalic fistula created 10 days ago. He has coolness in the ipsilateral hand, stiffness in his fingers, and swelling. Motor strength is normal, and two-point discrimination is intact. Capillary refill is normal. No radial pulse is palpable at the wrist.

Appropriate management would include:

A. Immediate ligation of the AV fistula to restore pulse at the wrist.
B. The distal revascularization and interval ligation procedure using saphenous vein creating a bypass from the brachial artery to the radial artery.
C. Banding of the outflow vessel creating at least a 1-cm wide area of narrowing and check for adequacy of flow limitation by assessing for forward flow in the radial artery with a color Doppler.
D. The patient elevating the arm whenever possible. Encourage use of the hand and see the patient back in a short interval.
E. An arteriogram to rule out a proximal arterial stenosis.

ANSWERS AND DISCUSSION

■ ANSWERS AND DISCUSSION FOR CHAPTER 117

Answer 117-1: B

Discussion 117-1

In keeping with DOQI guidelines, one should always offer the patient an autogenous access (AV fistula) over a prosthetic access (AV conduit shunt) if physical examination supports it. Moreover, preserving the remainder of the arm for future access if needed can best be accomplished by creating the access at the most distal, suitable position. Of the choices offered, (B) a radiocephalic direct autogenous access (Brescia-Cimino fistula) would be the most appropriate. E would be the next best choice. D might allow a forearm autogenous access when there would not otherwise be an opportunity for one, but this would require a duplex scan to evaluate its feasibility. Once a prosthetic AV shunt becomes necessary, the choices would then be A or C, in that order.

Answer 117-2: D

Discussion 117-2

In patients in whom a prior access has failed or there is reasonable suspicion that the major veins draining the arm may have been injured or jeopardized, further evaluation is required before placement of the next access. Although studies of anticoagulation (C) and (E) play a role in any vascular procedure when indicated by previous events, the situation here mandates thorough venous evaluation, and the most *sensitive* of these tests for detecting venous injury or disease is (D) bilateral venograms. The arteries are not usually the problem, so B is rarely needed. Many might start with (A) duplex scanning, which would suggest the location and size of venous outflow sites, but it would not reveal subtle endothelial damage from previous intravenous infusions or blood sampling, or subclavian vein narrowing from previous dialysis catheter placement.

Answer 117-3: C

Discussion 117-3

The DOQI was a National Institutes of Health committee and was established to unify practice patterns based on evidence-based data. Explicitly stated, the committee strongly supports the use of autogenous-based hemodialysis access and recommends that this mode of access creation be attempted in fully 50% of the hemodialysis population.

■ ANSWERS AND DISCUSSION FOR CHAPTER 118

Answer 118-1: C

Discussion 118-1

A. The venous transposition is an autogenous access, a category of access that should be considered as first-line treatment in 50% of patients according to the DOQI doc-

ument because of its superiority in patency and complication rate over prosthetic access.
B. It requires one anastomosis, after mobilization.
C. It is generally accomplished using the forearm or upper arm basilic vein, with anastomosis to the radial or brachial artery, respectively (correct answer).
D. It has excellent patency, close to other autogenous fistulas and superior to prosthetic shunts.
E. Venous transposition in the diabetic can be accomplished, especially in the upper arm, and is worth trying.

Answer 118-2: E

Discussion 118-2

Current hemodialysis access guidelines recommend against prosthetic access whenever autogenous access is possible. The surgeon should avoid use of the dominant extremity and favor the most distal accesses that can be created in the nondominant extremity. After a failed radiocephalic autogenous access in the nondominant arm, transposition of the forearm basilic vein to the radial artery in the same arm (E) would be the appropriate next step. A is in the dominant arm, B and D are prosthetic shunts, and C is a more proximal autogenous fistula, using transposition, than E, so they all would be less suitable choices following the strategy outlined.

Answer 118-3: A

Discussion 118-3

A. Your diagnosis should be distal steal. A steal phenomenon is occasionally observed after upper arm basilic transposition and most often results from creation of too generous an arteriotomy in the brachial artery. In this case, the created fistula flow steals from the distal arterial outflow below the anastomosis, so the radial artery pulse disappears and the hand becomes ischemic. Confirmation of the diagnosis is easily made by temporary digital compression of the fistula with reversal of physical symptoms and return of the radial pulse.
B. In the scenario presented, duplex scan is unnecessary.
C. The transposition/fistula has not clotted, so C would yield flowing blood not clot.
D. Correction of the steal is required to prevent progression of the critical ischemia with ischemic nerve dysfunction. Delay in correcting the problem, by observation under heparin anticoagulation, would be inappropriate.
E. In this scenario, digital subtraction would be unnecessary. Further studies, with duplex scan or arteriography, would only be indicated if the diagnosis of steal were in doubt or incorrect, but the presentation described is classic.

■ ANSWERS AND DISCUSSION FOR CHAPTER 119

Answer 119-1: E

Discussion 119-1

None of these modalities has demonstrated clear superiority over the others in outcome or efficacy. A and D are currently the most commonly used, and, although individual reports may suggest advantages of one over the other, there is no high level evidence of overall superiority, and under certain circumstances one may be a more appropriate choice than the others.

A. Surgical thrombectomy has the advantage of rapidly restoring patency, but evaluation of the underlying causative lesion is suboptimal using balloon catheters to detect narrowings. Depending on the lesion causing thrombosis, surgical revision or angioplasty may have more durable patency than PTA, but time to restart dialysis may be longer these with D.

B. Systemic thrombolysis is no longer used but was tried in the past. It is too slow to dissolve the clot and does not address the underlying cause. D has replaced it.

C. Percutaneous mechanical thrombectomy has been used to speed clot resolution in other settings, and some mechanical thrombectomy devices are able to remove firm arterial plugs as well as recent clot, but used alone it often does not completely remove the clot and thrombolysis has to be added. Reported experiences with it in this setting are few and have not presented evidence of superiority. It involves expensive equipment and has not shown advantages over CDT.

D. CDT has been used with increasing frequency, often with crossed catheter and pulse-spray techniques, to speed up clot resolution. Being done under angiographic control, it has the advantages of closer monitoring of clot dissolution and visualizing the underlying lesions. Unfortunately the narrowings seen may not give a durable response to balloon angioplasty. Its better preservation of access sites is offset by the greater cost of its repeated use, because recurrences after PTA are common.

E. In view of the lack of proven superiority of A or D, or a significant added benefit to C, the correct answer is E.

Answer 119-2: B

Discussion 119-2

A. Simple thrombectomy yields a poor outcome unless extrinsic manual compression or another mechanical cause can explain thrombosis of the access, and if performed through a transverse incision in the body of the graft, precludes visualizing and treating the underlying cause, which will be some distance away.

B. The most common cause for this graft's failure is the formation of neointimal hyperplasia at the venous outflow. Realizing that an adjunctive procedure (e.g., patch angioplasty or interposition bypass) will likely need to be performed after thrombectomy of the graft, the location of the incision for thrombectomy must be made to complement this need. Longitudinal graftotomy over the venous hood gives the best chance of visualizing the problem without compromising the choice between patch angioplasty and an interposition graft.

C. The problem is unlikely to be at the arterial end in this scenario.

D. Transverse graftotomy will not lend itself to patch angioplasty if this turns out to be the appropriate adjunctive procedure.

E. Anastomotic stenosis, requiring resection and reanastomosis, is an unlikely cause of failure of this access procedure.

Answer 119-3: D

Discussion 119-3

Techniques A, B, and C, in reverse order of frequency, are all used in the combined open and catheter-based approach to prosthetic access thrombectomy. This approach presents complementary advantages and utility regardless of the location of the underlying lesion(s). Thus, D is the correct answer.

■ ANSWERS AND DISCUSSION FOR CHAPTER 120

Answer 120-1: C

Discussion 120-1

Any one of these measures might be appropriate under certain circumstances, but A, B, and D would require special bleeding and clotting studies, and would not be undertaken as "shotgun" therapy. (E) Recombinant human erythropoietin is appropriate if the patient is anemic, but the patient is already on this drug at the usual dose and this would not address the underlying problem. However, recurrent bleeding or bleeding requiring prolonged pressure can often be a warning sign of venous outflow obstruction, and thus C is the correct answer.

Answer 120-2: A

Discussion 120-2

(A) Both hypothermia and hyperthermia can be seen in elderly or immunocompromised patients with access infections. Although the diagnosis of bacterial meningitis could be entertained after other sources are ruled out, the most likely source of infection would be the dialysis catheter. (B) Initiating broad-spectrum antibiotics while awaiting culture results, (C) obtaining blood cultures through the dialysis catheter and a peripheral stick, (D) administering insulin to combat the hyperglycemia, and (E) removing the catheter, which must be presumed to be infected and replacing it, are all appropriate measures. The removed catheter should also be directly cultured.

Answer 120-3: D

Discussion 120-3

A distal steal could cause the pulse distal to the fistula to not be palpable, but this takes time to develop after creating a fistula and would be unlikely in 10 days. *If* there was a *symptomatic* distal steal, one of the first three options could be entertained. A is the simplest and would suffice for most wrist fistulas. Its efficacy could be ensured by a response of pulse return with fistula compression (on the venous side to avoid compressing the radial artery). B is a more elaborate and sometimes necessary treatment for distal steal but is more commonly performed with proximally placed AV access. (C) The banding procedure was commonly performed in the past but has been abandoned. It is too difficult to achieve the correct degree of narrowing, even with duplex or other flow monitoring. However, D is the correct answer because mild symptoms of swelling, stiffness, and coolness are *common* after fistula creation. Most symptoms resolve within a few weeks. Patients should be seen at short-interval follow-up to check for symptom progression, which would warrant further investigation for other possible causes (anastomotic problems or distal steal). (E) Proximal arterial stenosis, from a technically flawed fistula creation, is an unlikely explanation, but it would be studied by duplex scan not arteriography.

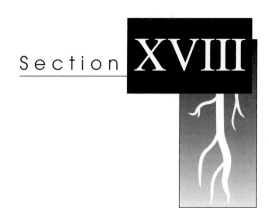

THE MANAGEMENT OF SPLANCHNIC VASCULAR LESIONS AND DISORDERS

STUDY QUESTIONS

■ QUESTIONS FOR CHAPTER 121

Question 121-1

Which of the following is not an important collateral pathway for the mesenteric arterial circulation?

A. The superior and inferior pancreaticoduodenal arteries.
B. The marginal artery of Drummond.
C. The "replaced" right hepatic artery arising from the superior mesenteric artery (SMA).
D. The superior and middle rectal arteries.
E. The Arc of Riolan.

Question 121-2

Splanchnic blood flow:

A. Increases significantly after eating because of a marked increase in hepatic artery blood flow.
B. Increases immediately after oral intake regardless of whether the nutrients are absorbed immediately.
C. Is reduced in response to decreases in extracellular volume by the direct action of angiotensin II.
D. Is maintained initially after blood loss by the release of vasopressin causing mesenteric vasodilation and venoconstriction.
E. Must be maintained above 300 mL/min/100 g of tissue to maintain mucosal integrity because intestinal mucosa has a limited ability to extract increased amounts of oxygen.

Question 121-3

Which of the following patients is most likely to have *symptomatic* mesenteric arterial occlusive disease?

A. A patient with greater than 80% SMA stenosis, a 50% celiac artery stenosis, a widely patent inferior mesenteric artery, and a previous transverse colectomy.
B. A patient with a celiac artery occlusion and a left hypogastric artery stenosis.
C. A patient with a greater than 90% celiac artery stenosis, a 50% superior mesenteric stenosis, and poorly developed pancreaticoduodenal collaterals.

D. A patient with a greater than 90% celiac artery stenosis, a 50% superior mesenteric stenosis, and an inferior mesenteric artery occlusion.
E. A patient with 50% to 60% stenosis of both the celiac artery and SMA and an inferior mesenteric artery occlusion.

Question 121-4

A 75-year-old female smoker, with a history of claudication and coronary artery disease, presents with a three-month history of postprandial abdominal pain that occurs after eating. Her discomfort is sometimes followed by diarrhea. She has not weighed herself, but she thinks she may have lost 5 pounds. What would be the *next* appropriate step in this patient's workup?

A. Mesenteric arteriogram.
B. Mesenteric duplex ultrasound.
C. Magnetic resonance arteriogram (MRA).
D. CT scan with oral and intravenous contrast.
E. Mesenteric duplex in fed and fasting states.

Question 121-5

Which of the following statements regarding mesenteric physiology is *correct*?

A. Shortly after a mixed-calorie meal, blood flow to the liver increases dramatically as a direct result of celiac and common hepatic artery vasodilatation.
B. During periods of intestinal hypoperfusion, the small intestine is able to extract increasing amounts of oxygen to keep overall oxygen consumption constant and preserve its integrity.
C. Vasopressin can be used therapeutically to mitigate the mesenteric vasoconstriction seen in cases of non-occlusive mesenteric ischemia.
D. Because of redundant collateral pathways, symptomatic chronic mesenteric ischemia is only seen when two of the three mesenteric vessels are occluded or critically stenotic.
E. The extrinsic neuro-hormonal control mechanism of splanchnic blood flow refers to the effects of the sympathetic nervous system, rennin-angiotensin axis, and adenosine on splanchnic vascular tone.

Question 121-6

A 70-year-old man is still in the hospital 9 days after a myocardial infarction and an emergency coronary artery bypass. He is about to be transferred out of the intensive care unit when he suddenly develops diffuse mid-abdominal pain. Which would be the *next best test* to confirm the diagnosis?

A. Emergent exploratory laparotomy.
B. Mesenteric duplex.
C. Mesenteric arteriogram with intra-arterial thrombolysis.
D. Bi-Phasic CT arteriogram (CTA).
E. Flat and upright KUB.

■ QUESTIONS FOR CHAPTER 122

Question 122-1

A 73-year-old woman presents to the emergency department at midnight with sudden onset of abdominal pain that began approximately 2 hours earlier. She denies other recent gastrointestinal symptoms. On physical examination her abdomen is unremarkable, lungs are clear, and heart sounds are irregularly irregular. An electrocardiogram reveals atrial fibrillation with a rate of 85, and laboratory studies are remarkable only for a white blood cell count of 24,000. What would be the next appropriate step in this patient's care?

A. Emergency abdominal arteriography.
B. Emergency computed tomographic angiography.
C. Duplex examination of the mesenteric vessels.
D. Operative exploration of the abdomen.
E. Immediate synchronized cardioversion.

Question 122-2

A previously healthy elderly patient with a long history of smoking is undergoing laparotomy for acute abdominal pain and suspected small bowel obstruction. You are consulted for the intraoperative finding of ischemic bowel. On examination, the bowel shows no signs of obstruction but is dusky from the ligament of Treitz to the mid-transverse colon. One area of distal jejunum is obviously infarcted. There is no gross spillage of enteric contents. The most likely diagnosis and appropriate therapy is:

A. Superior mesenteric thrombosis; bypass of the SMA using saphenous or femoral vein with resection of the distal jejunum.
B. Venous thrombosis; resection of the infarcted bowel and anticoagulation postoperatively.
C. Superior mesenteric embolus; resection of the distal jejunum and SMA embolectomy.
D. Nonocclusive mesenteric ischemia; resection of the distal jejunum, postoperative resuscitation, and second-look operation in 24 hours.
E. Nonocclusive mesenteric ischemia; begin an infusion of nitroprusside into the SMA through a catheter in one of its branches.

Question 122-3

An 81-year-old man is transferred from an outside facility for acute abdominal pain. He arrives in the emergency department with signs of peritoneal irritation, hypotension, and acidosis. After undergoing aggressive resuscitation, he is taken urgently to the operating room. On entering the abdomen, there is gross spillage of enteric content and infarcted bowel from the ligament of Treitz to the transverse colon. The *most appropriate* next step is:

A. Resection of the perforated segments of intestine, SMA bypass with saphenous vein, subsequent resection of remaining nonviable intestine, and second-look laparotomy in 24 hours.
B. Resection of perforated segments of intestine, SMA embolectomy, resection of remaining nonviable bowel, and second-look laparotomy in 18 hours.
C. Closure of the abdomen and institution of comfort measures.
D. Resection of all nonviable intestine, SMA bypass with saphenous vein, fluorescein dye assessment of remaining bowel, and resection where indicated.
E. Resection of the perforated intestine, SMA bypass with saphenous vein on-table angiography, and second-look laparotomy in 18 hours.

■ QUESTIONS FOR CHAPTER 123

Question 123-1

The primary mechanism for nonocclusive mesenteric ischemia is:

A. Thromboembolism.
B. Vasospasm.
C. Increased oxygen demand.
D. Mesenteric vasodilation.
E. Low cardiac output.

Question 123-2

Clinical settings considered to be associated with nonocclusive mesenteric ischemia include all of the following except:

A. Dialysis-dependent renal insufficiency.
B. Septic shock.
C. Cardiac failure.
D. Hepatitis.
E. Administration of digitalis-like drugs.

Question 123-3

Angiography in nonocclusive mesenteric ischemia demonstrates:

A. Normal mesenteric vasculature.
B. Diminished mesenteric venous outflow.
C. Pruning of mesenteric branch vessels.
D. Thrombosis of the SMA.
E. Dilation of distal mesentery artery branches.

■ QUESTIONS FOR CHAPTER 124

Question 124-1

A 55-year-old woman with an extensive smoking history, a 35-pound weight loss over the preceding 6 months, and postprandial pain is referred from her gastroenterologists for further evaluation and definitive treatment. She has undergone an extensive workup before referral that has included a computed axial tomography scan, an esophagogastroduodenoscopy, a colonoscopy, and a gall bladder ultrasound. She was found to have a gastric ulcer on the esophagogastroduodenoscopy, but the other diagnostic study results were essentially normal. Before her referral, she had a mesenteric duplex ultrasound study that showed probable high-grade stenoses (>70%) in both the celiac axis and SMA.

Of the following, which is *not likely* to be seen on a standard contrast arteriogram of the mesenteric vessels?

A. A high-grade orificial stenosis or occlusion of the SMA.
B. A large meandering artery that provides collateral flow between the inferior mesenteric and middle colic arteries.
C. Severe central aortic arterial occlusive disease with significant lesions in the celiac axis, SMA, and both renal arteries.
D. Severe stenoses or pruning of the distal SMA branches with multiple associated small aneurysms.
E. A large middle hemorrhoidal artery that provides collateral flow to the distal inferior mesenteric artery.

Question 124-2

A 75-year-old woman with several active medical problems including home oxygen-dependent chronic obstructive pulmonary disease and congestive heart failure (ejection fraction 30%) presents with chronic mesenteric ischemia with a typical history, and this is confirmed by a mesenteric duplex ultrasound study. A decision to proceed with diagnostic mesenteric arteriogram and possibly endovascular revascularization if possible was made.

Of the following, which is *the most appropriate* statement about the access for the diagnostic study and therapeutic endovascular procedure?

A. Access through the brachial artery is preferred because the celiac axis and SMA are actually closer relative to the femoral artery; therefore, proportionally shorter guidewires and catheters can be used.
B. One major advantage of the brachial artery access over the femoral approach is that it allows a larger maximal catheter sheath size without the need for open surgical exposure of the vessel.
C. Directing the catheters/guidewires into the descending thoracic aorta from the brachial artery is rarely associated with difficulty and does not subject the patient to potential risk from embolic events.
D. Femoral artery approach should only be used for diagnostic studies when the likelihood of endovascular intervention is very small because of the orientation of the mesenteric arteries relative to the aorta.
E. The vector forces of a catheter directed from the brachial artery are opposite to the angle of the mesenteric vessels; therefore, its pushability is compromised.

Question 124-3

A 55-year-old man, who is a heavy smoker (>100 pack-years) and has a very strong family history for atherosclerotic vascular occlusive disease, presents with postprandial abdominal pain and weight loss. A mesenteric duplex ultrasound demonstrates that *both* the celiac axis and SMA are

occluded at their orifices. These findings are confirmed by a diagnostic arteriogram.

Of the following, which is *not* an appropriate treatment plan?

A. Retrograde bypass from the proximal right common iliac artery to the SMA using a Dacron graft.
B. Antegrade bypass from the supraceliac aorta to both the celiac axis and SMA using a bifurcated Dacron graft.
C. Antegrade bypass from the supraceliac aorta to both the celiac axis and the SMA using the patient's own superficial femoral vein.
D. Total parenteral nutrition through a subcutaneous port with a catheter in the right subclavian vein and avoidance of oral intake, the only choice because of unreconstructable disease.
E. Balloon angioplasty and stenting of both the celiac axis and SMA using a balloon expandable stent.

■ QUESTIONS FOR CHAPTER 125

Question 125-1

A 27-year-old man is evaluated in the emergency department for worsening diffuse abdominal pain. He admits to similar discomfort "off and on" for approximately 3 weeks. He has had some diarrhea and has recently become anorexic. His heart rate is 98 beats/min, and his blood pressure is normal. He is distended but not particularly tender. His white blood cell count is 12,400. Other laboratory values suggest volume depletion. A CT scan suggests mesenteric venous thrombosis, and the bowel and mesentery appear thickened. As the surgical consultant you should recommend:

A. Low molecular weight heparin with outpatient conversion to warfarin and weekly office follow-up until asymptomatic.
B. Scheduling the patient for urgent abdominal exploration.
C. Hospital admission, coagulation studies for thrombophilic factors, anticoagulation with intravenous heparin, maintain n.p.o., intravenous fluids, and observation.
D. Arrangement with the interventional radiologist on-call to start transhepatic intramesenteric venous thrombolysis.
E. Hospital admission, stool and blood cultures, intravenous therapy to correct volume losses, and observation for development of peritoneal signs.

Question 125-2

A 34-year-old woman is admitted with acute onset of crampy abdominal pain and is diagnosed with mesenteric vein thrombosis (MVT). Exploration is undertaken, and a 26-cm of nonviable mid-jejunum is resected, with uneventful recovery. Thrombophilic studies return demonstrating factor V Leiden deficiency. Appropriate long-term management should include:

A. Three months of anticoagulation with warfarin and repeat thrombophilic panel 3 weeks after discontinuing the drug.
B. A diet with abundant leafy-green vegetables.
C. Life-long anticoagulation and consultation with a coagulation specialist.

D. Counseling with a geneticist for all her siblings and children regarding the risks of them or their progeny having factor V Leiden.
E. Vitamin B12 and folate supplements.

Question 125-3

An 84-year-old man is admitted from the emergency department with a diagnosis of subacute mesenteric venous thrombosis. The *most likely* underlying cause is:

A. Protein S deficiency.
B. Colonic neoplasm.
C. Crohn's disease.
D. Heparin-induced thrombocytopenia.
E. Schirmer-Hasselbach syndrome.

■ QUESTIONS FOR CHAPTER 126

Question 126-1

Clinically important (associated with variceal bleeding) venous collateral pathways to relieve portal venous hypertension include all of the following *except*:

A. Portal and splenic veins to the azygous/hemiazygous veins.
B. Retroperitoneal connections between pancreatic and colonic veins and the inferior vena cava.
C. Inferior mesenteric veins to middle and inferior hemorrhoidal veins.
D. Reopened umbilical vein connections to the internal mammary and inferior epigastric veins.
E. Small or large bowel veins to parietal peritoneal or subcutaneous veins through adhesions or ostomies.

Question 126-2

Appropriate management of a patient with portal hypertension presenting with acute upper gastrointestinal bleeding includes all of the following *except*:

A. Admission to the intensive care unit, monitoring of the hematocrit, and administration of appropriate volumes of crystalloid, blood, and clotting factors.
B. Emergency upper endoscopy.
C. Endoscopic variceal sclerotherapy or banding or emergency transjugular intrahepatic portosystemic shunt (TIPS) to prevent continued or recurrent bleeding.
D. Administration of vasopressin/nitroglycerin or octreotide to decrease portal venous pressure.
E. Preparation for an emergency surgical portosystemic shunt to definitively control the bleeding.

Question 126-3

Definitive therapy for variceal bleeding:

A. Is reserved for patients who have a second episode of bleeding and is necessary in less than 50% of patients.
B. Using chronic B-blockade reduces the likelihood of rebleeding by more than 80%.
C. Using endoscopic measures to control bleeding is preferred treatment because it is associated with a few long-term complications and is very effective, even in patients who have bled from gastric varices.
D. Using TIPS is associated with almost uniform initial success, but also a high rate of portosystemic encephalopathy and subsequent rebleeding because of occlusion of the shunt.
E. Using orthotopic liver transplantation is seldom done because of poor graft survival even if the patients stop drinking and is best reserved for those patients who fail chronic endoscopic therapy or surgical portosystemic shunt.

ANSWERS AND DISCUSSION

■ ANSWERS AND DISCUSSION FOR CHAPTER 121

Answer 121-1: C
Discussion 121-1

The collateral circulation of the mesenteric arterial system is extensive and includes the connections between the celiac artery and superior mesenteric arteries through (A) the superior and inferior pancreaticoduodenal arteries, the superior and inferior mesenteric arteries through the (B) marginal artery of Drummond, and occasionally (E) the Arc of Riolan and (D) the hypogastric and inferior mesenteric arteries through the superior and middle rectal arteries. Although (C) a replaced right hepatic artery arising from the SMA is the most common variant in the mesenteric circulation, it is not a collateral pathway.

Answer 121-2: C
Discussion 121-2

The control of splanchnic blood is complex and influenced by many factors.

A. After eating, splanchnic flow increases significantly by 45 minutes, primarily because of increased SMA flow while *hepatic artery flow remains relatively constant.*
B. Absorption of nutrients is necessary to initiate this increased flow.
C. In response to hypovolemia, splanchnic flow is significantly decreased primarily by the direct action of angiotensin II, causing vasoconstriction.
D. Splanchnic blood flow is also affected by vasopressin, which causes vasoconstriction (not vasodilation), which makes vasopressin a good treatment for bleeding caused by partial hypertension, but vasopressin does *not* maintain splanchnic flow after initial blood loss.
E. In response to hypoperfusion, mucosal integrity is maintained to blood flow rates of 30 mL/min/100 g of tissue (not 300 mL/min as in this incorrect answer) by the mucosal cells' ability to extract increasing amounts of oxygen.

Answer 121-3: A
Discussion 121-3

A. The majority of patients with symptomatic mesenteric arterial occlusive disease have multivessel disease, but the SMA is dominant and single-vessel disease involving the SMA can be symptomatic, particularly when collateral pathways such as the marginal Artery of Drummond and the Arch of Riolan in the left and transverse colon are interrupted, as they are in this case by a transverse colectomy. This prevents collaterals from the IMA compensating for a severe SMA stenosis, so this patient should be the most symptomatic.
B. In this case the SMA is patent and could compensate for celiac occlusion through collaterals. The left hypogastric might come into play as a collateral if the inferior mesenteric artery (IMA) was occluded.

C. Adequate flow would be obtained through the 50% SMA stenosis.
D. Same answer as C, although this patient is more dependent on no further SMA narrowing to avoid significant chronic mesenteric ischemia.
E. This patient, like the patient in D, would likely become symptomatic with further narrowing of the SMA.

Answer 121-4: B
Discussion 121-4

Although the overall incidence of chronic mesenteric ischemia is very low, it is much higher among patients with other evidence of peripheral vascular disease and not uncommon in women. Significant mesenteric stenoses may be present in up to 27% of that patient subgroup. Her clinical history is somewhat atypical however creating only a moderate index of suspicion.

A. Mesenteric arteriography is still the gold standard to confirm the diagnosis but is invasive, expensive and requires exposure to iodinated contrast (i.e., not a good choice for *next* step).
B. Mesenteric ultrasound is noninvasive, relatively inexpensive and in this situation is the best next test because of its high sensitivity and specificity. It does require an experienced technologist, however.
C. MRA spatial resolution (1mm^2) is not fine enough to provide adequate visualiztion of the mesenteric vasculature and does not yet have a routine role in the work up of CMI.
D. CTA provides excellent arterial reconstructions and confirms alternative diagnoses when the clinical diagnosis is in question, especially in more acute presentations. But it also requires iodinated contrast exposure, and is more expensive than B.
E. Postprandial mesenteric duplex does not add anything to the fasting study and, in fact, has a lower sensitivity and specificity.

Answer 121-5: B
Discussion 121-5

A. Hepatic arterial flow is low resistance and remains fairly constant during fed and fasting states. The postprandial increase in hepatic flow is largely the result of the dramatic increase in SMA and portal venous flow.
B. This is true down to a critically low flow rate of 30mL/min/100g of tissue.
C. Vasopressin (antidiuretic hormone) causes mesenteric arterial vasoconstriction and venorelaxation, which makes it useful in the medical treatment of variceal bleeding.
D. This is generally true but single vessel CMI does can and does exist when these collateral pathways may not have had time to develop (e.g., median arcuate ligament syndrome) or may have been interrupted by previous surgery. Single vessel CMI most commonly involves the SMA.

E. Extrinsic regulation of splanchnic blood flow is effected by the sympathetic nervous system, renin-angiotensin axis, and the pituitary in the form of vasopressin (antidiuretic hormone). Adenosine is an *intrinsic* metabolite of mucosal ischemia that causes vasorelaxation.

Answer 121-6: D

Discussion 121-6

Embolic acute mesenteric ischemia in the immediate post-MI, post CABG patient is only one of several possibilities to explain abdominal pain but needs to be ruled in/out promptly.

A. Emergent celiotomy for anything less than frank peritonitis is unwarranted and would expose the patient to a possible negative laparotomy.
B. Mesenteric duplex is often technically difficult in the non-fasted patient and will *not* identify other possible pathologies.
C. Diagnostic mesenteric arteriography would be a good choice to confirm the diagnosis of acute mesenteric thromboembolus. The efficacy of thrombolysis in the treatment of mesenteric embolus, however, has not been established and in this particular case is contraindicated because of the patients recent CABG.
D. Bi-Phasic CT arteriography would be the best overall choice to confirm the diagnosis of mesenteric thromboembolus. If performed with the addition of an oral negative contrast agent (i.e., water), early bowel wall edema may also be seen to support the diagnosis and confirm the distribution of bowel involvement. Importantly, alternative pathology can often be identified.
E. Abdominal plain films lack the sensitivity and specificity to identify any significant pathology in a timely manner.

■ ANSWERS AND DISCUSSION FOR CHAPTER 122

Answer 122-1: D

Discussion 122-1

The clinical scenario presented is characteristic for a patient with acute mesenteric ischemia caused by embolic occlusion of the SMA. Such emboli commonly have a cardiac source, particularly in patients with atrial fibrillation.

A. Imaging of the splanchnic arteries would be appropriate when the diagnosis is less certain than in this case. Time is of the essence. Intraoperative angiography in an angio-equipped operating room, *while preparing for surgery*, might be an option, but arranging for and obtaining an aortogram in the usual hospital in the early hours of the morning would waste valuable time.
B. When imaging is indicated, CT angiography with a new multislice imager *in preparation for exploration* is appropriate and takes less time than standard aortography in the radiology department. Nevertheless, exploration is indicated (see D).
C. Duplex interrogation takes time and expertise, the latter not being available at night in most hospitals.

D. Proper treatment of such a patient is prompt operative exploration because outcome directly correlates with the duration of bowel ischemia. The clinical scenario is characteristic enough for acute mesenteric ischemia caused by embolic occlusion of the SMA to warrant this. Pursuing diagnostic studies, at this time of night, increases the likelihood of significant bowel loss.
E. This can wait until after the bowel ischemia has been dealt with.

Answer 122-2: A

Discussion 122-2

Differentiation between thrombotic and embolic occlusion of the SMA intraoperatively can be challenging. However, differentiation is important because the exposure of the artery and subsequent reconstructive procedures are very different. The distribution of bowel ischemia provides an important clue, and examination of the SMA pulse will also help in the diagnosis, being absent in thrombotic SMA occlusion but palpable proximally in an embolus to the SMA.

A. The description here is typical of a thrombotic occlusion of an arteriosclerotic narrowing of the SMA, for the bowel is dusky from the ligament of Treitz to the mid-transverse colon. This requires a bypass that is best accomplished with an antegrade supraceliac aorta to SMA bypass using a longitudinal SMA arteriotomy.
B. Venous thrombosis produces purplish, edematous bowel, unlike the description here.
C. Most superior mesenteric arterial emboli spare the first branches of the SMA so that the proximal jejunum is usually well perfused, not ischemic as described. When the diagnosis is embolic occlusion, the SMA can be exposed at the base of the mesocolon and opened transversely (unlike thrombotic occlusion; see A).
D. Nonocclusive mesenteric ischemia usually presents with patchy bowel ischemia and often *also involves the colon.* This patient was previously healthy, rather than chronically ill with cardiac failure, as is the usual scenario with this diagnosis.
E. Same as D. This is not characteristic of *nonocclusive* mesenteric insufficiency.

Answer 122-3: C

Discussion 122-3

Infarction of the entire small bowel and right colon is incompatible with subsequent oral feeding and long-term survival. The colon does not tolerate drainage directly from the duodenum so that lifetime total parenteral nutrition with a defunctionalized colon and high-output duodenal fistula is the only option, an unsustainable condition in a patient this elderly. Therefore, C is the correct answer.

This patient has had an SMA thrombosis. Earlier in this progression, with a mixture of dusky and infarcted bowel being found at exploration, if the extent of the dusky bowel is sufficient to support life, an SMA bypass using saphenous vein might salvage the dusky bowel. The bowel can be reassessed after revascularization, but then anastomosing segments of bowel with borderline viability to preserve the maximum possible intestine, even with fluorescein dye assessment, can be treacherous, and because a second look is necessary anyhow, temporary ostomies might be preferable to anastomotic breakdown and more spillage.

ANSWERS AND DISCUSSION FOR CHAPTER 123

Answer 123-1: B

Discussion 123-1

A. By definition "nonoccusive" involves neither embolism nor thrombosis, although secondary thrombosis can be superimposed later as a secondary event.
B. Mesenteric vasospasm appears to be the primary mechanism for the development of nonocclusive mesenteric ischemia. Exactly what induces it is still a matter of conjecture. Mesenteric vasospasm has been seen on arteriography in these patients, and mesenteric infusions of vasodilators have been effective. The latter scenario has unfortunately been too infrequent.
C. Increased oxygen demand plays no role in the pathophysiology.
D. Vasodilatation plays no role; just the opposite is the case.
E. Many of the patients with this condition are seriously ill, and many have had periods of low cardiac output. Some are receiving drugs such as digoxin, and an experimental study in dogs once showed reduced intestinal flow in response to this drug, spawning a theory that digoxin-like drugs and low cardiac output were responsible, but this was not corroborated in primate experiments. It is clear, however, that reduced cardiac output with secondarily reduced mesenteric inflow could not produce this degree of ischemia alone, without vasospasm.

Answer 123-2: D

Discussion 123-2

A. Dialysis-dependent renal failure can result in episodic hypoperfusion and is a known risk factor for nonocclusive mesenteric ischemia.
B. Septic shock leads to hypovolemia and secondary mesenteric vasoconstriction through the actions of both angiotensin II and vasopressin.
C. Cardiac failure results in mesenteric vasoconstriction in response to hypoperfusion.
D. Hepatitis usually has little if any effect on mesenteric hemodynamics (correct answer).
E. Patients with cardiac failure are often given digitalis-like drugs, so there is at least a coincidental association here. A canine experiment study once claimed to show reduced intestinal flow with this drug, spawning a theory that this and low cardiac output were responsible, but this was never corroborated.

Answer 123-3: C

Discussion 123-3

Selective mesenteric angiography is both diagnostic and provides access for therapy in patients with nonocclusive mesenteric ischemia. A widely patent trunk of the SMA excludes thrombosis of the SMA, and this combined with *pruning of the SMA branches* defines the diagnosis. Treatment can then be initiated by infusion of papaverine through the diagnostic

catheter and should be continued for at least 24 hours. Therefore, C is the correct answer.

None of the other answers describe what is seen with this condition. A completely normal study excludes the diagnosis. Diminished venous outflow (B) can be seen in patients with mesenteric vasoconstriction (the primary cause of nonocclusive mesenteric ischemia), but this is a consequence rather than a cause of the disease. This finding in such patients is also not accompanied by contrast enhancement of the bowel wall and leakage of contrast into the bowel lumen as is seen with arteriography in patients with mesenteric venous thrombosis. (D) Thrombosis is not a primary finding. (E) Constriction rather than dilation occurs.

ANSWERS AND DISCUSSION FOR CHAPTER 124

Answer 124-1: D

Discussion 124-1

A. The celiac axis and SMA lesions are usually orificial, and the more distal extent of the vessels is spared or uninvolved. This usually holds true in the presence of a complete orificial occlusion even when the distal vessels are not seen with contrast arteriography.
B. The presence of well-developed collateral channels between the visceral vessels supports the diagnosis of mesenteric ischemia and attests to the hemodynamic significance of the ostial lesions. There is an extensive collateral network between the three visceral vessels and the internal iliac arteries. The celiac axis and SMA collateralize through the superior (celiac axis) and inferior (SMA) pancreaticoduodenal arteries with the direction of flow contingent on the location of the significant stenosis. The superior and inferior mesenteric arteries collateralize through both the meandering artery and the marginal artery of Drummond. The meandering artery is the most significant collateral vessel and connects the ascending branch of the left colic with the middle branch of the middle colic.
C. The mesenteric arterial occlusive disease from atherosclerosis is essentially an "aortic spillover." It is relatively common to see concomitant renal and mesenteric artery occlusive disease, and these findings support the concept of a "central aortic" atherosclerotic process. It is imperative that a lateral arteriogram be obtained at the time of the diagnostic study.
D. All the findings *in all of the answers except D* may be observed. Small visceral artery aneurysms are occasionally seen on arteriogram in the collateral branches, specifically the pancreaticoduodenal artery. These are presumably "flow"-related aneurysms, similar to those seen in the splenic artery in patients with portal hypertension, not mesenteric insufficiency. Involvement of the distal vasculature with occlusive lesion suggests a nonatherosclerotic process such as cocaine or ergot ingestion.
E. The inferior mesenteric artery communicates with the internal iliac artery through the hemorrhoidal branches and may represent a more important collateral than originally appreciated.

Answer 124-2: D

Discussion 124-2

Percutaneous access can be obtained through either the femoral or brachial arteries. The primary consideration for the particular approach should be the likelihood of a prior therapeutic intervention (with the exception of those patients with known anatomic limitations such as iliofemoral or subclavian artery occlusive disease). The femoral approach is more familiar to most surgeons; it is associated with a lower incidence of vascular injury, and it is *closer* to the target artery thereby allowing the use of proportionately shorter guidewires and catheters. However, it should only be used when the possibility of a therapeutic intervention is remote because of the orientation of the mesenteric vessels. Notably, the angle between the mesenteric vessels and the aorta is fairly acute and directed caudally. The vector forces of a catheter directed from the femoral artery are opposite to the angle of the mesenteric vessels, and therefore its pushability is compromised. Admittedly, these mechanical factors may be attenuated by the use of appropriate guiding catheters and stiffer wires. However, it may be difficult if not impossible to cross a tight mesenteric artery stenosis with this approach, and guidewire access may be permanently lost during a crucial step of the procedure. Therefore, D is the correct answer.

The brachial approach overcomes these limitations for approaching the celiac and superior mesenteric arteries and is the obvious choice. It is mandatory in patients with severe aortoiliac occlusive disease. However, the other answers, which all relate to it (A, B, C, E), contain *incorrect statements*. The change in catheter mechanics from the cephalad approach is sufficient to overcome the increased physical distance/need for *longer* devices and allows greater pushability for target vessel engagement. Additional disadvantages of the brachial approach (other than those cited as advantages of the femoral approach) include the limited maximum sheath size possible without use of a surgical cutdown (7F for men and 6F for women), risk of embolic stroke, and difficulty gaining access to the descending thoracic aorta in patients with a tortuous arch. Although aortic access may be easily obtained from either brachial artery, the *left* brachial approach is preferred because of the risk of carotid embolization with prolonged catheterization across the innominate artery.

Answer 124-3: D

Discussion 124-3

All patients with chronic mesenteric ischemia should undergo revascularization. The goals of treatment are to reduce pain, prevent bowel infarction, and allow patients to regain their weight and restore their nutritional reserves. Despite the theoretic appeal, there is likely no role for chronic parenteral alimentation and noninterventional therapies even in patients who are relatively high risk because of their other comorbidities. So D is the proper answer. Admittedly, the postprandial pain can be relieved by not eating, and total parenteral nutrition may allow the patients to regain their weight and restore their nutritional status. However, the potential for bowel infarction is not alleviated, and lifetime dependence on total parenteral nutrition is not very practical

in terms of convenience, expense, and the risk of catheter-related complications.

The optimal means of revascularization for patients with chronic mesenteric ischemia has been actively debated for the past few decades, and this debate has become more intense with the emergence of the endovascular approach. So the other options (A, B, C, E) are all to be considered. The pivotal questions are the type of revascularization (endovascular vs. open) and the type/configuration of open revascularization. Endovascular treatment has a tremendous appeal for patients with chronic mesenteric ischemia because it is less invasive and has the potential to reduce morbidity, mortality, length of hospital stay, and cost. However, the long-term outcome after endovascular treatment remains unclear and is a major concern given the patient's life expectancy and the potential catastrophic complications associated with thrombosis of a stented vessel.

The ongoing issues with regard to the open revascularization for patients with chronic mesenteric ischemia include the type of revascularization, number of vessels to be revascularized, and optimal conduit. The techniques of reimplantation, endarterectomy, and bypass have all been successfully used, and each possesses theoretic advantages. However, mesenteric bypass, either antegrade from the supraceliac aorta or retrograde from the infrarenal aorta/common iliac artery, has emerged as the most common treatment with the current debate being the specific configuration. The theoretic advantages of the antegrade bypass include the fact that supraceliac aorta is frequently uninvolved with atherosclerosis and that the limbs of the graft follow a direct path and have prograde flow. The theoretic advantages of the retrograde bypass include the fact that infrarenal aorta/common iliac artery is easier/faster to expose and generally more familiar to most vascular surgeons. Furthermore, there is less hemodynamic instability and potential for distal embolization with the *infrarenal* aortic/iliac clamp application. Major disadvantages of the retrograde bypass are the obligatory course of the graft and its potential to kink, which is even more problematic for vein conduits. Both prosthetic and autogenous conduits have been used with the various mesenteric bypass procedures, although reports comparing the long-term patency rates for the two different conduits have been inconclusive.

■ ANSWERS AND DISCUSSION FOR CHAPTER 125

Answer 125-1: C

Discussion 125-1

The presumptive diagnosis from this scenario is subacute mesenteric vein thrombosis (MVT).

A. Outpatient management with low molecular weight heparin and then warfarin would risk missing an insidious progression to necrotic bowel.
B. Exploration does not appear necessary in the described patient with mild to moderate abdominal signs and symptoms.
C. Patients with subacute MVT should be studied for both inherited and acquired thrombophilias immediately be-

fore starting anticoagulation so as not to confound the test results. As soon as those studies have been drawn, the patient should be started on intravenous heparin plus fluids to restore fluid loses, kept n.p.o., and observed in the hospital for resolution or progression. If the patient develops signs and symptoms of peritonitis, he or she should be taken to the operating room for exploration.

D. There are no data to support treatment of this condition by transhepatic intramesenteric venous thrombolysis.

E. Coagulation studies rather than cultures should be drawn, as in C.

Answer 125-2: C

Discussion 125-2

A. Three months of anticoagulant therapy is insufficient, and repeating the studies off warfarin will add nothing.

B. This diet is not known to benefit those with factor V Leiden deficiency (see also E).

C. A patient with a significant thrombotic event found to have a factor V Leiden deficiency should take lifelong anticoagulation. Consultation with a hematologist knowledgeable about this type of thrombophilia would be helpful in advising about the need for screening of first-degree relatives. There are various levels of this deficiency, and management of those with lower levels and without any history of thrombotic events does not mandate prophylactic anticoagulation.

D. A hematologist familiar with this condition can do this and arrange for appropriate screening of first-degree relatives, and manage their risk according to the results (see C).

E. Folate supplements are advised for homocystinemia, and vitamin B12 is advised for achlorhydria.

Answer 125-3: B

Discussion 125-3

A. Protein S deficiency should present with thrombotic problems earlier in life.

B. A malignancy-associated hypercoagulable state would be the most likely diagnosis in this older patient. A colonic neoplasm is the most likely underlying cause of those listed.

C. Crohn's disease would generally present at a much younger age.

D. Heparin-induced thrombocytopenia would generally not lead to mesenteric venous thrombosis and certainly would be a much less likely diagnosis.

E. Never heard of a syndrome with this name.

■ ANSWERS AND DISCUSSION FOR CHAPTER 126

Answer 126-1: B

Discussion 126-1

Obstruction of portomesenteric venous blood flow results in the development of abnormal portosystemic venous collaterals that when in clinically important areas can result in spontaneous life-threatening hemorrhage. The most important of these is (A) the portal/splenic vein connection to azy-

gous–hemiazygous veins in the mediastinum because these collaterals course through the submucosa of the duodenum and esophagus to form gastric and esophageal varices. (C) Connection from the mesenteric veins to the hemorrhoidal veins form rectal varices. (D) Connections between the reopened umbilical vein and the internal mammary/inferior epigastric veins form the "caplet medusae." (E) Important iatrogenic venous collateral connections in patients with portal hypertension include those in bowel and gastric adhesions to the parietal peritoneum and those around ileostomies and colostomies. Varices in all of these locations are subject to erosion and/or trauma resulting in potentially life-threatening hemorrhage. In contrast, although (B) retroperitoneal varices commonly develop in the face of portal venous hypertension, these are usually clinically silent unless a retroperitoneal procedure such as surgical repair of an aneurysm is attempted. Thus, B is the correct answer.

Answer 126-2: E

Discussion 126-2

Simultaneous resuscitation, diagnosis, and control of bleeding is the hallmark of optimal therapy of patient with variceal bleeding.

A. Monitoring in an intensive care unit and volume replacement with appropriate volumes of crystalloid and blood products should begin immediately.

B. This is followed by emergency upper endoscopy if at all possible because up to one third of patients have bleeding from a source other than varices.

C. Endoscopic sclerotherapy and/or banding, or an urgent/ emergency TIPS procedure can then be used to control bleeding or prevent early rebleeding.

D. Use of vasopressin or octreotide to reduce portal venous pressure is also of value because both these agents reduce blood loss and early variceal rebleeding.

E. In contrast, emergency operative therapy has largely been abandoned because of excessive postoperative mortality. Thus, E is correct.

Answer 126-3: D

Discussion 126-3

A. Incorrect. Definitive therapy is indicated in essentially all patients who have an episode of variceal bleeding because more than 70% of patients will have rebleeding with a greater than 75% mortality associated with each episode of rebleeding.

B. Incorrect. Chronic beta-blocker therapy has been shown to reduce rebleeding, but approximately 50% of patients treated with chronic beta-blockers alone will experience rebleeding.

C. Incorrect. Chronic endoscopic sclerotherapy/banding is very effective in limiting rebleeding in patients with esophageal varices and less effective in treating gastric varices. However, it is associated with a cumulative long-term risk of esophageal stricture, ulceration, reflux, and perforation and is contraindicated in patients who live a significant distance from a medical center.

D. Correct. TIPS is initially successful in more than 90% of patients, but, because of the large shunt initially created using a 10-mm stent, it is associated with approximately a 25% incidence of portosystemic encephalopathy. In addition, the failure rate from thrombosis associated with rebleeding is approximately 50% in most large series in the first year of follow-up. Use of covered stents may improve this patency rate, but that remains to be proven.

E. Incorrect. Orthotopic liver transplant is very effective in those patients who stop drinking with graft survival of approximately 80% at 2 years. In patients who are candidates for orthotopic liver transplant, TIPS should be used for recurrent bleeding because both chronic endoscopic sclerotherapy/banding and surgical portosystemic stent procedures may alter anatomy to an extent such that orthotopic liver transplant is not possible.

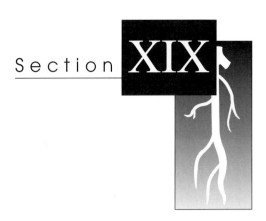

Section **XIX**

THE MANAGEMENT OF RENOVASCULAR DISORDERS

STUDY QUESTIONS

■ QUESTIONS FOR CHAPTER 128

Question 128-1

The most effective measure for the prevention of contrast-induced nephropathy includes pretreatment with:

A. Mannitol.
B. Diuretics.
C. Dopamine infusion.
D. Saline infusions.
E. Fenoldopam.

Question 128-2

The use of magnetic resonance angiography (MRA) as a diagnostic modality to evaluate renal artery stenosis (RAS):

A. Is best done without the use of contrast agents.
B. Can overestimate or underestimate the degree of stenosis.
C. Has poor sensitivity, even with gadolinium enhancement.
D. Must be supplemented with conventional arteriography before any intervention.
E. Is poor at detecting proximal renal artery lesions.

Question 128-3

Helical computed tomographic angiography (CTA) for the identification of RAS:

A. Involves minimal amounts of contrast material.
B. Has a lower resolution than MRA.
C. Is limited by the presence of arterial calcification.
D. Has poor sensitivity for RAS.
E. As with MRA, it cannot be used for the evaluation of stented renal arteries because of significant artifact.

■ QUESTIONS FOR CHAPTER 129

Question 129-1

The most common type of fibromuscular disease (FMD) of the renal arteries in adults is:

A. Intimal hyperplasia.
B. Medial hyperplasia.
C. Medial fibroplasias.

D. Perimedial dysplasia.
E. Developmental stenosis.

Question 129-2

Renal artery FMD can present to physicians in other ways than the detection of hypertension on routine examination. These include all of the following *except* which of the following:

A. Lethargy, easy fatigability.
B. Abdominal or flank bruit.
C. Hypertensive retinopathy.
D. Headache.
E. Advanced growth and development (for age).

Question 129-3

Which of the following statements regarding the endovascular treatment of renal FMD is *not* true?

A. Balloon angioplasty is usually successful.
B. Stenting is not usually required for long term relief of FMD stenoses.
C. Endovascular treatment is not as successful in those associated with neurofibromatosis.
D. Endovascular treatment is not as successful in children as it is in adults.
E. Endovascular treatment is more successful in those with intimal hyperplasia than it is in those with medial fibroplasias.

■ QUESTIONS FOR CHAPTERS 130

Question 130-1

The single most predictive characteristic of renovascular hypertension is:

A. Age.
B. Gender.
C. Ethnicity.
D. Severity of hypertension.
E. Presence of abdominal bruit.

Question 130-2

Ischemic nephropathy is characterized by each of the following *except*:

A. Severe hypertension.
B. Renal and extrarenal atherosclerosis.
C. Bilateral renal artery disease.
D. Slow decline in renal function.
E. Renal artery occlusion.

Question 130-3

Given severe hypertension, renal insufficiency, and bilateral renovascular disease, the patient with the *least* chance for beneficial blood pressure or renal function response to intervention is a:

A. Child aged less than 5 years.
B. White adult.
C. Black adult.
D. Diabetic adult.
E. Dialysis-dependent adult.

Question 130-4

Indications for empiric renal artery intervention in combination with open aortic repair include all the following, *except:*

A. Severe (>80%) unilateral RAS with severe hypertension.
B. Moderate (60%–80%) bilateral RAS with severe hypertension.
C. Severe (>80%) unilateral RAS without significant hypertension.
D. Severe (>80%) unilateral RAS with severe hypertension and renal insufficiency.
E. Severe (>80%) bilateral RAS with severe hypertension and dialysis-dependent renal failure.

■ QUESTIONS FOR CHAPTER 131

Question 131-1

Important adjuncts in the performance of endovascular renal artery revascularization include all of the following *except*:

A. Periprocedural administration of low-dose dopamine.
B. Periprocedural administration of antiplatelet agents.
C. Preprocedural hydration.
D. Preprocedural administration of acetylcysteine.
E. Procedural administration of heparin.

Question 131-2

Endovascular renal artery revascularization can be facilitated by all of the following *except*:

A. Use of guide catheters or sheaths for secure renal artery access.
B. Use of femoral artery access contralateral to the lesion to be treated.
C. Use of brachial access for downsloping renal arteries.
D. Primary stenting of renal artery occlusive lesions.
E. Use of oblique angiographic views.

Question 131-3

A 68-year-old patient with severe hypertension, a serum creatinine of 2.3 mg/dL, and bilateral high-grade renal artery stenoses is scheduled for endovascular renal artery revascu-

larization. What is the *most* appropriate imaging method or modality to guide intervention in this individual?

A. Use of ionic, hyperosmolar iodinated contrast.
B. Use of nonionic, low osmolarity iodinated contrast.
C. Use of gadopentate dimeglumine.
D. Use of intravascular ultrasound.
E. Use of intraoperative transcutaneous ultrasound.

■ QUESTIONS FOR CHAPTER 132

Question 132-1

The preferred conduit for renovascular repair in children is:

A. Autogenous vein.
B. Dacron graft.
C. Polytetrafluoroethylene graft.
D. Autogenous artery.
E. Cryopreserved vein.

Question 132-2

The best method of open repair for ostial atherosclerosis involving four renal arteries is:

A. Multiple bypass with saphenous vein.
B. Multiple bypass with hypogastric artery.
C. Transrenal thromboendarterectomy.
D. Transaortic thromboendarterectomy.
E. Multiple reimplantations.

Question 132-3

Contraindications to renal artery thromboendarterectomy include:

A. Bilateral RAS.
B. Transmural calcification of the perirenal aorta.
C. Occlusive disease of the perirenal aorta.
D. Occlusive disease of the infrarenal aorta.
E. Preocclusive (99%) stenosis of the renal artery.

■ QUESTIONS FOR CHAPTER 133

Question 133-1

The *most common* clinical presentation for renal arteriovenous malformation (AVM) is:

A. Flank pain.
B. Hematuria.
C. Hypertension.
D. High-output heart failure.
E. Abdominal mass.

■ QUESTIONS FOR CHAPTER 134

Question 134-1

A 70-year-old man with a history of atrial fibrillation presents with left flank pain over several hours. His temperature is 37.8°C. Serum creatinine is 1.8 mg/dL, and urinalysis demonstrates only hematuria. The most likely diagnosis is:

A. Renal artery thrombosis.
B. Aortic dissection.

C. Renal artery dissection.
D. Renal artery embolus.
E. Glomerulonephritis.

Question 134-2

In the scenario described in question 134-1, the most appropriate diagnostic test is:

A. Contrast-infused abdominal computed tomography (CT) scan.
B. Abdominal duplex ultrasound scan.
C. Angiography.

D. Intravenous pyelogram.
E. Nucleotide renography.

Question 134-3

Which of the following is *not* a typical characteristic of renal vein thrombosis?

A. Hypercoagulable state.
B. Nephrotic syndrome.
C. Renal arterial occlusive disease.
D. Hematuria.
E. Hypovolemia.

ANSWERS AND DISCUSSION

■   ANSWERS AND DISCUSSION FOR CHAPTER 128

Answer 128-1: D

Discussion 128-1

No data currently exist to support the routine use of (A) mannitol, (B) diuretics, or (C) low-dose dopamine as prophylaxis against contrast-induced nephropathy in angiography or endovascular interventions near the renal arteries.

(D) Preprocedural hydration with saline infusions and the administration of acetylcysteine have been proven effective in ameliorating the nephrotoxic effects of iodinated contrast.

(E) The use of dopamine agonists such as fenoldopam has not been shown to affect contrast-induced nephrotoxicity either.

Answer 128-2: B

Discussion 128-2

MRA can demonstrate vascular anatomy and generate an image that is similar in appearance to that obtained by conventional angiography.

Three-dimensional MRA, *with gadolinium-enhancement* (A), has become the standard in renal artery magnetic resonance imaging. Rather than image individual protons in flowing blood, this method allows direct visualization of the contrast agent filling the lumen, much like conventional angiography.

However, to accurately assess *the actual degree of stenosis*, it is necessary to examine the nonreformatted axial images, because the reformatting process, although it produces visually satisfying images, can often lead to overestimation or underestimation of the degree of stenosis. Therefore, *answer B is correct.*

(C) In the majority of series, MRA sensitivity is near 100%, which makes it an excellent screening tool for suspected ischemic nephropathy secondary to atherosclerotic disease of the main renal artery, including *(E) proximal renal artery lesions.*

(D) Additional contrast arteriography is usually unnecessary before the actual intervention.

Answer 128-3: C

Discussion 128-3

Helical CT has emerged as a promising technique for identifying RAS.

A. For arterial imaging, *a full dose* of intravenous iodinated contrast is injected through a peripheral vein. After an appropriate delay to allow passage of the contrast into the renal arterial circulation, a series of thin cuts are taken throughout the aorta at the level of the renal arteries. Rapid acquisition of data afforded by spiral CT allows multiple images to be made precisely at the moment when the contrast medium passes through the renal vessels. A number of technical variables must be optimized if the renal arteries are to be adequately imaged by spiral CT. Several of these parameters (collimation, table speed, and pitch) determine the interval at which cuts are acquired. These variables are adjusted so that sections are taken at 2- to 3-mm intervals.

B. Helical CT does *not* have a lower resolution than MRA. Adjusting the variables affords a resolution of approximately 0.5 mm (whereas that for MRA is 1–1.5 mm).

C. The major hindrance of helical CT is arterial calcification, *so (C) is the correct answer.* Atherosclerotic disease can be inferred by the presence of calcium, but the degree of stenosis cannot be gauged accurately.

D. Although helical CT has been less widely studied than MRA or duplex ultrasound, a number of centers with experience in helical CT have produced favorable results *with reasonable sensitivity.*

E. *Unlike MRA,* helical CT can be used to assess the patency of renal arteries that have been treated with endoluminal stents.

■   ANSWERS AND DISCUSSION FOR CHAPTER 129

Answer 129-1: C

Discussion 129-1

A. Intimal hyperplasia accounts for about 5%
B. Medial hyperplasia accounts for about 1%
C. Medial fibroplasia accounts for the vast majority, close to 85%, and is characterized by the familiar "string of beads" appearance.
D. Perimedial dysplasia may be a variant of (C), occurring in patients who are younger on average. It lacks the aneurysms between narrowings which give the "string of beads" appearance.
E. Developmental stenosis are less frequent and appear in much younger patients.

Answer 129-2: E

Discussion 129-2

A. Both adults and children can present with lethargy and easy fatigability.
B. Abdominal or flank bruit may be heard in renal FMD
C. FMD hypertension, if not discovered by blood pressure checks, can be spotted as hypertensive retinopathy seen on routine eye exams.
D. The hypertension of FMD, like other forms of hypertension can cause persistent headaches.
E. Advanced growth and development (for age) is *not* seen in children with FMD; rather failure to thrive may precipitate further evaluation by a pediatrician.

Answer 129-3: E (because it is not true)

Discussion 129-3

A. Balloon angioplasty alone is usually successful, and (B) stenting is not usually required for most renal FMD.
B. Discussed in answer A.
C. Those stenoses associated with neurofibromatoses do *not* respond as well to balloon angioplasty.

D. Endovascular treatment is not as successful in children as it is in adults, although the difference is less striking with the increased availabilty of smaller sized catheters, but the constellations of lesions seen in children differs from those seen in adults and they are not as amenable as a group to PTA.

E. Actually intimal hyperplasia is not as amenable to renal artery PTA as the more common medial fibroplasias, so this statement is *not* true.

■ ANSWERS AND DISCUSSION FOR CHAPTER 130

Answer 130-1: D
Discussion 130-1

A. Severe hypertension at the, extremes of age has a high probability of being renovascular in cause, but the *severity* of the hypertension is key, so this answer is a close second as the most predictive characteristic. With the exception of infants less than 1 year of age, the majority of children with severe hypertension have a secondary cause.

B. When *all patients* with renovascular hypertension are considered, there are no gender differences, even though medial fibroplasia occurs almost exclusively in women. Intimal fibroplasia of children and developmental or hypoplastic lesions occur without gender difference.

C. Earlier reports describing clinical experience with renovascular disease from the 1960s and 1970s suggested a low incidence of renal artery disease in African-Americans; however, recent population-based studies have demonstrated *no ethnic differences*. Differences in the prevalence of renovascular disease associated with severe hypertension reflect differences in severe hypertension within different ethic groups. In this latter regard, African-Americans, as a group, demonstrate more severe essential hypertension, and thereby secondary causes are less frequent.

D. The *single most predictive characteristic* of renovascular hypertension in all age groups is the severity of hypertension. It should be remembered that the severity of hypertension is untreated high blood pressure, not the difficulty in controlling blood pressure with medication. This latter value is probably best approximated in contemporary practice by noting the highest known blood pressure.

E. Although the presence of an abdominal bruit in a young female patient with severe hypertension correlates highly with the presence of renovascular disease, the presence or absence of bruit alone is not predictive.

Answer 130-2: D
Discussion 130-2

A. Renal artery disease contributing to renovascular renal insufficiency (i.e., ischemic nephropathy) is most commonly associated with severe hypertension. In fact, the more severe the hypertension, the greater the renal function benefit from operative intervention.

B. Patients with ischemic nephropathy frequently demonstrate both renal and extrarenal atherosclerosis.

C. Ischemic nephropathy that is correctible for recovery of renal function frequently involves both renal arteries or a renal artery to a solitary kidney.

D. The rate of decline in renal function before intervention correlates with the presence of renovascular disease, but rapid decline is more characteristic, *not a slow rate*. In addition, a rapid decline in renal function is associated with improved renal function recovery after intervention.

E. Approximately half of patients found to have severe renal insufficiency and ischemic nephropathy demonstrate a renal artery occlusion.

Answer 130-3: D
Discussion 130-3

A. Traditionally, children have been considered spared from ischemic nephropathy associated with renovascular disease. However, when prediction equations derived especially for children are considered, the estimated glomerular filtration rate in children with renovascular hypertension is frequently decreased. This group, however, demonstrates a significant rate of recovery.

B and C. Ethnicity has no influence on recovery of renal function.

D. Among the characteristics listed, diabetes introduces the greatest uncertainty in recovery of renal function. This uncertainty has no apparent relationship with the type of diabetes, insulin dependence, the duration of diabetes, or the presence of proteinuria.

E. Although authors have cited the severity of renal function as a limitation to renal function recovery, if a patient progresses to dialysis-dependence rapidly, with bilateral RAS or occlusion, approximately 75% of these patients can be removed from dialysis dependence with complete renal revascularization.

Answer 130-4: C
Discussion 130-4

A. Severe hypertension with severe unilateral RAS is perhaps the most common indication for empiric-combined repair.

B. When moderate stenosis is found angiographically, in combination with *severe* hypertension, there is a high rate of blood pressure benefit from empiric repair.

C. Severe angiographic disease in the absence of hypertension is of uncertain benefit and should not be performed.

D. Although the renal function recovery associated with severe hypertension and a unilateral renal artery lesion is less than that of a combined lesion, a high proportion of patients can be expected to have benefit in blood pressure and one third will have improved renal function.

E. Patients with severe bilateral RAS and severe hypertension, with rapidly deteriorating renal function to the point of dialysis-dependent renal failure, have a 75% change of renal function recovery with complete renal revascularization.

■ ANSWERS AND DISCUSSION FOR CHAPTER 131

Answer 131-1: A
Discussion 131-1

Important adjuncts for the performance of endovascular renal revascularization include (B) the periprocedural use of antiplatelet agents and (E) the administration of heparin during the procedure to minimize the formation of intraoperative thrombi and reduce the short-term risk of thrombosis. The use of these agents is supported by extensive data from the literature. (C) Preprocedural hydration and (D) administration of acetylcysteine are used to ameliorate the nephrotoxic effects of iodinated contrast, and their efficacy in this setting is well documented. No data currently exist to support the routine use of (A) low-dose dopamine in endovascular renal intervention.

Answer 131-2: D
Discussion 131-2

Secure access to the renal artery is essential for endovascular treatment and can be facilitated by several device and access alternatives.

A. Preshaped complex curve guide catheters and guide sheaths are indispensable for the provision of secure, low friction access to allow for the passage and accurate placement of angioplasty catheters and stents.
B. In cases of unilateral intervention, positioning of such catheters can also be facilitated by accessing the contralateral femoral artery. This allows the natural tendency of the catheter to track up the contralateral aortic wall to facilitate the engagement of the renal ostia.
C. For downsloping renal arteries, cannulation from a femoral approach may be extremely challenging or even impossible. However, brachial artery access is useful in this situation.
D. Primary stenting of renal artery lesions assists in the management of *ostial* renal lesions to avoid the common problems of elastic recoil, residual stenosis, and dissection, *but it is not necessary for the treatment of the other occlusive lesion causing renovascular disease.*
E. Secure access to the renal arteries and proper endovascular treatment can also be facilitated by the use of oblique views that take into account the direction of origin of the ostia.

Answer 131-3: C
Discussion 131-3

In patients with baseline excretory renal insufficiency, the choice of contrast agent for necessary procedural imaging is critical.

A and B. The use of iodinated contrast agents is potentially nephrotoxic and should be minimized or avoided, if possible.
C. The use of gadopentate dimeglumine (or carbon dioxide) offers a non-nephrotoxic alternative but with slightly less resolution. These agents are frequently used to localize and cannulate the renal arteries with small doses of iodinated contrast then used to more precisely plan and carry out the intervention. Staged interventions are frequently used to minimize contrast exposure as well.
D. Intravascular ultrasound can provide valuable information in planning and postprocedure assessment, but it is not currently an effective imaging alternative for the accurate positioning and performance of endovascular renal intervention.

E. Transcutaneous ultrasound has diagnostic screening value, and its intraoperative use has some value in open surgical revascularization, but neither play a useful role in guiding endovascular renal artery revascularization.

■ ANSWERS AND DISCUSSION FOR CHAPTER 132

Answer 132-1: D
Discussion 132-1

A. Autogenous vein as a renal conduit in children routinely demonstrates enlargement but rarely progresses to frank aneurysmal degeneration.
B and C. When autogenous artery is unavailable for reconstruction in the young child and when renal artery diameter measures *at least 4 mm in diameter*, prosthetic grafting with polytetrafluoroethylene (or Dacron) is an acceptable choice of conduit. However, it is not the preferred conduit for renovascular repair in children.
D. In children, autogenous artery for renal artery reconstruction is the preferred conduit. A technically satisfactory renal artery reconstruction with autogenous artery would be expected to provide lifetime patency. Preoperative imaging, however, should include the pelvic circulation to exclude simultaneous disease of the hypogastric artery, which is used most commonly. It may be possible to reimplant the renal artery, if it is long enough after dissecting it free, rather than construct a bypass, avoiding one anastomosis.
E. Cryopreserved vein graft is not a preferred conduit for renovascular repair in either children or adults.

Answer 132-2: D
Discussion 132-2

A and B. Multiple renal artery bypass for four renal arteries involved by ostial atherosclerosis is a suboptimal method of reconstruction.
C. Transrenal thromboendarterectomy fails to address the ostial atherosclerosis that contributes to 98% of atherosclerotic lesions leading to critical RAS or thrombosis.
D. Transaortic thromboendarterectomy for ostial renal artery atherosclerosis is a preferred method for treatment, especially when multiple renal arteries are involved. The disease should end within 1 cm of the renal artery origin by palpation. Like endarterectomy at other locations, transaortic thromboendarterectomy is contraindicated by aortic degeneration and transmural calcification.
E. Multiple reimplantations are rarely possible in cases of atherosclerotic renal artery disease and would represent a suboptimal method of repair for multiple renal arteries.

Answer 132-3: B
Discussion 132-3

A. Using either a trapdoor approach or a high anterior aortotomy, transaortic thromboendarterectomy can be performed on both renal arteries.
B. Transmural calcification of the perirenal aorta is a contraindication to transaortic thromboendarterectomy (as is aneurysmal disease of the perirenal aorta). Transmural

calcification can be detected by gentle palpation of the vessel, which may feel like a fine-grade sandpaper. If thromboendarterectomy is undertaken in this instance, multiple defects are frequently created within the adventitia.

C. Occlusive disease of the perirenal aorta is not a contraindication for thromboendarterectomy. In fact, the RAS contributing to occlusion is frequently aortic in origin, spilling over to involve the ostium of the renal artery.

D. Occlusive disease of the infrarenal aorta is not a contraindication to transaortic thromboendarterectomy of the perirenal portion. Transaortic thromboendarterectomy is a useful adjunct when a combined aortic repair is planned for infrarenal occlusive disease.

E. Preocclusive high-grade stenosis of the renal artery is not a contraindication for transaortic thromboendarterectomy. As long as the renal artery atheroma ends within 1 cm of the renal artery origin, the technique is useful. However, transaortic thromboendarterectomy and all other methods of renal artery reconstruction should be monitored with intraoperative imaging to ensure technical satisfaction. In this latter regard, intraoperative renal duplex sonography is particularly useful.

■ ANSWERS AND DISCUSSION FOR CHAPTER 133

Answer 133-1: B

Discussion 133-1

Although most AVMs are asymptomatic, of those producing symptoms, 72% present with (B) hematuria. Back or flank pain (A) can also lead to the diagnosis of AVM, but when caused by AVM it is usually secondary to renal colic associated with hematuria. (C) Renin-mediated hypertension can also occur and be an indication for treatment but is less common than hematuria. (D) High-output heart failure is rarely observed, only with giant AVM. (E) AVMs rarely are palpable.

■ ANSWERS AND DISCUSSION FOR CHAPTER 134

Answer 134-1: D

Discussion 134-1

A. Renal artery thrombosis is typically associated with preexisting advanced atherosclerotic disease of the aorta and branches rather than with atrial fibrillation. It may be clinically silent if adequate collaterals have developed, but if symptomatic, it will often manifest as severe hypertension with acute oliguric renal failure, not this picture.

B. Aortic dissection is marked by other typical stigmata, such as severe hypertension, more generalized back or abdominal pain, and possibly other organ ischemia. Often, aortic dissection may be clinically silent in terms of pain referable to the ischemic kidney, but might result in acute hypertension. The patient population affected

by this disease process is younger than the typical patient with renal artery embolism.

C. Primary renal artery dissection is a rare occurrence that most commonly affects younger women with fibromuscular disease. This can also be clinically silent, but once again may manifest itself with severe, difficult-to-control hypertension. It is not typically associated with atrial fibrillation.

D. Renal artery embolus most commonly originates from the heart and is typically associated with atrial fibrillation. Common presenting symptoms include acute flank pain, back or abdominal pain, hypertension, hematuria, and nausea and vomiting. Arteriography provides a definitive diagnosis.

E. Although some symptoms of glomerulonephritis may mimic the presentation of renal artery thrombosis, the associated history of advanced age, atrial fibrillation, and acute onset of symptoms favor a diagnosis of renal artery embolus.

Answer 134-2: C

Discussion 134-2

A. Although CT scan, using advanced CTA technology, can demonstrate an embolic occlusion of the renal artery (the presumed diagnosis), this test is time consuming, limited in its availability, is technique- and phase-dependent, and requires extensive processing to render the study easily interpretable. Time is of the essence here. In addition, although it can demonstrate decreased perfusion to the affected kidney, collateral vessels may be difficult to see, and the presence of atherosclerotic changes within the adjacent juxtarenal aorta may suggest an alternative diagnosis of renal artery thrombosis superimposed on atherosclerotic occlusive disease. This test exposes the patient to potentially nephrotoxic contrast.

B. An abdominal duplex scan has limited utility in the setting of acute abdominal or flank pain where visualization of the renal artery is limited by bowel gas and abdominal or flank tenderness. In addition, the resolution of duplex ultrasonography is not usually adequate to demonstrate an embolus in the main renal artery or one of its branches.

C. Arteriography is the gold standard in the diagnosis of acute renal artery embolism. It frequently demonstrates an abrupt occlusion of the renal artery or multiple emboli within branches with limited collateralization. Bilateral emboli or emboli to additional visceral vessels may be seen. Arteriography demonstrates not only the diagnosis of renal artery occlusion but also the degree of atherosclerotic disease. The pattern of collateral blood flow to the distal renal artery can help differentiate between renal artery embolus and thrombosis.

D. Intravenous pyelography may reveal absent or poor function depending on the degree of renal artery obstruction, but this test provides no anatomic information and is not definitive for renal artery embolism.

E. Renal nuclear medicine studies may demonstrate impaired renal perfusion in the setting of renal artery embolism but provide no anatomic information and, like (A), will delay the definitive diagnosis in a setting in which such a delay will affect renal salvage.

Answer 134-3: C

Discussion 134-3

A and B. Renal vein thrombosis occurring in patients with nephrotic syndrome is typically associated with a hypercoagulable state in combination with an element of dehydration. The hypercoagulable state typically results from the loss of low molecular weight proteins in the urine, decreased antithrombin III levels, and thrombocytosis.

C. Renal arterial occlusive disease is not associated with renal vein thrombosis. Renal vein thrombosis most commonly occurs in neonates with dehydration and patients with nephrotic syndrome.

D. Hematuria, proteinuria, flank pain, and impairment of renal function are common manifestations of renal vein thrombosis.

E. Dehydration and intravascular volume contraction contribute to stasis in the renal vein, predisposing to thrombosis.

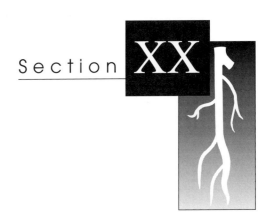

Section **XX**

THE MANAGEMENT OF EXTRACRANIAL CEREBROVASCULAR DISEASE

STUDY QUESTIONS

■ QUESTIONS FOR CHAPTER 135

Question 135-1

All of the following can be accepted as true examples of transient ischemic attacks (TIAs) *except*:

A. Transient loss of vision in the upper field of one eye.
B. Transient numbness in one arm.
C. Transient episode of dizziness and lightheadedness clearing completely in 1 hour.
D. Transient episode of garbled speech.
E. Transient loss of strength in the left arm and left leg.

Question 135-2

Which of the following statements regarding the timing and frequency of hemispheric TIAs preceding a hemispheric stroke is correct?

A. Antecedent TIAs most often occur within 24 hours of the stroke event.
B. TIAs occur at least 1 year before the stroke event in the majority.
C. Antecedent TIAs occur in multiple distributions before the final stroke.
D. Antecedent TIAs occur in only 30% to 50% of those patients ultimately having a stroke.
E. Antecedent TIAs closely mimic the subsequent stroke, except that they resolve within 48 hours.

Question 135-3

Territorial transient ischemic events are best explained by:

A. Reduced blood flow secondary to a hemodynamically significant carotid stenosis.
B. Emboli of arterial origin.
C. Transient vasospasm after hemorrhage under a plaque.
D. A hypercoagulable state causing platelet deposition.
E. Emboli of cardiac origin.

Question 135-4

The *first published* report of carotid endarterectomy (CEA) is attributed to:

A. Eastcott, Pickering, and Robb.
B. DeBakey.

C. Carrea, Molins, and Murphy.
D. Javid.
E. Wiley.

■ QUESTIONS FOR CHAPTER 136

Question 136-1

Symptoms indicating an ischemic event caused by atherosclerotic disease of the left internal carotid artery (ICA) most likely include:

A. Neglect of stimuli presented to the left side of the body.
B. Diplopia.
C. Denial of blindness.
D. Monocular visual disturbance.
E. Gaze deviation to the right.

Question 136-2

Which of the following statements regarding the treatment of an acute cerebral infarction is *true*?

A. Tissue plasminogen activator (t-PA) should be given within 12 hours after acute onset of ataxia, if the head computed tomography (CT) shows no intracranial hemorrhage and the neurologic examination results are otherwise within normal limits.
B. Elevated blood pressures should be normalized aggressively.
C. Aphasic patients should be kept *non per os* until they have a formal swallowing evaluation.
D. The majority of patients with acute infarction should be treated with intravenous (IV) heparin to prevent stroke progression.
E. Seizures at the onset of acute stroke symptoms are not a contraindication to initiating t-PA treatment if the patient presents within 3 hours of symptom onset.

Question 136-3

Which of the following is a *true* statement regarding the management of patients with ischemic stroke?

A. Transcranial Doppler (TCD) studies performed in the early postoperative period after CEA can help identify patients at high risk for cerebral infarct.
B. Cerebral angiography should be performed in all patients before CEA.
C. Patients with ischemic infarcts should routinely be evaluated for cardioembolic events by transesophageal echocardiogram.
D. Diplopia, vertigo, and imbalance indicate a dissection of the ipsilateral ICA.
E. In patients with asymptomatic carotid stenosis, TCD studies of the middle cerebral artery rarely detect emboli.

■ QUESTIONS FOR CHAPTER 137

Question 137-1

The Circle of Willis:

A. Is simply a "catch-all" term applied to a highly variable collection of intracranial collateral vessels.
B. Is often incomplete and thus of unpredictable value in protecting the intracranial circulation from the potential ischemic effects of a single-vessel carotid artery occlusion.
C. Reliably protects the intracranial circulation from the potential ischemic effects of a single-vessel carotid artery occlusion.
D. Is an embryonic structure that closes at, or shortly after, birth.
E. Is a network of venous channels draining the cerebral cortex.

Question 137-2

Carotid/cerebral arteriography:

A. Is essential in determining whether a carotid lesion warrants surgical endarterectomy.
B. In the setting of occlusive atheromatous carotid artery disease should be reserved for situations in which the clinical diagnosis is in question and the results of noninvasive imaging are inconclusive.
C. Does not add appreciable risk to the workup and treatment of occlusive atheromatous carotid artery disease.
D. Need not include intracranial views in situations in which there is no suspicion of intracranial vascular disease.
E. Is the one area of the body where current digital imaging technology is still insufficient to adequately examine the smaller vessels of the brain.

Question 137-3

Stroke:

A. Is essentially an "all-or-nothing" phenomenon because the period of viability for brain tissue is so short that there is no practical way to undo the effects of an ischemic insult.
B. Must be treated with catheter-directed thrombolysis to achieve the desired effect.
C. Is the common term for ischemic cerebral infarction.
D. Is caused by in situ thrombosis of the carotid arteries in the setting of a preexisting stenotic lesion.

E. Will likely be viewed in the future as the cerebral analog of myocardial infarction, that is, a treatable and potentially reversible emergency.

Question 137-4

Relative to the arteriographic evaluation of proximal ICA stenoses:

A. The lack of a demonstrable widening at the carotid bulb indicates the presence of significant atheromatous plaque within that region, and thus can represent a carotid stenosis.
B. Internal carotid stenosis is expressed as the ratio of the diameter of the stenosis as seen in the projection that shows the most severe degree of narrowing compared with the diameter of the adjacent normal vessel segment.
C. Internal carotid stenosis is always expressed as a percentage narrowing of the cross-sectional area of the vessel at the site of the stenosis compared with the cross-sectional area of the adjacent normal vessel segments because the ratio of these areas is a far more accurate measurement of flow impediment than a single-view diameter measurement.
D. Always requires selective angiography in addition to nonselective aortic arch arteriography.
E. Selective angiography presents no additional risk when compared with nonselective aortic arch angiography.

■ QUESTIONS FOR CHAPTER 138

Question 138-1

A 72-year-old man experiences a single episode of right arm paralysis for 10 minutes with a complete recovery. Carotid duplex ultrasound examination reveals a left carotid occlusion and 50% to 79% stenosis of the right carotid artery. At this point, appropriate management of this patient should be:

A. Antiplatelet agents and follow-up carotid duplex of right carotid artery stenosis every 6 months.
B. Urgent right CEA.
C. Thrombolysis of left carotid artery.
D. Confirmatory testing of carotid occlusion with computed tomographic angiography (CTA), magnetic resonance angiography (MRA), or angiography.
E. CT scan of the head.

Question 138-2

CEA may be safely carried out on the basis of a duplex scan, without angiography, if which of the following conditions are met:

A. Ongoing quality assurance program has been carried out in the vascular laboratory.
B. Common carotid artery (CCA) stenosis is suspected.
C. The distal ICA is visualized well and free of disease.
D. All of the above.
E. A and C.

Question 138-3

A 70-year-old woman has sudden onset of left arm and leg weakness lasting 2 hours. She has a history of coronary artery disease and has stable angina, hypertension, renal insufficiency, and hypercholesterolemia. Of the following, the most appropriate next diagnostic test is:

A. Cerebral (aortic arch and four vessel) angiography.
B. Duplex scan of the carotid arteries.
C. Duplex scan of the renal arteries.
D. Cardiac stress test.
E. None of the above.

■ QUESTIONS FOR CHAPTER 139

Question 139-1

Stroke-in-evolution is best managed by:

A. Systemic anticoagulation.
B. Emergency CEA.
C. Heparin, aspirin, and blood pressure control with nitroprusside.
D. Barbiturate coma, intubation, and hyperventilation to produce hypocapnia.
E. An IV bolus of a thrombolytic agent.

Question 139-2

Which of the following indications for CEA *in symptomatic patients* has been supported by and confirmed by randomized trials?

A. Single focal TIA with greater than 70% stenosis.
B. Multiple focal TIAs with greater than 50% stenosis and ulceration.
C. Previous mild ipsilateral stroke with greater than 50% carotid stenosis and a large ulcer.
D. Evolving stroke with greater than 70% stenosis.
E. Global symptoms with greater than 70% carotid stenosis and uncorrectable vertebrobasilar disease.

Question 139-3

Presuming an ipsilateral carotid lesion is technically suitable for CEA, which of the following situations would *not* be considered a contraindication to proceeding directly with that operation?

A. An intercurrent illness that will materially shorten the patient's life expectancy.
B. A major acute stroke that has not begun to recover neurologically.
C. A major completed stroke without significant neurologic recovery.
D. An acute stroke with recovery of a minor to moderate neurologic deficit between 2 and 6 weeks afterward.
E. An episode of amaurosis fugax 6 months before coronary artery bypass recently scheduled because of severe angina, but with no other carotid or vertebral occlusive lesions seen angiographically.

■ QUESTIONS FOR CHAPTER 140

Question 140-1

The immediate combined stroke and death rate after carotid angioplasty and stenting (CAS), based on available literature, is closest to which of the following:

A. 0%–1%.
B. 2%–3%.
C. 5%.
D. 7%–10%.
E. >10%.

Question 140-2

The incidence of restenosis after carotid CAS is typically reported as between 5% and 10% at 18 to 24 months after intervention. Of the following, which has *not* been associated with an increased risk of restenosis after CAS?

A. Elevated levels of C-reactive protein after CAS.
B. CCA diameter less than 7 mm.
C. Incomplete stent apposition.
D. Female gender.
E. Residual stenosis after CAS.

Question 140-3

CAS has been advocated for use in patients believed to be at high risk for CEA. The Stenting and Angioplasty with Protection in Patients at High Risk for Endarterectomy (SAPPHIRE) trial randomized high-risk patients to either CAS or CEA on the basis of a number of specific risk criteria, criteria likely to be used to determine the appropriateness of and reimbursement for CAS. Inclusion (high-risk) criteria for the SAPPHIRE study included all of the following *except*:

A. Age >65 years.
B. Lesions below the clavicle.
C. Restenosis after CEA.
D. Positive cardiac stress test result.
E. Recent myocardial infarction.

■ QUESTIONS FOR CHAPTER 141

Question 141-1

Which of the following statements about vertebrobasilar ischemic symptoms is true?

A. The presence of orthostatic hypotension (with a 20 mm Hg systolic pressure decrease on standing) excludes a patient from further workup of the status of the vertebrobasilar arteries.
B. A brain CT scan is used to rule out the presence of ischemic infarcts in the posterior circulation.
C. In labyrinthine disease when the patient's head is turned suddenly, the inertial changes result in symptoms after a 2- to 3-second delay accompanied by nystagmus, whereas in vertebral artery (VA) compression, symptoms occur without any delay as the head is rotated.
D. A 24-hour electrocardiogram (ECG) (Holter monitoring) is an unnecessary part of the evaluation of patients with TIA of vertebrobasilar distribution.
E. Magnetic resonance imaging (MRI) is equivalent to late-generation CT for demonstrating brain stem infarction.

Question 141-2

With respect to indications for reconstruction of the vertebral artery (VA), which of the following statements is correct?

A. In patients with orthostatic hypotension (decrease of 20 mm Hg systolic on standing), symptoms should be corrected by medical treatment and reconstruction of a severely stenosed or occluded dominant VA is not indicated.
B. When a critically diseased VA is reconstructed in patients with extensive vascular disease and occluded (or severely diseased but unreconstructable) internal carotid arteries, the presence of large, disease-free, posterior communicating arteries does not improve outcomes.
C. The morbidity from combined, concomitant, carotid, and VA repair is the sum of the morbidities observed in carotid and vertebral reconstructions performed at separate times.
D. In VA reconstructions performed for low-flow symptoms, only severely obstructed (>75% luminal narrowing) and clearly dominant or single VAs undergo operation.
E. In patients with an embolic source in a VA or subclavian artery, a normal VA in the opposite side is sufficient to supply adequate blood flow into the basilar artery and obviates repair of the diseased side.

Question 141-3

Regarding arteriographic evaluation of the vertebral arteries, the following statements are true *except*:

A. The most common congenital anomaly is the left VA arising from the aortic arch proximal to the left subclavian artery.
B. The most common atherosclerotic lesion of the VA is severe stenosis of its origin.
C. The second segment of the vertebral artery (V_2), which extends from C_6 to C_2, is the segment of the VA most commonly compressed by osteophytes.
D. V_2 is the second most common site for atherosclerotic involvement of the VA.
E. V_3, which extends from the top of C_2 to the atlantooccipital membrane at the base of the skull, is the segment most frequently affected by dissection due to fibromuscular dysplasia and/or trauma.

Question 141-4

A technique *most* commonly used for surgical reconstruction of the VA to treat vertebrobasilar ischemia caused by low flow is:

A. Transposition or bypass of the V_1 segment.
B. Cervical sympathectomy, as a concomitant procedure to improve bypass flow and avoid associated vasospasm.
C. Bypass to the V_4 segment.
D. Bypass to the V_2 segment.
E. Bypass to the V_3 segment from the subclavian artery.

Question 141-5

Brain infarction in the vertebrobasilar territory is most often caused by:

A. Thrombosis superimposed on a severe atherosclerotic lesion in the primary or secondary branches of the VA or basilar artery.

B. A low-flow condition (from chronic stenoses or occlusion of the VAs) particularly affecting the watershed areas.
C. Embolization from an atheromatous/dissecting lesion of the VA.
D. Embolization from a carotid bifurcation atheroma through a large posterior communicating artery.
E. An episode of transient hypotension.

Question 141-6

A patient with type 2 diabetes and well-controlled hypertension presents with dizziness that is triggered or aggravated by standing. MRI results of the brain are normal. Arteriogram shows 90% stenosis of the left VA, 40% to 60% stenoses of both carotid arteries, and a normal right VA. The *next* step in management should be:

A. Auditory-evoked potentials.
B. Angioplasty of left VA stenosis.
C. Surgical correction of left VA stenosis.
D. Medical evaluation of orthostatism.
E. Stenting of the narrowest carotid artery.

Question 141-7

A 50-year-old woman has positional vertigo that occurs 1 to 2 seconds after maintaining rotation-extension of the head with the patient sitting up and takes up to 10 seconds to relieve once the normal position of the head is reestablished. The most appropriate *next* step in management is:

A. Ear, nose, and throat evaluation.
B. Duplex of the carotid-vertebrals with head in neutral and rotated position.
C. Dynamic arteriogram in supine position with craniocaudal head compression.
D. Cardiac electrophysiologic evaluation.
E. MRI of the brain.

■ QUESTIONS FOR CHAPTER 142

Question 142-1

A 40-year-old hypertensive woman presents with an asymptomatic carotid bruit and is found to have severe fibromuscular dysplasia of the ICA. What is the most appropriate next step in management?

A. Balloon angioplasty of the ICA.
B. Balloon angioplasty and stent placement of the ICA.
C. Carotid exploration with graded probe dilatation of the ICA.
D. Evaluation of the renal arteries.
E. Anticoagulation.

Question 142-2

A 50-year-old woman with asymptomatic carotid fibromuscular disease (FMD) has been followed with annual carotid duplex scans. She presents to the emergency department with a very severe headache and decreased consciousness. Cooperation with the neurologic examination is difficult, but she appears to be developing some upper extremity weakness. What is the most likely cause of the patient's condition?

A. Internal carotid dissection caused by FMD.
B. Cerebral embolus from internal carotid narrowings caused by FMD.
C. Lacunar infarct caused by hypertension.
D. Rupture of cerebral aneurysm.
E. Coincidental presentation of brain tumor.

Question 142-3

A patient presents with focal motor TIAs and is found to have ipsilateral carotid FMD. Which of the following descriptions of diagnostic study findings is most likely?

A. Carotid duplex shows an 80% to 99% carotid bifurcation stenosis.
B. Head CT shows an arteriovenous malformation involving the intracranial vessels.
C. MRA shows critical stenosis in the distal CCA and proximal ICA.
D. Carotid arteriography shows multiple narrowings of the mid- to distal extracranial ICA.
E. Carotid arteriography shows an 85% stenosis of the ICA.

■ QUESTIONS FOR CHAPTER 143

Question 143-1

A 60-year-old woman has a pulsatile mass at the base of the neck on the right side. She thinks it has grown since her primary care doctor discovered it 6 weeks ago. Although she has no history of cardiovascular disease, her risk factors include hypertension, obesity, and elevated serum cholesterol.

Which one of the following recommendations for management is best?

A. Establish the diagnosis using duplex ultrasound.
B. Obtain either an MRA or CTA because of the location of the lesion.
C. Obtain a cardiac risk assessment, because the most likely diagnosis, a brachiocephalic artery aneurysm, will require a median sternotomy for its repair.
D. Advise that surgical treatment will be required to prevent rupture of this atherosclerotic aneurysm.
E. Advise endovascular repair with stents and/or (possibly) coils.

Question 143-2

A 25-year-old man is involved in a single-vehicle automobile accident during which he was wearing a seat belt. The paramedics report that he had temporary loss of consciousness and then was not moving his left upper extremity. He has a large laceration on his forehead, moves his left upper extremity on command with good strength, and smells of alcohol. He is hemodynamically stable and has a normal chest x-ray film. An MRI/MRA ordered by the emergency department physician shows only a 1.0-cm aneurysm of the distal right ICA near the base of the skull. Which of the following is the most appropriate management?

A. Perform a carotid angiogram in preparation for interposition graft repair of the aneurysm.
B. During the angiogram, perform trial carotid occlusion and measure carotid back-pressure in preparation for carotid ligation.

C. Treat the aneurysm by filling it with coils at the time of angiography.
D. Perform cerebral angiography to confirm the aneurysm size and location and then treat the patient with antiplatelet agents and order a follow-up angiogram in 3 to 6 weeks.
E. Initiate antiplatelet therapy with clopidogrel, follow the aneurysm with duplex ultrasound, and intervene only for documented aneurysm enlargement.

Question 143-3

Two years after a CEA performed for a symptomatic high-grade stenosis, a 79-year-old woman is found to have a 4-cm pulsatile mass beneath her cervical scar. She is afebrile and has a normal white blood cell count. Which of the following represents the most appropriate management?

A. Because the most likely diagnosis is atherosclerotic aneurysm of the distal CCA, repair with either an interposition vein or prosthetic graft.
B. If the original operation was performed with a vein patch, treat her with anticoagulants to prevent possible embolization and stroke.
C. If the original operation was performed with a prosthetic patch, treat with IV antibiotics for at least 6 weeks and possibly longer.
D. Despite her age, if a prosthetic patch was used in the initial operation, perform an autogenous reconstruction now without a trial of antibiotics.
E. Regardless of the type of patch used in the initial operation, her age mandates endovascular treatment with a covered stent rather than open surgical repair.

■ QUESTIONS FOR CHAPTER 144

Question 144-1

Regarding carotid artery tortuosity, coils and kinks, which of the following statements is *not* true?

A. Bilateral carotid coiling is more common in children than adults.
B. Carotid kinks are four times more common in women.
C. Kinks may cause intermittent symptoms of cerebral insufficiency with turning of the head.
D. Most symptomatic kinks not associated with atherosclerosis can be corrected by arteriopexy, and resection/reanastomosis techniques to shorten the involved carotid artery are unnecessary.
E. In symptomatic patients with kinks associated with atherosclerosis, the kink is best corrected at the time of CEA.

Question 144-2

Regarding the carotid body and carotid body tumors, which of the following statements is *not* true?

A. The carotid body is derived from both mesodermal and neural crest elements.
B. The carotid body is composed of nonchromaffin cells, and its stimulation has no endocrine or hemodynamic effects.
C. Carotid body tumors can be familial and are more commonly bilateral in this case.

D. Malignant carotid body tumors can be locally invasive, spread to lymph nodes, and metastasize to distant locations.
E. Most of the blood supply of a carotid body tumor comes from the external carotid artery rather than the ICA.

Question 144-3

A 57-year-old pipe smoker underwent a standard right radical neck dissection followed by 5000 rad external irradiation 4 years ago for a carcinoma of the floor of the mouth lateral to the tongue. Four nodes in the upper neck were positive. He presents with multiple, frequent (crescendo) TIAs involving the right hemisphere. Arteriography shows a fusiform, slightly irregular narrowing involving the right CCA and ICA, which is 80% of diameter at its tightest point. The right external carotid is patent. The left carotid arteries have no significant narrowing. His blood pressure is normal, but his lactic dehydrogenase and total cholesterol are significantly elevated. He now smokes only cigarettes. The skin of his right neck is atrophic and pigmented, but the carotid artery can be easily seen pulsating under the surgical scar. Careful head and neck examination shows no signs of recurrent or metastatic disease. A thallium scan shows normal early and late distribution.

Which is the most appropriate treatment of his symptomatic carotid stenosis?

A. Right CEA with Dacron patch closure.
B. Resection of the narrowed carotid segment followed by an interposition vein graft. Neck closure with a myocutaneous flap.
C. Ligation of the common carotid low in the neck and depend on collateral flow.
D. Carotid stenting, using an emboloprotective device.
E. Antiplatelet therapy plus statins.

■ QUESTIONS FOR CHAPTER 145

Question 145-1

You are called by the nursing staff about a patient who underwent a CEA 2 hours ago. The patient was neurologically intact at the completion of your procedure. The only problem he has had since the procedure is hypertension. The nurse tells you that the patient is having some difficulty breathing. What is the *first* cause to exclude?

A. Pulmonary embolism.
B. Myocardial infarction.
C. Cranial nerve injury.
D. Cervical hematoma.
E. Congestive heart failure.

Question 145-2

A patient undergoes an uncomplicated right CEA and appears to be neurologically intact at the completion of the procedure. You are called to the recovery room 1 hour later because the patient has a new neurologic deficit involving the left side of his body. Which of the following would be the appropriate initial diagnostic study?

A. Head CT scan.
B. Electroencephalograph (EEG).
C. Carotid duplex.
D. TCD.
E. Head MRI.

Question 145-3

You have planned staged bilateral carotid endarterectomies 1 week apart. The first procedure is uncomplicated. What would be the most important diagnostic study to perform before the second procedure?

A. Head CT scan.
B. Carotid duplex.
C. EEG.
D. ECG.
E. Laryngoscopy.

Question 145-4

A 60-year-old man has a left hemispheric TIA and is found to have a 99% left carotid stenosis and an occluded right internal carotid. The patient undergoes an uncomplicated left CEA and is discharged on the first postoperative day. You receive a call 4 days later because the patient has developed a severe left-sided headache. What is the most likely diagnosis?

A. Hyperperfusion syndrome.
B. Migraine headache.
C. Ischemic stroke.
D. Greater auricular neuropathy.
E. Cerebral vasospasm.

ANSWERS AND DISCUSSION

■ ANSWERS AND DISCUSSION FOR CHAPTER 135

Answer 135-1: C

Discussion 135-1

TIAs refer to episodes of transient loss of function in the distribution of either the carotid or VA as it affects the hemisphere or one of its lobes, brain stem, or eye, as in A, B, D, and E. Symptoms often related to transient global ischemia, such as (C) dizziness and lightheadedness, are most often related to transient decreases in cardiac output or blood pressure and do not relate directly to arterial occlusive disease of the cerebral circulation.

Answer 135-2: D

Discussion 135-2

TIAs are an important warning sign of extracranial arterial occlusive disease and the risk of subsequent stroke. The majority of strokes occur as the initial event, emphasizing the importance of an asymptomatic carotid lesion as a potential marker for subsequent stroke risk.

A. They do *not* "most often" occur within 24 hours before the stroke.
B. They do *not* occur 1 year before the stroke "in the majority."
C. They characteristically occur in *the same distribution* as the stroke.
D. A retrospective review of patients who have had a stroke indicated that only 30% to 50% of those individuals had experienced any form of transient cerebral ischemia before the stroke event. This is the correct statement.
E. Although they *may* mimic the stroke, they often have milder symptoms and symptoms may differ (e.g., amaurosis fugax before a hemiplegic stroke), and by accepted definition, must resolve before *24 hours* to qualify as a TIA.

Answer 135-3: B

Discussion 135-3

A. Although high-grade stenoses are normally associated with neurologic events, TIAs are not a hemodynamic event, that is, related to transiently flow decreases caused by a carotid stenosis.
B. TIAs are secondary to the plaque burden associated with a lesion that results in fragmentation of atheromatous debris or platelet aggregation and secondary embolization from irregular or ulcerated surfaces. The evidence for the repetitive nature or stereotypic presentation of transient ischemic events is based on the concept of laminar blood flow. Thus, when a particle is introduced from the surface of an atherosclerotic plaque in the flowing blood, particles within that particular portion of the flow stream will inevitably end up in the same distribution and terminal vessel of the intracranial circulation.
C. Subplaque hemorrhage may be associated with increased carotid narrowing or disturb the overlying atheromatous

debris or platelet aggregates, but *associated vasospasm does not play a major role in TIAs*, similar to that theorized for coronary artery disease.
D. Platelet deposition clearly occurs and platelet aggregates may embolize, causing a TIA, but hypercoagulable states have rarely been implicated in this process.
E. Emboli of cardiac origin must be considered in someone presenting with TIAs, but they are not "territorial" since this term means they characteristically have the same cerebral arterial distribution, which cardiac emboli do not.

Answer 135-4: C

Discussion 135-4

A. The landmark publication by Eastcott, Pickering, and Robb in the *Lancet* in 1954 first called attention to the possibility that direct repair of a carotid artery would be helpful in alleviating neurologic symptoms. However, their operation consisted of a resection and reanastomosis rather than endarterectomy.
B. Debakey claims to have performed the first CEA in 1956. However, it was not published until he reported a 19-year follow-up of the "first case" in 1975.
C. The Argentinean surgeons, Carrea, Molins, and Murphy, published their experience with three CEAs in 1955. In their article they described the operations as being performed in 1953, but they withheld publication until they had at least a 2-year follow-up.
D. Javid and Julian reported sizable early experiences with CEA, and Javid was responsible for the first specially designed shunt for maintaining flow during CEA, but they did not publish the first reported case.
E. Edwin J. Wiley was a pioneer in developing endarterectomy as a technique in the United States after seeing it performed in Portugal, but he did not perform or publish the first report of CEA.

■ ANSWERS AND DISCUSSION FOR CHAPTER 136

Answer 136-1: D

Discussion 136-1

A. Because the left ICA perfuses the left cerebral hemisphere, neglect, if any, would be on the right, not on the left, side of the body.
B. Diplopia is related to brain stem abnormalities because of the lesions affecting three, four, and/or six cranial nerves, which are perfused by the vertebral basilar system.
C. Denial of blindness is a bilateral vertebral occipital lobe phenomenon and relates to the two posterior cerebral arteries that supply the occipital lobes. The posterior cerebral artery generally arises from the termination of the vertebral basilar system, but in approximately 2% it arises from the ICA, so that a stroke in this distribution could possibly result in hemi-neglect. However, *denial* means lack of insight and is dignified with the name of

Anton's syndrome. Such people are unaware that they are blind and will deny it if asked. This does *not* occur with carotid artery lesions or unilateral posterior cerebral artery occlusions.

D. Correct answer. The ophthalmic artery is one of the first intracranial branches of the ICA, and it occasionally may be the landing site of an embolus from the carotid artery, which would then produce either transient or permanent monocular visual disturbance. This is also a herald for embolic phenomena to the brain more distally on the same side.

E. Gaze deviation to the right is lost with left-sided lesions. The rule is that gaze looks toward the side of the lesion.

Answer 136-2: C

Discussion 136-2

A. The weight of evidence shows that t-PA is the best mode of therapy for resolution of *clot* causing an ischemic event *if* its onset is documented to be *less than 3 hours* before administration. t-PA carries morbidity because of bleeding, but if there are no contraindications, such as previous gastrointestinal bleeding or blood dyscrasia, and brain imaging shows no hemorrhage, t-PA should be given. However this answer suggests an inappropriately long window of time for its use (i.e., 12 hours).

B. Treatment of elevated blood pressure depends on the degree to which it is elevated, but as a general rule it should *not* be lowered for the first 24 to 48 hours after the onset of a cerebral ischemic event. Lowering the blood pressure may actually augment the size of the ischemic lesion because of the lowered perfusion pressure.

C. This is the correct answer because in aphasic patients, deglutition may be impaired and aspiration could result.

D. There is no proof that heparin results in prevention of stroke progression, although it may be used to prevent the complications of bed rest, which include venous thrombosis.

E. Seizure represents a relative contraindication of the use of t-PA because of the possibility that recurrent seizures may cause injury and uncontrolled bleeding.

Answer 136-3: A

Discussion 136-3

A. TCD is a safe, noninvasive means for determining potential sources for infarction caused by microemboli from the site of the CEA. Unfortunately, it is not widely available, and a minority of patients will not have an adequate cranial window for the test. Nevertheless, this is a true statement.

B. In some situations angiography is needed but should not be performed on *all* patients, particularly if a tight carotid stenosis has been identified by ultrasound performed by reliable and trained technicians.

C. Transesophageal echocardiogram requires cooperation from the patient with the passage of a long tube through the esophagus that can worsen neurologic deficits in patients who are having a progressive stroke. Transthoracic echocardiography should suffice for most patients. Patent foramen ovale can be considered, but in most elderly people it is not a source for cerebral vascular episodes caused by emboli.

D. Diplopia, vertigo, and imbalance suggest abnormality in the vertebral basilar system, not the carotid artery.

E. Even in patients thought to have "asymptomatic" stenosis, TCD studies often detect the presence of microemboli.

■ ANSWERS AND DISCUSSION FOR CHAPTER 137

Answer 137-1: B

Discussion 137-1

A. The Circle of Willis is a well-defined group of intracranial arteries (anterior and posterior communicating arteries) that effectively forms an arterial manifold that balances the inflow coming from the ICA and VA with the outflow to the anterior, middle, and posterior cerebral arteries.

B. However, only 20% of individuals actually have the "textbook" symmetric Circle of Willis; hypoplasia of one or more components occurs in most individuals. Thus, the ability of the Circle of Willis to supply flow to the brain in the event of a carotid or VA occlusion depends on whether the necessary arterial segment of the Circle is intact and is thus impossible to predict in advance.

C. See discussion of answer B; the protection provided by the Circle of Willis cannot be termed "reliable."

D. It is *not* an embryonic structure that closes at or shortly after birth.

E. It is *not* a network of *venous* channels; it is a connecting collateral pathway between intracerebral arteries.

Answer 137-2: B

Discussion 137-2

A. Current duplex ultrasound, MRA, and high-resolution multislice helical CTA are modalities that are now capable of providing high-resolution images of the extracranial carotid arteries that are of sufficient diagnostic quality to determine whether a lesion warrants surgical intervention in most patients. Therefore carotid/cerebral arteriography is no longer *essential* for such decisions.

B. However, in situations in which the images from these modalities are inconclusive, because of poor quality as the result of body habitus, poor techniques, poor patient cooperation, metallic implants, and so forth, contrast angiography can still be of value, but it can now be reserved for such situations.

C. Carotid/cerebral arteriography is a relatively low-risk diagnostic modality, but certainly not as risk free as noninvasive imaging. Although the risk of major complications in carotid angiography is generally less than 1% to 1.5%, this is still significant because it comes close to the risk of endarterectomy in the hands of experienced surgeons and thus materially impacts the risks involved in the diagnostic and therapeutic care of such patients.

D. Views of the proximal intracranial circulation are a standard part of carotid angiography in the setting of occlusive atheromatous disease (A) because the proximal intracranial carotid circulation is a common site of atheromatous occlusive disease and (B) the adequacy of cross-filling of the contralateral anterior circulation can have a significant impact on surgical decision making, especially in the hands of surgeons who do not routinely operate using carotid bypass shunts.

E. Digital imaging has become the de facto standard in angiographic imaging and provides resolution sufficient for all practical diagnostic purposes, including visualization of the smaller cerebral vessels.

Answer 137-3: E

Discussion 137-3

A. This is not true. Although collateral circulation in the brain is limited, it is most often sufficient to allow a substantial portion of the compromised region of the brain to remain viable for as much as 3 to 6 hours. Thus, the outcome of stroke can be affected by *early* treatment. See discussions below.

B. Catheter-directed thrombolysis, *but also high-dose IV thrombolysis*, administered as soon as possible after it has been determined that the event is an ischemic, rather than a hemorrhagic, stroke can effectively reverse much if not all of the effects of the cerebral vascular event. Although some investigators may argue the advantages of catheter-directed thrombolysis over the IV administration, logistic factors such as the availability of appropriate specialist physicians and facilities favor the use of IV thrombolysis except in situations in which the required personnel and facilities are readily available in a timely manner.

C. Stroke is a term that refers to both ischemic and hemorrhagic cerebral vascular accidents.

D. Although stroke was once thought to be caused by thrombotic occlusion of underlying carotid stenoses, angiographic and ultrasound examinations performed in connection with acute stroke intervention over the past decade have shown that the majority of ischemic strokes are the result of embolic occlusion rather than in situ thrombosis. New methods of differentiating early ischemic stroke from hemorrhagic events using MRI are being actively investigated; however, the differentiation is still routinely made by CT in which an intracranial hemorrhage appears as a high-density lesion early on, as opposed to *early* ischemic stroke, which generally does not change normal appearance of the brain.

E. For the reasons outlined in this discussion, it seems highly likely that stroke will eventually be viewed as a analog of myocardial infarction, requiring similar emergency triage and treatment with similar expectation of success.

Answer 137-4: B

Discussion 137-4

A. Although "flattening" or "effacement" of the expected broadening in the proximal ICA known as the carotid bulb does indeed indicate the presence of pathologic material occupying what would otherwise be vessel lumen, it does not actually constitute a hemodynamically significant impediment to flow, and thus does not constitute a carotid stenosis.

B. Because catheter-based angiography is, at least for the present, a planar projection technique, the generally accepted convention for expressing the severity of angiographically demonstrable stenoses is the ratio of the diameter of the stenosis as seen in the projection that shows the most severe degree of narrowing compared with the diameter of the adjacent normal vessel segments in that same projection. This was used in the landmark North American Symptomatic Carotid Endarterectomy Trial.

C. Although it is certainly true that the ratio of the cross-sectional area compared with the cross-sectional area at the site of a stenosis compared with the cross-sectional area of adjacent normal vessel segments is a far more accurate measurement of the hemodynamic significance of a stenosis than a single-plan diameter ratio, this is *not* the customary method of expressing the severity of stenotic lesions seen on angiography. As three-dimensional computer reconstruction techniques for display of conventional catheter-based angiography become more widely available and high-resolution multislice CTA gains wider acceptance, the cross-sectional area ratio will become much easier to calculate on a routine basis. When that happens, the current worst diameter convention may well be abandoned in favor of the more accurate cross-sectional ratio measurement.

D. Although selective angiography may indeed be necessary to evaluate the cervical and proximal intracranial carotid arteries, high-quality nonselective aortic arch angiography in at least two oblique projections is often sufficient to evaluate these vessels without the need for selective catheterization.

E. There is an added risk of embolization inherent in selective carotid angiography, albeit relatively low. Thus, consideration should always be given first to how well the nonselective arteriogram satisfies the need for diagnostic evaluation before simply proceeding with selective catheterization and angiography.

■ ANSWERS AND DISCUSSION FOR CHAPTER 138

Answer 138-1: D

Discussion 138-1

A. The currently accepted and effective treatment for hemispheric TIA, which this patient clearly experienced, is CEA. However, this patient had a *left* hemispheric TIA and has an apparent *left* carotid occlusion, a situation that would not allow endarterectomy. Confirmation of a duplex-detected occlusion is indicated because this is an area that duplex scan, on occasion (~3%), may not distinguish between a very tight stenosis versus an occlusion. Thus, if the patient is otherwise an appropriate candidate for CEA, one would not want to exclude that treatment option simply on the basis of one duplex scan. There may be situations, with the left carotid occlusion a certainty, in which option "A" would be selected in a high-risk patient.

B. There is no indication for *urgent* treatment of the asymptomatic, contralateral carotid stenosis. Evaluation and treatment can be carried out in an elective fashion.

C. There are no data to support this course of action. It might expose the patient to a higher risk of embolism and stroke.

D. Because of an approximate 3% risk of error by duplex scan (calling an occlusion when a very tight stenosis occurs), confirmatory studies are appropriate. In most cases, with today's refined imaging techniques, noninvasive studies with CTA or MRA can be used, avoiding the stroke risk of angiography, although a weakness of MRA is its tendency to overcall tight stenoses. This situation emphasizes the need for individual vascular laboratories to validate and correlate their own results.

E. Although in the past a CT head scan may have been ordered "in case" the clinical event that was thought to be a TIA was actually a stroke, this might then affect treatment options. In this particular scenario, with a very typical TIA being described, CT scan results are unlikely to have any impact on subsequent decision making regarding appropriate treatment.

Answer 138-2: E

Discussion 138-2

A. CEA without arteriography can be safely performed if the following criteria are met: (1) vascular laboratory duplex accuracy is known (ongoing quality assurance); (2) duplex scan is technically adequate; (3) vascular anomalies, kinks, or loops are not present; (4) CCA is free of significant disease; and (5) distal ICA is free of significant disease.

B. CCA stenosis would actually be an indication for arteriography.

C. See criterion (4) in "A" above.

D. B is incorrect.

E. This is the correct answer. A and C are (1) and (4), respectively, in the criteria cited in the discussion of A.

Answer 138-3: B

Discussion 138-3

A. Arteriography is an invasive test and caries a risk of stroke of approximately 1%. It should not be the first-line diagnostic test in a patient with cerebrovascular symptoms because, with appropriate noninvasive testing, it may be completely avoided.

B. The patient has had a clear-cut TIA. A common cause of this problem is carotid bifurcation disease that can be effectively treated with CEA. Carotid duplex is a noninvasive test that can accurately diagnose carotid disease and guide therapy. It is the correct answer.

C. Although the patient's hypertension may eventually merit evaluation, the acute symptoms take precedence. Like many patients with symptomatic carotid disease, this patient may have widespread atherosclerosis, and renovascular hypertension is a possibility that should be evaluated *after* the acute problem.

D. Appropriate evaluation should start with determining the source of the patient's TIA. Subsequent evaluation, particularly if surgical options are selected, may justify cardiac stress testing, based on clinical indications.

E. "B" is the correct answer, making E wrong.

■ ANSWERS AND DISCUSSION FOR CHAPTER 139

Answer 139-1: B

Discussion 139-1

Patients who present with stroke-in-evolution or the stuttering and progressive neurologic deficit represent a particularly high-risk group of patients for permanent neurologic deficit or death. A variety of nonsurgical approaches, including those listed in answers A, C, D, and E, have been tried and have *not* been shown to significantly improve on the outcome *in the particular scenario of stroke-in-evolution*. Thrombolytic therapy, either delivered by IV bolus (E) or catheter directed, has had some success with strokes caused by thrombosis of certain cerebral arteries, when administered early, but the arterial location and completeness of the thrombus formation are important considerations in its success. The carotid lesion responsible for stroke-in-evolution is best treated by CEA, performed as an emergency (B). Emergency CEA, when combined with good medical management and strict control of postoperative blood pressure, has been shown to have a major impact in improving the prognosis of this disadvantaged group of patients.

Answer 139-2: A

Discussion 139-2

All of these indications have been supported by reports based on retrospective data analysis, the Rand panel, and the guidelines of the Joint Council of North American Vascular Surgery Societies, and are generally widely accepted, but only (A) single focal TIA associated with a greater than 70% carotid stenosis, has been confirmed by a prospective randomized clinical trial (North American Symptomatic Carotid Endarterectomy Trial).

Answer 139-3: D

Discussion 139-3

A. An intercurrent illness that will materially shorten the patient's life expectancy is an accepted contraindication.

B. Major acute strokes without any neurologic recovery, with the possible exception of those occurring in the hospital where progression from stenosis to occlusion has been promptly documented, are considered a contraindication to CEA.

C. CEA cannot be expected to significantly improve patients with a major completed stroke without significant neurologic recovery.

D. Although it was once believed that one *must* wait 6 weeks after any acute stroke before proceeding with CEA, this was based on earlier empiric retrospective observational data. More recent experiences suggest it is safe to proceed earlier in those with minor to moderate strokes with earlier complete recovery, particularly if the carotid lesion is a threatening one, for example, a critically tight stenosis. This is now a correct answer.

E. Although amaurosis fugax, as prima facie evidence for the need for CEA, has been recently debated, a remote episode should not take precedence over a clearly indicated coronary bypass. In addition, although CEA has commonly been performed before elective coronary bypass, it more often is performed first in those with recently symptomatic and/or bilateral carotid disease with poor collateral circulation, unlike this scenario.

■ ANSWERS AND DISCUSSION FOR CHAPTER 140

Answer 140-1: C

Discussion 140-1

Early results of CAS, using relatively crude guidewires, balloons, and stents, were less than 10%. With improvements in device technology, refinements in the technique of CAS, and better patient selection, and possibly emboloprotective devices, the combined risk of stroke and death is approximately 5%, This estimate is based on more than 17,000 procedures reported in the peer-reviewed medical literature. Thus, C is currently the correct answer.

Answer 140-2: B

Discussion 140-2

A number of factors, including (A) elevated C-reactive protein levels 48 hours after CAS, (C) incomplete stent apposition, (D) female gender, and (E) residual stenosis (and age >75 years) have been associated with recurrent stenosis. Carotid artery diameter (B) has not been identified as a risk factor for restenosis.

Answer 140-3: A

Discussion 140-3

The SAPPHIRE trial compared the results of CEA and CAS in patients with carotid stenosis considered to be at increased risk for CEA based on a number of criteria.

These included:
Local/anatomic factors
Previous ipsilateral CEA (Answer C)
Severe tandem lesion
Cervical radiation treatment
Contralateral carotid occlusion
High cervical lesion (at least C_2)
Lesion below the clavicle (Answer B)
Contralateral laryngeal palsy
Medical comorbidities:
Chronic oxygen therapy
Resting $Po_2 \leq 60$ mm Hg
Baseline hematocrit $\geq 50\%$
Forced expiratory volume in 1 second or diffusing capacity of lung for carbon monoxide $\leq 50\%$ predicted
Open heart surgery <6 weeks
Myocardial infarction <4 weeks (Answer E)
Angina Canadian Cardiovascular Society class III/IV
Congestive heart failure class III/IV
Ejection fraction <30%
Abnormal cardiac stress test (Answer D)
Age >80 years, not >65 years as (A), which is therefore the correct answer

■ ANSWERS AND DISCUSSION FOR CHAPTER 141

Answer 141-1: D

Discussion 141-1

A. Known systemic causes of vertebrobasilar ischemic symptoms include orthostatic hypotension, overzealous antihypertensive therapy, arrhythmias, malfunction of pacemakers, anemia, brain tumor, and subclavian steal. A 20 mm Hg systolic pressure decrease on standing is an arbitrarily chosen criterion for diagnosis of orthostatic hypotension. However, the presence of orthostatic hypotension does not exclude a patient from further workup because orthostatic hypotension may be the mechanism that triggers symptoms of ischemia in patients with less-than-critical stenoses in the vertebrobasilar system.

B. A CT scan resolves poorly small brain stem infarcts, because of scatter from the dense bone that surrounds this part of the brain.

C. Inner ear problems may cause symptoms of vertebrobasilar ischemia. Patients may also present with similar posterior TIA on turning their heads. The latter occurs when osteophytes compress the dominant VA in its second (V_2) portion. However, in labyrinthine disease, sudden inertial changes (as when shaking the head) will result in immediate symptoms. In VA compression, it takes a few seconds to experience symptoms, and these appear even though the head is rotated slowly. (The opposite of Answer C.)

D. Some patients with vertebrobasilar ischemic symptoms caused by arrhythmias may recognize the association of palpitations with the appearance of their symptoms, the latter being secondary to a transient decrease in cardiac output (because of the arrhythmia). The patient may not have experienced palpitations or recognized their association with ischemic brain symptoms. A 24-hour ambulatory ECG (Holter monitoring) should be obtained in patients being evaluated for vertebrobasilar TIA before the symptoms are incorrectly attributed to coexisting VA lesions.

E. Brain stem infarctions are often missed by the CT scan because they tend to be small and the resolution of the CT scan in this area is poor (see B, above). MRI is *superior* (not equivalent) to CT scan in demonstrating these lesions.

Answer 141-2: D

Discussion 141-2

A. Patients with symptoms of vertebrobasilar ischemia *and* orthostatic hypotension may or may not have concomitant VA stenosis or occlusion. In some patients the postural decrease of arterial pressure can be corrected by readjustment of antihypertensive medication, by antiarrhythmic drugs, by insertion of a pacemaker, or by pressure stockings. If the patient does not respond to medical treatment, reconstruction of a stenosed or occluded VA may be needed to render the patient asymptomatic.

B. An indication for reconstruction of a critically diseased VA occurs when one or both carotid arteries are occluded and the patient experiences low-flow cerebral ischemia. In this group, the presence of large posterior communicating arteries increases the likelihood that reestablishing normal vertebrobasilar inflow will correct the symptoms.

C. Patients undergoing concomitant internal carotid and VA repair experience *greater* morbidity than the aggregate of complications from separate carotid and VA reconstructions.

D. Correct answer. Similar to lesions in the carotid artery, VA reconstructions should be performed when the lumen is severely stenosed (i.e., >75% luminal narrowing). This applies to a clearly dominant or single VA. A potential indication for concomitant VA repair involves patients with severe carotid lesions who also have severe disease of the origin of the dominant or single VA *on the same side* as the planned carotid operation. Treatment of these patients is controversial, but concomitant VA reconstruction (usually vertebral carotid transposition) can readily be performed through a single incision after CEA.

E. In patients with embolic sources in one VA or the subclavian artery, the source of the embolus is corrected regardless of the status of the opposite VA.

Answer 141-3: D

Discussion 141-3

A. The most common anatomic variant of the vertebral artery is an origin arising from the aortic arch just proximal to the left subclavian artery. Less commonly, the right vertebral artery takes origin from the innominate or right common carotid artery.

B. The most common atherosclerotic lesion of the vertebral is severe stenosis of its origin. This lesion may be missed in standard arch views because of supraimposition of the subclavian over the first segment of the vertebral artery. Oblique projections may be helpful in this instance, along with recognition of poststenotic dilatation of the first centimeter or two of the vertebral artery. While redundancy and kinks are common, only the most severe are associated with hemodynamic significance.

C. The most common pathology of the V_2 segment is extrinsic compression by osteophytes. Selective subclavian injections are required to evaluate the V_2 segment, which extends from C_6 to the top of the transverse process of C_2. In patients with symptoms prompted by neck rotation, the V_2 segment must be evaluated with angiograms taken with the neck in right or left rotation. The vertebral, artery may be perfectly normal in one projection and occluded in the other by extrinsic compression.

D. V_2 is *not* the second most common site for atherosclerotic involvement of the VA; it is rarely affected by atherosclerosis.

E. The V_3 segment, which extends from the top of the transverse process of C_2 to the atlanto-occipital membrane at the base of the skull, is the section most frequently affected by dissection due to fibromuscular dysplasia and/or trauma. Importantly, when the vertebral artery is occluded proximally, it usually reconstitutes at the V_3 segment via the occipital connection, a collateral linking the occipital artery with the vertebral artery at this level. Because of this collateral, the distal vertebral and basilar arteries usually remain patent despite proximal VA occlusion.

Answer 141-4: A

Discussion 141-4

Most reconstructions of the VA attempt to relieve either an orificial stenosis (V_1 segment) or disease/occlusion of its intraspinal course (V_2 segment) by bypassing above it to the V_3 segment.

A. Transposition of the VA into the CCA is the most frequent type of reconstruction. It has all but replaced the subclavian to vertebral bypass, which was popular in the 1970s. Nevertheless, the latter is still useful when a contralateral carotid occlusion increases the risk of clamping the single carotid supply during a transposition operation. Inadequate length of the VA for transposition also may require a subclavian-vertebral bypass procedure. Subclavian VA endarterectomy has been virtually abandoned because it is technically more difficult and involves dissection and control of the proximal subclavian, a maneuver that can be problematic on the left side from a cervical incision.

B. Cervical sympathectomy is *not* a part of VA surgery. Injury to the sympathetics (Horner syndrome) may result from dissection of the proximal VA without identification and sparing of the sympathetic fibers that cross it.

C. The V_4 segment is surgically inaccessible.

D. Direct access to the V_2 segment is difficult because of the short distance between the transverse processes between C6 and C2 where the VA can be exposed. When a bypass is planned it is done at the level of C2-C1 (V_3 segment) because (1) it bypasses all the potential sites of compression in the cervical spine, (2) it is the wider space between transverse processes and at this level (C1-C2) an adequate length of VA is available, and (3) it is the level at which the VA is generally reconstituted when its proximal portion is thrombosed.

E. Bypass to the V_3 segment is usually with autogenous vein from the carotid (not the subclavian) artery. Alternative V_3 segment reconstructions can involve transposing the external carotid artery or a large occipital artery to it.

Answer 141-5: C

Discussion 141-5

A. Intrinsic disease and superimposed thrombosis of primary or secondary branches can be presumed to be the cause of an ischemic infarct only in a minority of cases. The fact that most infarcts of the vertebrobasilar territory are embolic has been shown by the postmortem studies of Castaigne, Amarenco, and many others.

B. Infarction in the vertebrobasilar territory generally follows the distribution of the secondary or tertiary branch that was occluded by the embolic particle. The mapping of infarctions in the vertebrobasilar territory does not correspond to the areas of watershed flow between the carotid and vertebrobasilar systems.

C. Embolization is the most common mechanism of infarction in the posterior circulation as demonstrated in postmortem studies. In a symptomatic patient, once the source of infarction in the VA is removed, further brain infarction does not occur. Embolization is also the mechanism that causes infarctions in patients with dissection of the VA. Dissection of the VA is a rare event, but, when it occurs, it is usually followed by a brain infarction in 60% to 90% of patients. This infarction usually develops 1 to 2 weeks after the local symptom of neck pain that occurs when the dissection starts.

D. This rare mechanism can only be presumed in embolization of the posterior cerebral arteries. It has not been described in the territory of the basilar artery and VA.

E. An episode of transient hypotension could only in rare circumstances be implicated as the cause of a discrete infarction in the vertebrobasilar territory.

Answer 141-6: D

Discussion 141-6

A. Auditory-evoked potentials are valuable in the evaluation of demyelinating diseases but useless in the evaluation and topographic localization of ischemic disease of the brain stem or cerebellum.

B. A unilateral severe lesion with a normal contralateral VA is seldom, if ever, the cause of low-flow symptoms. There is no indication for intervention.

C. Same as B. There is no indication for intervention.

D. The common causes of orthostatism (e.g., antihypertensive medications, venomotor paralysis in diabetics, and anemia) must be sought and treated.

E. Same as B. There is no indication for intervention.

Answer 141-7: C

Discussion 141-7

A. Cochleovestibular pathology manifests by dizziness/vertigo with rapid short motions (shaking). Gentle rotation that triggers symptoms after a brief delay indicate compression of a critical vertebral supply and subsequent ischemia (low-flow) of the territory it supplies.

B. Duplex of VAs gives fragmentary information, and the signal is usually lost during manipulation of the neck.

C. The arteriogram must be performed in supine position reproducing the normal weight of the head on the cervical spine by exerting craniocaudal compression while maintaining rotation. The patient must experience symptoms during the arterial injection that shows compression of the dominant vertebral supply. Only in this circumstance can a cause and effect be established.

D. A baroceptor mechanism inducing hypotension and vertebrobasilar symptoms could only be implicated if there was extrinsic compression of the neck (over the carotid) when the symptoms were elicited. Cardiac electrophysiology to rule out arrhythmias would not be the next best step.

E. Patients with low-flow symptoms generally have normal MRI scan results.

■ ANSWERS AND DISCUSSION FOR CHAPTER 142

Answer 142-1: D

Discussion 142-1

A. No. The patient is asymptomatic from a cerebrovascular standpoint, and the presence of carotid FMD alone is

not an indication for intervention. There are few natural history studies, but available data suggest that serious neurologic symptoms in more than 5 years of follow-up will develop in less than 5% of patients with carotid FMD.

B. As in A, the patient is asymptomatic from a cerebrovascular standpoint, and the presence of carotid FMD alone is *not* an indication for intervention.

C. As in A, the patient is asymptomatic from a cerebrovascular standpoint, and the presence of carotid FMD alone is *not* an indication for intervention.

D. There is a high likelihood that the hypertension in this woman is caused by FMD of the renal arteries, which coexists in 8% to 40% of patients with carotid FMD. In this case, the presence of hypertension in a 40 year old, *the renal arteries should be fully investigated.* If renal artery FMD is present, balloon angioplasty should be performed.

E. Answer E is not correct in that there is no evidence to support the use of anticoagulants in this condition. One might consider the empiric use of antiplatelet agents for patients with asymptomatic carotid FMD, but there is no solid evidence for its use either.

Answer 142-2: D

Discussion 142-2

A. Carotid dissection occurs with increased frequency in patients with FMD. This may cause neck pain and headache, but it is less likely than a ruptured cerebral aneurysm to cause this particular clinical picture.

B. Most cerebral symptoms from FMD will be that of TIA or stroke, *not headache and decreased consciousness.*

C. A lacunar infarct is *not* likely to present with this clinical picture. In addition, hypertension was *not* part of the presentation.

D. Patients with carotid FMD should also be evaluated for the possibility of cerebral artery aneurysms, which coexist in 10% to 50% of patients with carotid FMD, and may be much more threatening to the patient than the carotid FMD itself. This patient's presentation, with headache, decreased consciousness, and neurologic deficit, is more suggestive of cerebral hemorrhage than any other cerebral vascular event, so the patient should undergo immediate CT scan of the brain to look for hemorrhage, followed by urgent cerebral arteriography.

E. Answer E is least likely of all. There is no association between FMD and brain tumors, and this would be an abrupt presentation for a brain tumor.

Answer 142-3: D

Discussion 142-3

A. The FMD lesion is not at but usually well above the carotid bifurcation, high enough that duplex scan may miss it.

B. This is unlikely; there is not the prominent association between carotid FMD and arteriovenous malformations as there is with intracerebral aneurysms.

C. A lesion in this location is not typical of FMD (see D).

D. This is the correct answer. Carotid FMD typically starts in the ICA a few centimeters distal to its origin and involves the extracranial ICA as far up as the base of the skull. This location makes duplex studies unreliable because this portion of the ICA may not be visualized.

E. The lesion in E is possible but is *less likely* than the lesion described in D, which is found in 85% of cases of carotid FMD. In the minority (≤15%) of carotid FMD cases a single tight web-like narrowing at the origin of the ICA is found. The treatment of carotid FMD is based on the presence of associated symptoms (e.g., TIAs), *not* on the degree of stenosis.

■ ANSWERS AND DISCUSSION FOR CHAPTER 143

Answer 143-1: A

Discussion 143-1

A. One of the most common findings misdiagnosed as a carotid aneurysm is a dilated tortuous right subclavian or proximal CCA. It is most common in older, obese, hypertensive women, is of little clinical significance, and can be correctly identified by duplex ultrasound. It is not uncommon for patients to perceive that the "aneurysm" has enlarged once they are made aware of its existence.

B. Duplex ultrasound can readily see this condition despite the proximity to the clavicle. CTA and MRA will display the tortuosity to better advantage, but neither is necessary to make the diagnosis.

C. Brachiocephalic aneurysms cannot be safely treated through a cervical incision and therefore would require median sternotomy for their repair. *If* this were the lesion in question, cardiac risk assessment (in contrast with "cardiac clearance") would be appropriate at some point before intervention because of her cardiovascular risk factors.

D. Atherosclerosis *is* the most common cause of extracranial aneurysms and the CCA *is* the most frequently involved vessel, but *the most common location is at the distal portion (bifurcation) of the CCA.* Surgery might well be appropriate for this lesion, but not a dilated tortuous right subclavian or proximal CCA.

E. Endoluminal repair is appropriate treatment for *some* aneurysms, that is, those involving the distal extracranial ICA, and also for some more proximal lesions as well, but this patient's kinked and tortuous artery requires no specific treatment.

Answer 143-2: D

Discussion 143-2

Size and location are the keys to managing this traumatic lesion.

A. MRA permits the noninvasive diagnosis of this traumatic aneurysm. This aneurysm is small, and some of these small ones do not enlarge or cause symptoms. Therefore, angiography is not routinely *necessary in the emergency setting.* Because this lesion is located at or near the skull base, interposition grafting will be technically challenging and require special maneuvers, resulting in risks that may not have to be taken.

B. Performance of carotid trial occlusion and measurement of carotid back-pressure are useful adjuncts before open surgical treatment of distal carotid lesions, but carotid ligation of this aneurysm would be a last resort.

C. Coiling with or without an accompanying stent has been used successfully to treat these lesions but may not be necessary in the described scenario.

D. As mentioned above, small traumatic aneurysms of the distal ICA do *not* have a uniformly bad natural history. Some remain stable for years, and therefore all do not require interventional treatment. The safest course for this patient is antiplatelet therapy and follow-up angiography.

E. The location of this aneurysm is typical of this type of trauma, but that location makes it unlikely to be suitable for follow-up evaluation by duplex ultrasound.

Answer 143-3: D

Discussion 143-3

A. The most likely diagnosis in this case is *not* an atherosclerotic aneurysm but a pseudoaneurysm at the endarterectomy site. Because infection of a prosthetic patch is a probability, use of a prosthetic interposition graft would be *inappropriate.*

B. Embolization is a frequent cause of symptoms from carotid aneurysms; the size of this one is an indication for surgical (not anticoagulant) treatment because this lesion probably represents degeneration of the patch.

C. If a prosthetic patch had been used, the most likely diagnosis is an *infected* pseudoaneurysm. This will not likely be successfully treated with antibiotics alone, even if the organism is of low virulence.

D. A "mycotic" carotid pseudoaneurysm, caused by infection of a prosthetic patch, requires debridement of all the prosthetic material and adjacent involved arterial wall. Sometimes the resulting defect can be closed with an autogenous patch, but interposition grafting may be required. Either way, prosthetic materials must *not* be used. If the organism is a methicillin-resistant *Staphylococcus aureus*, aggressive debridement of adjacent tissues is required and muscle flap coverage should be considered.

E. Age is not, per se, a contraindication for primary or secondary carotid procedures. In addition, if she had a prosthetic patch, and therefore a likely infection, a covered stent would be ill-advised.

■ ANSWERS AND DISCUSSION FOR CHAPTER 144

Answer 144-1: D

Discussion 144-1

A. Coiling *is* more common in children than adults. Coiling is caused by carotid redundancy and is quite common in infants, decreasing with age and growth. Bilateral coiling in children suggests it persists because of a lack of sufficient carotid straightening with the descent of the heart into the chest and subsequent skeletal elongation.

B. Carotid kinks *are* four times more common in women. This increased predominance in women may explain the greater frequency with which older hypertensive women, in contrast with men, are thought to have carotid aneurysms when they actually have tortuous carotid or subclavian vessels.

C. Kinks may cause intermittent symptoms of cerebral insufficiency with turning of the head. When focal neurologic deficits can be reproduced by head motion, one should suspect a carotid kink. Although positional testing using noninvasive tests might be helpful in identifying hemodynamically significant kinking, the incidence of false-positive studies has not been established. Thus, definitive diagnosis of carotid kinking requires four-vessel cerebral arteriography. Multiple views are necessary, with patients in neutral, flexion, extension, and rotation positions. It is most important that the arteriogram be performed with the head in a position thought to produce neurologic symptoms.

D. Simple surgical tethering of the elongated redundant, and tortuous kinked or coiled carotid artery (arteriopexy) is inadequate treatment because it does not correct the redundancy.

E. Kinking of the carotid can cause flow disturbances, and the kink may be associated with focal atherosclerosis. Bifurcation atherosclerosis may result in kinking at the upper end of the plaque in patients with elongated, redundant carotids. Thus, problems may occur in assigning symptoms to one or the other. The best solution is to correct the kinking at the time of CEA. This may be achieved by using a long patch angioplasty or a variety of techniques involving resection and reimplantation, preferably with wide oblique anastomoses. Reanastomosing the internal carotid lower on the common carotid is a technique well suited to the carotid eversion technique of CEA.

Answer 144-2: B
Discussion 144-2

A. The carotid body is derived from both mesodermal elements of the third branchial arch and neural elements originating from the neural crest ectoderm. These neural crest cells further differentiate into forerunners of paraganglionic cells.

B. The carotid body is responsive primarily to hypoxia and, to a lesser degree, to hypercapnia and acidosis. Stimulation of the carotid body produces an increase in respiratory rate, tidal volume, heart rate, blood pressure together with vasoconstriction, and production of circulating catecholamines. In addition, approximately 5% of carotid body tumors are endocrinologically active, and the same percentage show positive chromaffin staining.

C. Carotid body tumors may be sporadic or familial. In the more common *sporadic* form, there is a 5% incidence of bilateral carotid body tumors. In the *familial* form, transmitted by an autosomal dominant pattern, there is a 32% incidence of bilateral tumors. Screening of family members is strongly recommended for early detection, because the ease of resection is related to size of the tumor.

D. Local growth and encroachment on surrounding structures creates the greatest problem in successfully resecting carotid body tumors. A minority (5%–50%) is found to be malignant but mostly by histologic criteria. The metastatic rate is approximately 5%. However, malignant carotid body tumors can metastasize to regional lymph nodes, and metastases have also been described to the kidney, thyroid, pancreas, cerebellum, lungs, bone, brachial plexus, abdomen, and breast.

E. A carotid body tumor may be fed by microscopic vessels from the adventitia of the ICA, but most of its inflow comes from the external carotid artery and its branches. This is the reason for the strategy to free it from the ICA first, taking advantage of the fact that, although it might be wrapped around this artery, there is usually an opening posteriorly and the tumor can be freed from it by dissecting in the adventitial plane using magnifying glasses and a bipolar cautery tip to control the small adventitial feeders. Once freed from the internal carotid, the origin of the external carotid artery is exposed, clamped, and divided, at which point the carotid body tumor loses its vascularity and shrinks dramatically, making the final dissection relatively easy.

Answer 144-3: D
Discussion 144-3

The carotid narrowing is most likely caused by radiation arteritis, although radiation-induced acceleration of atherosclerosis may contribute. Any of the options listed *might* succeed, and all have been reported in this setting.

A. Radiation arteritis obliterates cleavage planes making the usual CEA technique difficult if not impossible. Dissecting through the scarred neck increases the risk of cranial nerve injury and primary healing may be a problem, risking exposure of the prosthetic patch.

B. This option would also involve a difficult dissection but would require greater exposure and have a risk of injury. Kinking of the vein graft is a reported complication. A myocutaneous flap closure is an attractive but difficult adjunct, with the ipsilateral sternocleidomastoid muscle missing.

C. Ligation of the common carotid might be tolerated in terms of overall cerebral perfusion, but it would not exclude the diseased segment with the external carotid still patent.

D. One of the accepted indications for stenting of a carotid stenosis is a hostile, irradiated neck. Emboloprotective devices are a useful adjunct, particularly in the face of multiple TIAs. The choice of stent and its diameter and length will be important considerations in opening up this irradiation-induced narrowing.

E. Antiplatelet therapy and statins may well be indicated in this patient over the long term but are unlikely to eliminate the threat of crescendo TIAs.

■ ANSWERS AND DISCUSSION FOR CHAPTER 145

Answer 145-1: D
Discussion 145-1

Any of these problems could arise after CEA, but this question focuses on *which should be excluded first*:

A. Pulmonary embolism would be unlikely, particularly so soon after CEA, a short procedure performed under heparinization. Such patients usually have a history of, and are known to be at risk for, venous thromboembolism.

B. Myocardial infarction is the leading cause of death after CEA, and although myocardial ischemia can be present without chest pain, chest pain would be more likely if the MI were large enough to lead to heart failure or rhythm problems leading to difficulty breathing. ECG monitoring would likely detect some evidence of myocardial ischemia or arrhythmia.

C. Cranial nerve injuries are not uncommon after CEA and can lead to difficulties with phonation, swallowing, and speech, but these nerve injuries, when unilateral, rarely present with difficult breathing as the first manifestation. The fact that the patient developed the symptoms after being intact for 2 hours after the procedure also goes against a cranial injury, which should have been evident at the completion of the procedure.

D. After CEA performed under heparinization, a patient with postoperative hypertension is at risk of developing a cervical hematoma. More to the point, if this is the cause of breathing difficulty, it represents a serious danger and must be evacuated quickly. Tracheal deviation and swelling from the hematoma may make intubation very difficult. Cervical hematoma with airway compromise can be a fatal complication. Therefore it is *the first diagnosis to exclude.*

E. Congestive heart failure can develop in patients with underlying heart disease after surgery, particularly if excessive IV fluids are administered. This complication would be unlikely so soon after a procedure like CEA, and the treatment does not usually require the same degree of immediacy as airway compromise from a cervical hematoma.

Answer 145-2: C
Discussion 145-2

A. A head CT scan might show a hemorrhagic but not an ischemic infarct 1 hour old. It would take time to get and would *not* be the most appropriate *initial* study.

B. An EEG might be abnormal in this patient but would not lead to the diagnosis of why he has a left-sided deficit.

C. In this scenario one first needs to rule out thrombosis of the right CEA site. This would mandate immediate reoperation. In most centers a carotid duplex can be obtained rapidly, and the finding of a widely patent reconstruction can preclude the need for repeat anesthesia and exploration. On the other hand, if a duplex study cannot be obtained rapidly or is nondiagnostic, reexploration to document patency of the endarterectomy site should be performed. Thrombectomy and restoration of flow can result in reversal of the neurologic deficit.

D. TCD results would be abnormal if there were ongoing embolic events and might show flow disturbances in the face of total carotid occlusion, but it is not a first-line test in this scenario. It currently is more of a research tool in studying CEA or is used for intraoperative monitoring to determine the need for shunting. It does not provide direct information about the endarterectomy site.

E. A head MRI shares similar objections to a head CT scan (see A), but it is even more difficult to obtain in this setting. Neither are first-line decision-making diagnostic studies in this setting.

Answer 145-3: E
Discussion 145-3

There are findings on the first four of these studies that could conceivably affect the decision to proceed with the second side, and these are mentioned for the sake of completeness, but these would be unusual and not common enough to make any of them the correct answer (which is E).

A. A head CT scan conceivably could show a postoperative cerebral infarct, but it would be unlikely to have been occult, clinically.

B. A carotid duplex, with one carotid stenosis relieved, might show lower carotid velocities suggesting a lesser lesion on the opposite side, but it is hoped that the indications for the second CEA are based on more than a borderline finding on the original duplex scan. Occult occlusion would be unlikely.

C. An EEG would have little bearing on the decision and likely would not have been obtained in the first place.

D. An ECG, if it showed unexpected acute changes that represent an occult cardiac event, might well affect the decision to proceed with the second side.

E. The reason laryngoscopy is important in this scenario is that recurrent nerve injury at the first CEA could produce occult unilateral vocal cord paralysis. The same complication on the opposite side 1 week later could lead to bilateral cord paralysis and respiratory obstruction requiring tracheotomy, a risk one would not be willing to take. A delay might show that the cord paralysis was not permanent, but a reversible injury. The contralateral CEA can await this surveillance.

Answer 145-4: A
Discussion 145-4

A. Headache in this scenario means a hyperperfusion syndrome until proven otherwise. It is important to pick up this clue and institute preventative measures before more serious symptoms develop in the patient: agitation, disorientation, seizures, and cerebral hemorrhage, often in that order. Hyperperfusion syndrome is most common in the face of preexisting severe bilateral carotid obstruction as was described in the case scenario. The syndrome most commonly peaks 3 to 7 days after the procedure and thus often after the patient has been discharged.

B. Migraine headache would be unlikely in this setting and is not an emergency.

C. Stroke may be associated with headache, but would have other signs. More important, headache can be a warning sign of impending hemorrhagic stroke in some situations (see A).

D. Greater auricular neuropathy is not a likely diagnosis and not as threatening as the correct answer (see A).

E. Cerebral vasospasm is not a likely cause of headache, but the subsequent vasodilation can produce migraine headaches. Neither is a likely or worrisome diagnosis in the setting described.

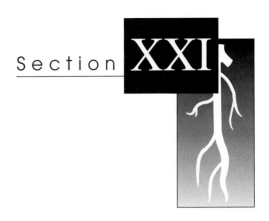

THE MANAGEMENT OF VENOUS DISORDERS

STUDY QUESTIONS

■ QUESTIONS FOR CHAPTER 147

Question 147-1

Which of the following statements regarding risk factors for deep venous thrombosis (DVT) and/or pulmonary embolism (PE)—in combination, venous thromboembolism (VTE)—is *not* true?

A. It is associated with malignancy and is greater in those undergoing chemotherapy or pelvic surgery for malignancy.
B. It is associated with oral contraceptives (OCs), but the progestins in third-generation ACs carry a much lower risk than second-generation OCs.
C. It is associated with multisystem trauma.
D. It is associated with hospitalization and further increased by associated recent surgery.
E. Increasing age and male gender are independent risk factors for VTE.

Question 147-2

Which of the following inheritable conditions is *not* associated with an increased incidence of DVT?

A. Protein C deficiency.
B. Protein S deficiency.
C. Resistance to activated protein C (factor V Leiden).
D. Mutation in position 20201 in the prothrombin gene.
E. Decreased plasminogen activator inhibitor-1.

Question 147-3

Certain DVT characteristics (e.g., location), treatments, or associated risk factors have been shown to significantly affect the severity of the postthrombotic sequelae. Which of the following do *not*?

A. Time from thrombosis to complete recanalization.
B. Rethrombosis of femoropopliteal DVT (i.e., recurrent DVT).
C. Proximal location of the DVT.
D. Treatment of femoropopliteal DVT with catheter-directed thrombosis (CDT).
E. Uninvolved distal segment located below a proximal segment involved with DVT.

■ QUESTIONS FOR CHAPTER 148

Question 148-1

Regarding the clinical diagnosis of DVT, which of the following statements is *not* true?

A. The diagnosis of DVT on the basis of signs and symptoms is inaccurate.
B. If prior DVT, malignancy, bed rest, edema, and cyanosis are combined, they have a positive predictive value of more than 90%.
C. It is easier to diagnose DVT on clinical grounds in inpatients than in outpatients.
D. Eighty percent of patients with DVT have at least one known risk factor.
E. The absence of calf swelling combined with absence of known risk factors can rule out DVT in more than 90% of inpatients and outpatients.

Question 148-2

Regarding duplex ultrasonography (DS) for DVT, which of the following statement is *not* true?

A. It is the most widely used imaging study to detect DVT.
B. A majority of studies show negative results.
C. Incompressibility is the most objective criterion in diagnosing DVT by duplex scan (DS).
D. Color flow ultrasonography significantly improves the diagnosis of calf vein DVT.
E. If the vascular diagnostic laboratory (VDL) is closed at night it is not appropriate to administer heparin on the basis of clinical suspicion.

Question 148-3

D-dimer (D-d) levels and pretest probability (PTP) scores (based on risk factor and clinical findings) have been used to limit the need for duplex scan (DS) without reducing the certainty of diagnosis. In that regard which of the following statements is *not* true?

A. If the PTP score is "high," a DS is not necessary.
B. If the PTP score is "moderate," a negative D-d rules out DVT.
C. If the PTP score is "low," a negative D-d excludes DVT.
D. If the PTP score is "low," a positive D-d mandates a DS.
E. Speed and high specificity of the D-d method are important in the D-d method used.

■ QUESTIONS FOR CHAPTER 149

Question 149-1

When spinal anesthetics are used, the initial dose of low molecular weight heparin (LMWH) should be given at which time:

A. One to 2 hours post-spinal anesthesia.
B. Four hours post-spinal anesthesia.
C. Two hours preoperatively.
D. Twenty-four hours post-spinal anesthesia.
E. Not given for 1 week.

Question 149-2

LMWH has which one of the following advantages over unfractionated heparin?

A. It is less expensive.
B. It does not cause heparin-induced thrombocytopenia (HIT).
C. It requires only periodic measurements of anti-Xa activity.
D. It does not cause osteoporosis.
E. It can be given by once daily subcutaneous injection without laboratory monitoring.

Question 149-3

The current management of patients who develop HIT and require ongoing anticoagulation involves the use of which one of the following:

A. LMWH.
B. Arvin (Ancrod).
C. Initiation of warfarin therapy.
D. Argatroban or lepirudin.
E. Plasmapheresis.

■ QUESTIONS FOR CHAPTER 150

Question 150-1

Which one of the following statements related to the choice between catheter-induced thrombolysis (CDT) and anticoagulant therapy (ACRx) alone, in the treatment of acute DVT, is *true*?

A. The potential benefits of CDT relate primarily to a reduction in the severity of the postthrombotic sequelae, and this applies to all levels of proximal lower extremity DVT (i.e., involvement of iliac, femoral, and popliteal segments).
B. The benefits of CDT only apply to DVT up to 14 days after onset of the current episode.
C. The benefits of CDT over ACRx have been measured in terms of restored and maintained patency, not by DS or other noninvasive tests of segmental venous reflux or by venous severity scoring.
D. Quality of life (QOL) has not been shown to be one of the benefits of CDT.
E. The advantages of CDT have been shown in two randomized prospective controlled trials.

Question 150-2

Which of the following statements about percutaneous mechanical thrombectomy is *true*?

A. Five devices are now approved by the Food and Drug Administration (FDA) for use in DVT.
B. The newer devices do not require adjunctive CDT.
C. They are intended to speed up clot removal by reducing the thrombus load.
D. They all are based on the same basic design principle.
E. Hemolysis and hematuria are not associated problems.

■ QUESTIONS FOR CHAPTER 151

Question 151-1

In acute iliofemoral DVT, all of the following are *potential* benefits of early thrombus removal, *except*:

A. Thrombus extension is prevented.
B. Recurrent DVT is prevented.
C. PE is prevented.
D. Progressive swelling of the leg with phlegmasia cerulea dolens is prevented.
E. May-Thurner syndrome is prevented.

Question 151-2

Regarding the choice between thrombus removal and anticoagulant therapy alone, in which of the following patients is thrombus removal *not* indicated?

A. A 30-year-old woman who develops iliofemoral DVT immediately after delivery.
B. A 75-year-old man in poor general health with stage III prostate cancer who develops venous gangrene caused by iliofemoral DVT.
C. A 55-year-old man who develops iliofemoral DVT after a long-distance air flight.
D. A 70-year-old previously healthy woman who develops phlegmasia cerulea dolens.
E. A 55-year-old man who develops a painful pale swollen leg (phlegmasia alba dolens) 5 days after surgery for colon cancer.

Question 151-3

In a 45-year-old man with acute iliofemoral DVT, which of the following treatments is *least* likely to prevent the postthrombotic syndrome?

A. Ambulatory treatment: elastic leg compression bandaging with LMWH followed by warfarin.
B. Hospital admission, bed rest, leg elevation, and intravenous heparin followed by warfarin.
C. CDT followed by ACRx.
D. Percutaneous mechanical thrombectomy with or without local thrombolysis followed by ACRx.
E. Surgical open thrombectomy followed by ACRx.

■ QUESTIONS FOR CHAPTER 152

Question 152-1

All of the following are approved indications for IVC filter placement *except*:

A. Chronic PE in a patient with pulmonary hypertension and cor pulmonale.

B. Recurrent pulmonary thromboembolism in a patient with subtherapeutic anticoagulation.

C. Intracerebral hemorrhage in a trauma patient with iliofemoral DVT.

D. A free-floating iliofemoral DVT with tail greater than 5 cm.

E. A patient with recurrent septic embolism.

Question 152-2

Concerning vena cava filters, which of the following statement is *false*?

A. The only prospective randomized trial of vena cava filter efficacy concluded that filters are more effective than anticoagulation alone to prevent PE in the first 12 days.

B. Temporary filters are generally used, particularly in Europe, to protect against pulmonary thromboembolism during endovenous procedures, such as CDT or percutaneous mechanical thrombectomy.

C. Retrievable filters, by definition, are placed within the vena cava but attached to the body extracorporeally by a sheath or wire.

D. Migration, vena cava occlusion, and insertion site thrombosis are potential complications associated with vena cava filter placement.

E. Retrievable filters may be ideal for use in young trauma patients or patients who have undergone orthopedic procedures, patients whose need for PE prophylaxis is short in duration and risk of bleeding from anticoagulation is high.

Question 152-3

Concerning vena caval filter insertion in patients with malignant disease, which of the following statement is *false*?

A. Patients with malignancy have 3.6 times the risk of PE than patients without cancer.

B. Patients with cancer and DVT are at higher risk of bleeding from anticoagulation than patients with DVT and without a malignancy.

C. The presence of a malignancy is a contraindication to vena cava filter placement in a patient with DVT and contraindications to anticoagulation.

D. Patients with cancer who seem to be at higher risk for PE are those with newly discovered metastasis, a history of PE, and multiple episodes of neutropenia.

E. PE is the presenting symptom of newly metastatic disease in 55% of patients with cancer.

■ QUESTIONS FOR CHAPTER 153

Question 153-1

Superficial thrombophlebitis:

A. Carries little risk to the patient.

B. Can usually be treated with bed rest and warm compresses.

C. Indicates antiplatelet therapy.

D. Is an indication for saphenous vein ligation at the groin.

E. Is an indication for duplex ultrasound scans (DS).

Question 153-2

Migratory phlebitis is associated with all of the below *except*:

A. Pancreatic carcinoma.

B. Buerger's disease.

C. Periarteritis nodosa.

D. Penile Mondor's disease.

E. Behçet's disease.

Question 153-3

PE associated with superficial venous thrombosis:

A. Is virtually nonexistent.

B. Is more likely in patients in whom the process approaches the groin.

C. May approach 20% to 22% in some series.

D. Is most common in suppurative phlebitis.

E. Requires pulmonary scanning for all patients.

■ QUESTIONS FOR CHAPTER 154

Question 154-1

Chronic ambulatory venous hypertension causes a persistent inflammatory injury secondary to extravasation of which of the following:

A. Macromolecules like fibrinogen and red blood cells.

B. Lymphocytes.

C. Macrophages.

D. Collagen.

E. Fibronectin.

Question 154-2

The dermal fibrosis observed in patients with late-stage chronic venous insufficiency (CVI) is primarily regulated by what cytokine:

A. Interleukin-1.

B. Tumor necrosis factor-alpha.

C. Transforming growth factor (TGF)-beta-1.

D. Basic fibroblastic growth factor.

E. Keratinocyte growth factor.

Question 154-3

All of the following contribute to the development of varicose veins *except*:

A. Morbid obesity.

B. Vein wall degeneration secondary to venous thrombosis.

C. Autosomal dominant gene with variable penetrance.

D. Dietary factors.

E. Conversion of smooth muscle cells from a contractile phenotype to a secretory phenotype.

■ QUESTIONS FOR CHAPTER 155

Question 155-1

The clinical classes of the (Clinical, Etiologic, Anatomic, and Pathophysiologic [CEAP]) classification of chronic venous disorders includes all of the following except:

A. Lipodermatosclerosis.

B. Healed leg ulcer with deep venous reflux on duplex scan.

C. Lipedema.

D. No abnormalities on clinical examination.

E. Telangiectasis or reticular veins.

Question 155-2

Symptoms of CVI worsen in specific circumstances. Which of the following is true?

A. Clinical signs of chronic venous stasis in the lower leg are associated with progression to leg ulceration.

B. Increasing age is associated with the increasing severity of CVI.

C. Increasing obesity is associated with more severe symptoms of CVI.

D. Although a leg ulcer from CVI can be healed with conservative measures, it will eventually recur.

E. Ulcer recurrence is much more frequent in patients with postthrombotic syndrome than in those with primary valvular incompetence.

Question 155-3

In North America, routine diagnostic evaluation of venous disease and assigning patients to the CEAP classification requires several tests. Which of the following is *not* required for routine evaluation of patients with chronic venous disorders?

A. Clinical examination including a standing evaluation.

B. Duplex examination evaluating valvular competence of deep and superficial leg veins.

C. Duplex examination evaluating valvular competence of superficial leg veins.

D. Air plethysmography.

E. Infrainguinal duplex examination evaluating patency of deep veins.

Question 155-4

The severity of chronic venous disease is assessed with several disease specific and general instruments. Which of the following has been subject to validation and has sufficient correlation to be valuable (>0.7) in assessing the severity of the disease?

A. Clinical Severity Score (18-point).

B. Nottingham Health Profile.

C. Venous Clinical Severity Score (30-point).

D. Venous Segmental Disease Score (10 points each for obstruction/reflux).

E. Short Form-36.

■ QUESTIONS FOR CHAPTER 156

Question 156-1

A weak, arthritic 80-year-old man presents with a large superficial ulcer at the medial malleolus. The surrounding skin is atrophic and pigmented, and there is subcutaneous fibrosis. He is unable to perform dressing changes or apply a compression stocking on his own. What is the best therapeutic option for this patient?

A. Hospital admission for wound care.

B. Unna boot dressing changed weekly by a health care professional.

C. Oral antibiotics and bed rest with elevation.

D. Continuation of the use of compression stockings, using application aids.

E. Application of Stanozolol to ulcer and advice for the patient to stay off his feet as much as possible.

Question 156-2

A 55-year-old woman with chronic venous edema has been treated with compression therapy for 9 months. Duplex evaluation confirmed her deep venous system incompetence, but she has a patent and competent saphenous vein. She wears compression stockings and elevates her legs three times daily but has noticed worsening of her edema over the past month. A lower extremity duplex scan is negative for a new DVT. What is the most appropriate next step in patient management?

A. Start her on diuretic therapy.

B. Begin Unna boot applications.

C. Start her on pentoxifylline.

D. Replace her old stockings.

E. Obtain ascending and descending venography and consider deep vein valve reconstructive venous surgery.

Question 156-3

A 68-year-old man presents with a large ulcer over the left medial malleolus with significant lower extremity edema. The ulcer is very painful and has been present for the past 6 months. It is increasing in size despite compression therapy with an Unna boot. His left ankle-brachial index (ABI) is 0.30. What is the most appropriate *next* step in patient management?

A. Continue the current therapeutic regimen.

B. Perform contrast or CT lower extremity arteriography with run-off visualization, with plans for arterial reconstruction.

C. Administer oral antibiotics.

D. Apply an Apligraf skin substitute.

E. Strip the great saphenous vein and perform subfascial endoscopic perforator vein surgery (SEPS).

■ QUESTIONS FOR CHAPTER 157

Question 157-1

Although the diagnosis of varicose veins can be made by inspection, precision in locating refluxing vein segments is best achieved by using:

A. Air plethysmography with patient standing.

B. Continuous wave Doppler probe, with patient standing.

C. Venous plethysmography, with patient sitting.

D. Duplex scan, with patient standing.

E. Magnetic resonance venography (MRV), with patient supine.

Question 157-2

Surgery for varicose veins is followed by a tendency for late recurrence. Of the choices listed below, which gives the best long-term results?

A. Proximal greater saphenous vein ligation.

B. Proximal greater saphenous vein ligation, with ligation and division of all proximal tributaries.

C. Proximal greater saphenous vein ligation with adjunctive sclerotherapy.

D. Proximal greater saphenous vein ligation, ligation and division of all proximal tributaries, with adjunctive sclerotherapy.

E. Proximal great saphenous vein ligation, with ligation, division of all proximal tributaries, and saphenous stripping.

Question 157-3

The CEAP classification has become useful worldwide because it is clinically descriptive. Which of the following testing methods should be done for CEAP class 1 venous disorder?

A. Air plethysmography.

B. Ankle venous pressure.

C. Duplex ultrasound of lower extremity veins.

D. Descending contrast venography.

E. None of the above.

■ QUESTIONS FOR CHAPTER 158

Question 158-1

Which of the following statements is the *most accurate* regarding the evaluation of incompetent calf perforating veins (ICPVs)?

A. The evaluation of calf perforator incompetence is based on the identification of venous flow from the superficial to the deep venous system.

B. Ascending phlebography has been shown to be superior to duplex scanning (DS) in the diagnosis of ICPVs.

C. Ascending phlebography has a high rate of false-negative findings in determining the presence or absence of ICPVs.

D. Physical examination (PE), using a tourniquet, is an accurate enough method of screening for the presence of ICPVs.

E. Physical examination, using a handheld Doppler, is the most accurate method of diagnosing the presence of ICPVs.

Question 158-2

Which statement concerning the anatomy of the perforating veins is *false*?

A. Perforating veins connect the superficial to the deep venous system, either directly to the main axial veins (direct perforators) or indirectly to muscular tributaries or soleal venous sinuses (indirect perforators).

B. The term "communicating veins" refers to interconnecting veins within the same system.

C. Perforating veins of the foot are valveless and paradoxically direct flow from the deep to the superficial venous system.

D. In the mid- and distal calf the most important direct medial perforators originate directly from the greater saphenous vein.

E. The mid- and upper posterior tibial perforators (*Cockett II* and *III* perforators) are located 7 to 9 cm and 10 to 12 cm proximal to the lower border of the medial malleolus.

Question 158-3

Which of the following statements concerning SEPS (subfacial endoscopic perforator surgery) is *false*?

A. During the SEPS procedure CO_2 is insufflated into the superficial posterior subfascial space.

B. Paratibial fasciotomy is *not* required to interrupt important medial calf perforators (Cockett perforators).

C. There are single-port and double-port techniques for performing SEPS.

D. During the procedure the pressure in the subfascial space is maintained at 15 to 30 mm Hg.

E. A thigh tourniquet is helpful to decrease bleeding and enlarge the working space in the subfascial area.

■ QUESTIONS FOR CHAPTER 159

Question 159-1

Reported surgical experience has shown that:

A. Descending venography has essentially a one-to-one direct correlation with the status of the valve (presence, absence, incompetence) observed during surgery.

B. DVT (the postthrombotic syndrome) is a destructive process leaving venous valves that do not allow an in situ repair.

C. Primary deep venous valvular incompetence does not lead to vein wall thickening as seen with the postthrombotic syndrome.

D. The postthrombotic syndrome can lead to vein wall thickening without valve cusp involvement leaving a valve for in situ repair.

E. Primary and secondary deep venous valvular incompetence have essentially mutually exclusive morphology.

Question 159-2

A patient presents with a 5-cm venous ulcer located at the medial malleolus. Conservative management with compression therapy and correction of superficial venous reflux has not prevented recurrence of the ulcer. Noninvasive studies confirm segmentally isolated deep venous incompetence. The descending venogram demonstrates reflux through the femoral and profunda femoris veins with apparent preserved proximal valves in both. At operation, you discover an incompetent proximal femoral vein valve but no obvious profunda femoris valve. What is your most logical operative approach? In situ repair of the femoral vein valve *and*:

A. Ligation of the profunda femoris vein.

B. Transposition of the profunda femoris vein.

C. Axillary valve transplantation to the profunda femoris vein.

D. Intimal flap reconstruction of a valve for the profunda femoris vein.

E. Cryopreserved allograft valve transplantation to the profunda femoris vein.

Question 159-3

You have recommended an internal valvuloplasty for your patient with a recurrent venous ulceration and isolated femoral vein incompetence with a valve clearly visualized on descending venography and duplex evaluation. The patient previously underwent ablation of the incompetent saphenous veins and the SEPS procedure. What should you tell the patient is his/her risk of experiencing clinically significant DVT at the time of operation and the prospects for long-term ulcer healing without recurrence at 5 years?

A. DVT, 1% to 2%; healed ulcer, 70%.
B. DVT, 1% to 2%; healed ulcer, 50%.
C. DVT, 5% to 10%; healed ulcer, 70%.
D. DVT, 15% to 20%; healed ulcer, 90%.
E. DVT, 25% to 30%; healed ulcer, 70%.

■ QUESTIONS FOR CHAPTER 160

Question 160-1

In evaluating symptomatic postthrombotic patients with obstruction of the iliac veins, which of the following tests is the *most* useful to plan a procedure?

A. Arm/foot or femoral/central venous pressure differential.
B. Ascending venography with bilateral femoral vein injections to visualize the occluded segment(s) and assess any inferior vena cava (IVC) involvement.
C. Descending venography to evaluate any additional infrainguinal reflux.
D. Color duplex examination for obstructions and incompetence of the femoropopliteal veins.
E. Strain-gauge outflow plethysmography.

Question 160-2

Which of the following statements is *false* concerning diagnostic criteria for the patient undergoing venous bypass for chronic obstruction?

A. Venous pressure studies and phlebography are mandatory preoperative evaluations.
B. Phlebographic demonstration of venous obstruction with large, profuse collaterals is a contraindication for bypass surgery.
C. A femoral pressure gradient between limbs at supine rest that exceeds 2 mm Hg indicates a significant iliofemoral obstruction in the limb with elevated pressure.
D. An arm/foot venous pressure differential at rest of more than 4 mm Hg and a foot venous pressure elevation with reactive hyperemia of more than 6 mm Hg are indicative of hemodynamically significant venous obstruction.
E. Hemodynamic measurements are abnormal whenever phlebographic obstruction is observed.

Question 160-3

Which of the following statements is *false* regarding operative techniques unique to bypass grafts in the venous system?

A. Bypass conduits interposed in the venous system should be longer than the excised vein segment.
B. Bypass conduits may be either autogenous or prosthetic.
C. Adjunctive arteriovenous fistulas (AVFs) can improve long-term patency of both autogenous and prosthetic venous bypass conduits.
D. Adjunctive AVFs are usually closed within the first year, usually within 6 months.
E. Traumatic injury to the femoral vein distal to the profunda femoris vein must always be repaired.

■ QUESTIONS FOR CHAPTER 161

Question 161-1

A 45-year-old machine operator has had increasing right lower extremity swelling, severe aching pain, and leg pigmentation for 3 years. He had deep vein thrombosis after an appendectomy 25 years ago. Duplex Doppler of the lower extremity showed axial deep reflux. Transfemoral venogram now shows a patent but irregular iliac vein with several focal 50% stenoses, and there is no proximal resting pressure gradient, between the IVC and the femoral vein.

What is the most appropriate *next* step in the treatment?

A. Apply a below-knee medical compression stocking of 30 to 40 mm Hg.
B. Perform a femorofemoral vein bypass ("Palma procedure") with a ringed polytetrafluoroethylene (PTFE) graft.
C. Percutaneously insert a stent-mounted valve into the distal femoral vein.
D. Perform an axillary vein transfer to the proximal femoral vein.
E. Perform a balloon dilation and stenting of the iliac vein.

Question 161-2

A previously healthy 35-year-old mother of three is experiencing daily severe aching pain of the left lower extremity with intermittent swelling of the leg. Moderate varicosities of the calf are seen. She has used over-the-counter support stockings for several years, but they no longer help. Duplex scan of the lower extremity shows a 4-mm wide refluxing great saphenous vein, and photoplethysmography records a refilling time of 25 seconds.

What is the most appropriate *next* step in the management of this patient?

A. Laser obliteration of the great saphenous vein.
B. Medical compression stockings (30–40 mm Hg) for daily use.
C. Ipsilateral multiplane transfemoral venogram.
D. CT scan of the pelvis to exclude pelvic mass.
E. Stab avulsions of nontruncal varicose veins of the calf.

Question 161-3

Moderate cross-pelvic collaterals through the internal iliac vein with filling of the ascending lumbar vein are seen during a transfemoral ascending venogram with the patient supine. It is being performed to evaluate lower extremity pain and swelling. The venogram shows no obvious obstruction of the iliofemoral segment.

Which of the following statements is the proper response to these findings?

A. This is a normal finding.
B. A multiplane venogram or an intravascular ultrasound (IVUS) study should be performed.
C. A femoral vein-central vein pressure gradient should be measured, with and without leg exercise, to exclude a significant obstruction.
D. The patient must have inhaled at the time of contrast dye injection.
E. Because no obstruction of the iliac segment is visualized, a descending venogram should be performed.

■ QUESTIONS FOR CHAPTER 162

Question 162-1

Which one of the following statements concerning contrast venography of patients with superior vena cava (SVC) syndrome is *false*?

A. A combined transfemoral and internal jugular access is an option to access central veins.
B. Bilateral access is obtained first through both the right and left basilic veins.
C. When there is an SVC occlusion with extension of acute thrombus into both brachiocephalic veins, the subclavian vein must not be traversed with catheters and wires to avoid the risk of a PE.
D. For chronic venous occlusions the best way to traverse the involved segment is to first pass a 5 French (F) angiographic catheter with a simple curve and a 0.035-inch steerable hydrophilic guidewire through it.
E. To traverse fibrotic occlusions of the subclavian and innominate veins, a coaxial system consisting of a 7F or 8F braided coronary guiding catheter fitted with an adapter can be used to allow placement of the 5F catheter and guidewire.

Question 162-2

Multiple options are available to stent central veins. Of the following statements, which one is *true* concerning different venous stents?

A. Balloon-expandable stents such as Wallstents are susceptible to plastic deformation when external, two-point compression is applied.
B. A Wallstent for the treatment of brachiocephalic vein stenosis and a Palmaz stent in the SVC *are* excellent choices.
C. The Gianturco Z-stent is an excellent balloon-expandable stent for large vein reconstructions.
D. The Palmaz stent is best because it is a longitudinally flexible, self-expanding, metal stent.
E. The advantage of the Wallstent is that it does not foreshorten as it is deployed the lumen of the vessel.

Question 162-3

A 37-year-old man presented with ascites, liver failure, bilateral leg swelling, and occasional hip and thigh pain after walking four or five blocks. Evaluation revealed high-grade segmental stenosis of the intrahepatic IVC associated with thrombosis of the hepatic veins (Budd-Chiari syndrome). His portal hypertension improved under medical management, but his leg swelling and venous claudication worsened, despite diuretics and compression garments. At this stage the best way to manage this patient is to:

A. Increase diuretics and add oral anticoagulation to decrease chances of deep vein thrombosis.
B. Perform thrombolysis of the hepatic veins.
C. Perform a cavoatrial bypass with a PTFE graft.
D. Stent the IVC lesion with a self-expanding Gianturco-Z stent.
E. Stent the IVC with Wallstents.

■ QUESTIONS FOR CHAPTER 163

Question 163-1

All of the following are true statements characteristic of primary venous leiomyosarcomas *except*:

A. These tumors involve the IVC more often than other central or peripheral veins.
B. The most common growth pattern is intraluminal.
C. The tumors occur more often in women than men.
D. Most tumors are discovered incidentally during other investigations.
E. They can occur in patients of all ages.

Question 163-2

A 54-year-old man presents with a 2-week history of cardiac palpitations and one "blackout spell." He also has vague right-sided abdominal discomfort and fullness and has microhematuria on urinalysis. A CT scan shows a 5-cm mass in the upper pole of the right kidney. The mass displaces the liver superiorly and abuts the IVC. A tissue plane is apparent between the tumor and the IVC. The suprarenal and retrohepatic segments of the vena cava are distended but do not fill with contrast. The most likely diagnosis is:

A. Adrenal cortical carcinoma with intracaval tumor thrombus.
B. Renal cell cancer with tumor thrombus extending into the vena cava and upward to the right side of the heart.
C. Pheochromocytoma.
D. Renal cell cancer with tumor thrombus extending 3 cm above the renal veins.
E. Retroperitoneal leiomyosarcoma with invasion of the vena cava.

Question 163-3

A 29-year-old man is referred for evaluation of a localized 6-cm retroperitoneal mass that invades the infrarenal segment of the IVC. A CT scan shows the tumor does not involve the vertebrae, aorta, or nerve roots. The right ureter is displaced laterally but is not obstructed. There is no adenopathy along the aorta or the suprarenal IVC. The metastatic workup shows negative results. He has no major medical comorbidity and is physically active without limitation. He has no lower extremity edema, and his renal function is normal. Ultrasonography and CT imaging show the infrarenal IVC is chronically occluded. There are dilated veins in the left side of the pelvis and along the left paravertebral region. The next step in management is:

A. Radiation and chemotherapy.
B. Needle biopsy of the mass with subsequent therapy directed by that result.
C. Resection of the tumor en bloc with the IVC with no graft replacement.
D. Resection of the tumor and vena cava, and replacement of the IVC with a femoral vein graft.
E. Only supportive treatment because the tumor is unresectable.

■ QUESTIONS FOR CHAPTER 164

Question 164-1

A 29-year-old woman presents with a 1-year history of progressive head and neck swelling, and a feeling of fullness in the head and neck that is exacerbated when she bends over or lies flat in bed. She sleeps on four pillows and has intermittent headaches and dizziness. She had several recent episodes of near-blackout spells. She has dilated neck veins and prominent upper chest venous collaterals; 6 months of oral anticoagulation and diuretics has not helped. Evaluation revealed SVC obstruction, but two separate attempts at angioplasty and stenting at another institution was unsuccessful. CT excluded malignancy. Which one of the following choices is *not* appropriate in the management of this patient?

A. Perform bilateral upper extremity venography and attempt again to cross the lesion with a guidewire.
B. Perform SVC reconstruction using an autologous internal jugular vein.
C. Perform SVC reconstruction using an externally supported PTFE graft.
D. Perform SVC reconstruction/bypass using the left femoral vein.
E. Perform SVC reconstruction using a spiral saphenous vein graft.

Question 164-2

A 67-year-old man presents with severe head and neck swelling, hoarseness, dilated subcutaneous veins on the upper chest, near-blackout spells, and weight loss. He has a 45-year history of smoking. Which of the following statements is *not true*?

A. The patient should have a chest CT scan and then start treatment for his mediastinal malignancy.
B. This patient likely has mediastinal malignancy, but relieving his SVC syndrome should be undertaken to avoid blindness and cerebral hemorrhage.
C. If stenting of the SVC is not possible, a bypass from the external jugular vein to the femoral vein using both saphenous veins is a reasonable alternative, to be performed after cancer treatment.
D. If the life expectancy is less than 1 year, direct reconstruction by median sternotomy should *not* be attempted.
E. Angioplasty and stenting of the occluded venous segments is a reasonable plan after cancer treatment has started.

Question 164-3

Which of the following statements concerning vascular grafts used in open surgical reconstruction for the SVC syndrome is *false*?

A. Spiral saphenous vein grafts have a reported 90% secondary patency rate at 5 years.
B. Externally supported expanded (e)PTFE grafts have a reported 2-year patency rate of 70%.
C. Femoral vein grafts should not be used for SVC reconstructions in patients with SVC syndrome.
D. Saphenous vein grafts are usually too small to use as venous conduits for the SVC syndrome.
E. Bovine pericardial patch has low thrombogenicity, and it is thus useful for venous reconstructions.

ANSWERS AND DISCUSSION

■ ANSWERS AND DISCUSSION FOR CHAPTER 147

Answer 147-1: B

Discussion 147-1

A. In Heit and colleagues' population-based case-control study, malignant neoplasm without chemotherapy carried an elevated odds ratio for VTE (4.05), but with chemotherapy this was 6.53. Other studies have shown an association in those with episodes of chemotherapy-induced neutropenia. Pelvic procedures for malignancy are also associated with an increased risk of DVT.

B. ACs are a recognized risk factor for DVT, one that is related to the dose of estrogen and the type of progestin. Reducing the estrogen dose to less than 50 μg has significantly decreased (not eliminated) this risk, but the progestins in third-generation ACs (progestin desogestrel, norgestimate, or gestodene) have been reported (twice) to have a twofold *higher* risk of VTE than second-generation ACs. Thus, this statement is false.

C. Major multisystem trauma has been associated with a significantly enough increased risk of VTE that it has spurred the prophylactic use of IVC filters.

D. Hospitalization is associated with a risk of VTE, and this is further increased if associated with recent surgery (odds ratio 7.98 increasing to 21.72).

E. Increasing age and male gender *are* independent risk factors for VTE, although the former may be multifactorial (acquired prothrombotic states increasing with age, higher levels of thrombin activation markers, and anatomic changes in soleal veins with increased stasis).

Answer 147-2: E

Discussion 147-2

Primary hypercoagulable states represent discrete genetic mutation. These include inherited deficiencies of naturally occurring anticoagulants (antithrombin III), (A) protein C, (B) protein S, (C) resistance to activated protein C (factor V Leiden), hyperhomocysteinemia, and several potential defects in fibrinolysis, among them dysplasminogenemia, hypoplasminogenemia, decreased synthesis or release of t-PA, and *increased but* not (E) *decreased* plasminogen activator inhibitor-1. Recently (D), a mutation in position 20201 in the prothrombin gene (G to A) has been associated with increased prothrombin levels and a thrombotic tendency.

Answer 147-3: D

Discussion 147-3

Longitudinal duplex studies of a large cohort of patients with DVT, reported in multiple publications over the years by Strandness, Meissner, and their associates has shed much light on the subject of this question.

A. Time from thrombosis to complete recanalization (as expressed as median lysis time) has been shown to affect the presence or absence of reflux in all lower extremity venous segments except the posterior tibial vein.

B. Rethrombosis significantly increased the eventual incidence of reflux in the mid- and distal superficial femoral and popliteal segments, and was greater, but not statistically significantly so, in the proximal superficial femoral and posterior tibial veins. It was not different in the common and deep femoral or greater saphenous veins. [Note the superficial femoral vein is now called the femoral vein, because it is a deep vein, to avoid confusion (and failure to treat) among primary care physicians.]

C. The worse outcome of proximal DVT versus calf vein thrombosis has been well established from the above mentioned and other studies.

D. Early spontaneous lysis and lack of rethrombosis have been shown to correlate with less reflux for the femoral and popliteal segments (see answers A and B). However, a large venous registry, although establishing a significant benefit, in terms of extended patency, from CDT for iliofemoral DVT, did *not* show a similar benefit for femoropopliteal DVT.

E. Uninvolved distal segments located below a proximal segment involved with DVT have been shown to develop a steadily increasing rate of reflux in the above-mentioned longitudinal DVT follow-up studies.

■ ANSWERS AND DISCUSSION FOR CHAPTER 148

Answer 148-1: C

Discussion 148-1

A. The diagnosis of DVT on the basis of signs and symptoms *is* notoriously inaccurate, and this has resulted in a deluge of referrals to VDLs for DS to "rule out DVT." In turn, many have tried to combine clinical findings with combinations of known risk factors to increase the accuracy of diagnosis and offload the VDLs with mixed success. The remaining answers reflect this effort.

B. Markel et al. combined prior DVT, malignancy, bed rest, edema, and cyanosis to achieve a positive predictive value of 94%.

C. Not true. It is the reverse; it is easier to diagnose DVT on clinical grounds in outpatients than in inpatients.

D. Markel et al. also showed that 80% of patients with DVT have at least one known risk factor; 40% had two and 10% had three.

E. Criado and Burnham found that when absence of calf swelling was combined with absence of known risk factors, they could rule out DVT with negative predictive values of 97% in outpatients and 92% in inpatients. This approach would have missed DVT in 3 of 610 outpatients and 15 of 916 inpatients—*in retrospect!*

Answer 148-2: E

Discussion 148-2

A. DS has long replaced venography as the most used diagnostic method. Other imaging techniques, for example, MRV, are improving, but are too expensive and play a secondary role.

B. Only 20% to 30% of studies are positive for the ipsilateral leg; 2% of studies are positive for the contralateral leg.
C. Incompressibility *is* the most objective criterion in diagnosing DVT by DS. However, it can be difficult to test for compressibility because of adjacent musculoskeletal structures in the superficial, iliac, and proximal upper extremity veins.
D. Color flow ultrasonography *does* significantly improve the diagnosis of calf vein DVT.
E. If the VDL is closed at night, *it is appropriate* to administer heparin on the basis of clinical suspicion. A study can be scheduled early the next morning and heparin can be stopped if the study result is negative. Stopping ACRx is appropriate if a technically adequate DS study is negative. Follow-up DS studies in this situation are not cost-effective. A single follow-up costs $390,000 per life saved, and a second follow-up study costs $3.5 million. However, by combining PTP scoring and D-d assays, this dilemma, and even the need for a DS, may be eliminated (see Question 148-3).

Answer 148-3: A
Discussion 148-3

A. If the PTP score is "high," a DS *is* necessary, but the intermediate step of getting a D-d is eliminated.
B. If the PTP score is "moderate," a negative D-d *does* rule out DVT. However, a positive D-d would dictate the need for a DS.
C. If the PTP score is "low," a negative D-d *does* exclude DVT and obviates the need to get a DS.
D. If the PTP score is "low," a positive D-d mandates a DS. It overrides the low PTP and acts as a safety net to avoid missing a subtle DVT in a patient without known risk factors.
E. If the D-d is going to function in these strategies as an exclusionary test it must *not* have a low specificity, and it must be available and give a prompt result to serve in its intermediary role. A number of rapid quantitative assays are now available that have a good combination of convenience, sensitivity, and specificity.

■ ANSWERS AND DISCUSSION FOR CHAPTER 149

Answer 149-1: D
Discussion 149-1

The FDA has suggested caution in using LMWH in association with regional anesthesia (spinal and epidural). There have been reports of spinal hematomas, some resulting in permanent neurologic deficits. The American Association of Regional Anesthesia has studied this, and their committee has issues guidelines. With spinal anesthesia, 24 hours should pass before LMWH administration, so (D) is the correct answer. A, B, and C are too soon, and E is much too conservative.

Answer 149-2: E
Discussion 149-2

A major advantage of LMWH over unfractionated heparin is that it can be given by a once daily subcutaneous injection without laboratory monitoring (E is correct). It is not (A) less expensive; although much of its higher cost is offset by savings in monitoring. It does *not* require periodic measurements of anti-Xa activity (C). It *can* cause HIT (B) and (D) osteoporosis.

Answer 149-3: D
Discussion 149-3

A. LMWH may well reduce the likelihood of recurrence of HIT, but this is not absolute protection.
B. Arvin (Ancrod) has not been approved for this use but is difficult to administer.
C. Warfarin therapy may be used but not until one of the other agents has been used for 3 or 4 days to suppress thrombin production. It is therefore useful mainly to avoid prolonged use of the other agents.
D. Argatroban or lepirudin has been approved for use in the United States and Canada and is the drug of choice here. Hirudin is also approved, and the heparinoid Danaparoid has been approved for compassionate use.
E. Plasmapheresis is not used for this indication.

■ ANSWERS AND DISCUSSION FOR CHAPTER 150

Answer 150-1: C
Discussion 150-1

A. The potential benefits of CDT relate primarily to a reduction in the severity of the postthrombotic sequelae in *iliofemoral* DVT, not DVT at more distal levels.
B. In the venous registry documenting the results of CDT, benefit was primarily shown for primary (first time) acute iliofemoral DVT, up to 10 days.
C. True; the benefits of CDT over ACRx have been measured in terms of restored and maintained patency and not by DS or other noninvasive tests of venous reflux, or Venous Severity Scoring.
D. An improved QOL *has been demonstrated* for CDT over ACRx, but this was shown for *initially successful* CDT. Tellingly the QOL for *failed* CDT was equivalent to ACRx.
E. The advantages of CDT over ACRx have *not* been shown in TWO randomized prospective trials. One trial, organized at the Temple University Medical School, did compare these two treatments in a prospective manner using a QOL instrument that showed benefit, but a major randomized control trial is needed. Fortunately, such a trial (the TOLEDO trial) is now in progress. Most of the proposed benefits of CDT have been based on observational studies without ACRx controls.

Answer 150-2: C
Discussion 150-2

A. *Five* devices have *not* been approved for this use, although at least that many are being used for this purpose off-label. Approval by the FDA has been mainly for hemodialysis access thrombosis for which the risk of endothelial damage and the size of thrombus are less.

B. All of the current devices depend on thrombolytic therapy to finish up and remove residual thrombus.

C. The clot burden in the DVT that has the most to gain from CDT, namely, iliofemoral DVT, is great, and CDT alone often takes 48 hours or more and is thus very costly. By quickly removing clot, percutaneous mechanical thrombectomy is intended to speed up the task of clot removal. However, procedure time has not yet been shown to be reduced.

D. Current devices are different in design and even in the underlying principle. Some apply the Venturi principle to create negative pressure to aspirate the clot, and others have high-speed rotating elements (such as a spiral wire) to disintegrate clot, with different methods of retrieving/removing the fragments, and so forth.

E. The risk of hemolysis and hemoglobinuria has been a concern with these devices, and they have been observed. It is a potential greater problem in those with preexisting renal insufficiency. Limits of use (time and infusate) and other measures have been recommended by the manufacturers to avoid this complication.

■ ANSWERS AND DISCUSSION FOR CHAPTER 151

Answer 151-1: E

Discussion 151-1

An acute iliofemoral venous thrombosis can extend proximally into the IVC and lead to IVC obstruction (A). If the iliac vein thrombus is not removed, the result is contralateral iliac DVT in many of cases. The thrombus can also extend distally with progressive swelling of the leg. (D) Distal extension of acute iliofemoral DVT leads to progressive swelling of the leg with increased intramuscular compartment pressures in the calf resulting in "phlegmasia cerulea dolens," literally a painful, blue swelling of the leg. This can then progress to venous gangrene and limb loss.

Persisting proximal obstruction leads to higher incidence of recurrent DVT (B). It can also cause valvular incompetence in distal deep veins not involved in the original DVT. Both of these conditions lead to an increased severity of the postthrombotic sequelae. Another potential benefit is a reduced incidence of PE, in that removed clot cannot embolize (C). Iliofemoral DVT has ventilation/perfusion lung scan-proven PE in 50% to 60% of the patients. Recurrent PE can lead to chronic pulmonary hypertension.

May-Thurner syndrome is an obstruction of the left common iliac vein that can lead to swelling of the leg with a higher risk for DVT. (E) It is a compression of the left common iliac artery by the right common iliac artery and is either congenital or acquired. Thrombectomy alone does not correct the chronic stenosis or occlusion seen in patients with May-Thurner syndrome who progress to develop iliofemoral DVT. Currently, residual stenosis of the left common iliac artery may be treated with percutaneous transluminal angioplasty and stenting.

Answer 151-2: B

Discussion 151-2

Early clot removal is intended to significantly reduce the severity of subsequent postphlebitic sequelae. As a general rule, it is indicated in active, relatively healthy patients with good longevity even if they have only phlegmasia alba dolens, but in elderly patients with serious intercurrent disease that will limit upright activity and longevity, it is indicated only to reduce the morbidity of phlegmasia cerulea dolens and prevent progression to venous gangrene. It is most effective in patients with iliofemoral DVT.

A. It is indicated in this relatively young woman with postpartum iliofemoral DVT. She is otherwise healthy with many years ahead. Percutaneous mechanical thrombectomy with or without localized thrombolysis is the first choice. If it fails, surgical thrombectomy with a temporary AV fistula (AVF) is a valid alternative. If intraoperative venogram shows residual obstruction of the left common iliac vein (May-Thurner syndrome), balloon angioplasty and stenting should be considered.

B. A 75-year-old man in poor general condition who has advanced cancer and has already developed venous gangrene because of iliofemoral DVT would not benefit from thrombus removal. The patient should be treated with ACRx.

C. A 55-year-old man who develops iliofemoral DVT after a long air flight should be treated with CDT, once the diagnosis is confirmed and the top end of the thrombus is determined with DS, MRV, or venography. If this approach is contraindicated or fails, one of the thrombectomy techniques is the next alternative. Because the patient developed this condition during a flight, risk factors for DVT should be investigated so that prophylactic measures can be instituted in the future.

D. Early clot removal is indicated in most patients with phlegmasia cerulea dolens. It is a serious condition with high intramuscular pressure in the calf compartments that can lead to venous gangrene. The leg should be elevated 30 to 45 degrees, intravenous heparin should be infused, and CDT should be instituted. If there is no prompt decrease in the swelling and the calf compartment pressure is increased, the patient should be taken to the operating room for fasciotomies of the calf compartments and surgical thrombectomy with a temporary AVF.

E. Phlegmasia alba dolens is a painful, white swollen leg resulting from acute iliofemoral DVT. After confirmation of the diagnosis by DS with determination of the top of the thrombus by MRV or contrast venogram, early clot removal by percutaneous mechanical thrombectomy could be attempted. If it fails, surgical thrombectomy is indicated. However, thrombolysis 5 days after major surgery is contraindicated (correct answer).

Answer 151-3: B

Discussion 151-3

A. Ambulatory treatment with LMWH followed by warfarin for 6 months is the standard treatment of choice in many countries today. European studies have shown a very low rate of fatal PE (<1%). If this treatment is combined with compression stockings (30–40 mm Hg), swelling and pain are controlled and the postthrombotic syndrome rate is significantly reduced.

B. Answer B has been the standard treatment and is still used in some places in the United States. A randomized controlled trial performed in Sweden on acute iliofemoral DVT showed that with anticoagulation alone there was residual iliac vein obstruction in 70% and valvular incompetence and pathologic calf muscle pump function in *all* patients after 5 years. Conservative therapy with anticoagulants in this manner may reduce PE and DVT recurrence, but it does little to reduce the severity of the postthrombotic sequelae.

Early thrombus removal offers the best chance of mitigating postthrombotic sequelae. It can be accomplished with (C) CDT, (D) percutaneous mechanical thrombectomy, and (E) open surgical thrombectomy. Obstruction alone is rarely sufficient to cause venous hypertension and mostly causes pain and swelling with activity. Valvular incompetence alone causes most of the "stasis sequelae" (pigmentation, lipodermatosclerosis, and ulceration). However, those with both obstruction and reflux have the most severe postthrombotic sequelae. The importance of the proximal obstruction has been well studied by the Strandness group in Seattle, who showed that initially uninvolved distal veins became incompetent over time. Other studies on the inflammatory response to DVT, indicating that it injures the venous wall and valves, support the need for early thrombus removal. Percutaneous mechanical thrombectomy, with or without local thrombolysis, has shown promising early clinical results. The effectiveness of surgical thrombectomy was documented in a Swedish randomized controlled trial with 10-year follow-up, which showed persisting patency of the iliac vein in 80% after thrombectomy with a temporary AV fistula, compared with 30% after conservative treatment with anticoagulation.

■ ANSWERS AND DISCUSSION FOR CHAPTER 152

Answer 152-1: B
Discussion 152-1

Recurrent pulmonary thromboembolism in the face of ACRx is an approved indication, *only if* that therapy was at therapeutic levels. So B is *not* an approved indication. IVC filters are indicated in patients with venous thrombembolism who have failed therapeutic levels of anticoagulation, complications of ACRx (usually bleeding), or a contraindication to ACRx (e.g., intracerebral hemorrhage in a trauma patient with iliofemoral DVT, answer C). (A) Chronic (multiple recurrent) PE in a patient with pulmonary hypertension and cor pulmonale *is* an approved indication. (D) A free-floating iliofemoral DVT with a tail greater than 5 cm is also an accepted indication. (E) Recurrent septic embolism, although listed as an approved indication, is a relative one, because recurrent septic emboli are often small and may pass by a filter, plus efforts need to be directed at the source of the sepsis where possible.

Answer 152-2: C (statement is incorrect)
Discussion 152-2

(A) The only prospective randomized trial of vena cava filter efficacy, the PREPIC (Prévention du Risque d'Embolie Pulmonaire par Interruption Cave) trial, also concluded that filters are more effective than anticoagulation alone to prevent PE in the first 12 days. This applied to preventing PE and

fatal PE. At 2 years the same advantages had barely lost statistical significance, but there was a significant greater risk of recurrent DVT. This may have spurred the development of temporary/retrievable filters. (C) This definition for retrievable filter is incorrect and should apply to *temporary* filters. Temporary vena cava filters are *by definition* placed into the vena cava and remain attached to the body extracorporeally by means of a sheath, catheter, or wire (e.g., Tempofilter II). Retrievable filters are *designed* to be removed and are placed in a manner identical to permanent filters. They are retrieved through a percutaneous approach at a later date (e.g., OptEase, Recovery, and Tulip). (B) Temporary filters are generally used, particularly in Europe, to protect against pulmonary thromboembolism during short interventions, for example, endovenous procedures such as CDT or percutaneous mechanical thrombectomy. (D) Migration, vena cava occlusion, and insertion site thrombosis *are* among the potential complications associated with vena cava filter placement. Tilting and caval penetration are others. (E) Retrievable filters may be ideal for use in young trauma patients and patients who have undergone orthopedic procedures, patients whose need for PE prophylaxis is relatively short in duration and risk of bleeding from anticoagulation is high.

Answer 152-3: C (statement is false)
Discussion 152-3

(C) The presence of malignancy in and of itself is not a contraindication to vena cava filter placement in a patient with cancer with DVT and contraindications to anticoagulation. The indications for placement of vena cava filters in patients with malignancy are identical to those for patients without cancer. However, patients with cancer have a much higher (3.6 times) risk of PE (A), and that risk has been shown to be significantly higher still in association with certain risk factors: newly discovered metastasis, history of PE, and multiple episodes of neutropenia (D). In fact, PE was the presenting symptom of newly metastatic disease in 55% of patients with cancer (E). They also have a higher risk of bleeding (B). Unfortunately such patients may have a very poor longevity outlook.

■ ANSWERS AND DISCUSSION FOR CHAPTER 153

Answer 153-1: E
Discussion 153-1

(E) It is best to estimate severity and extent of the process with DS and to detect DVT, which may be associated with superficial venous thrombosis, because this will change therapy. (A) Superficial thrombophlebitis *does* increase patient risk. (B) Warm compresses and bed rest suffice only for localized cases. (D) High ligation is necessary *only* in patients in whom the process approaches the saphenofemoral junction; stripping is unnecessary in the acute phase. (C) Antiplatelet drugs are not indicated.

Answer 153-2: D
Discussion 153-2

(D) Penile Mondor's disease is a local process involving the dorsal penile vein. The others, A, B, C, and E, all relate to migratory phlebitis or are associated inflammatory states.

Answer 153-3: C

Discussion 153-3

(C) The occurrence of PE varies but approaches low double digits in some series. A is therefore incorrect, (B) PE may also occur when the process involves the *lower* venous segments, likely entering the deep system through lower major perforators.

■ ANSWERS AND DISCUSSION FOR CHAPTER 154

Answer 154-1: A

Discussion 154-1

Venous hypertension is transmitted to the exchange vessels of the microcirculation. Macromolecules like fibrinogen and red blood cells extravasate and cause a persistent inflammatory injury (A). It has been demonstrated that macromolecules like fibrinogen and alpha-2 macroglobulin and red blood cells are forced out of the microcirculation (extravasated) into the interstitium. Unlike white blood cells, red blood cells do not have the capacity to reenter the circulation. Once forced into the interstitium, they begin to degrade. Degrading red blood cells and macromolecules are potent inflammatory mediators that lead to white blood cell activation. Inflammatory mediators attract leukocytes that initiate a cascade of events that lead to tissue remodeling, fibrosis, and senescence. Compression stockings decrease venous hypertension and inhibit the extravasation of macromolecules and red blood cells and therefore mitigate the inciting inflammatory injury.

None of the others, like (B) lymphocytes, (C) macrophages, (D) collagen, or (E) fibronectin extravasate and cause chronic inflammatory responses.

Answer 154-2: C

Discussion 154-2

Dermal fibrosis is mediated by (C) the cytokine TGF-beta-1. Extensive data indicate that macrophages and mast cells release TGF-beta-1, which binds to dermal fibroblasts. Fibroblasts regulate tissue remodeling by synthesis of collagen, regulation of metalloproteinases, differentiation into myofibroblasts, and extracellular matrix contraction. All of these processes are regulated by TGF-beta-1. TGF-beta-1 is present in pathologic amounts in the dermis of patients with severe CVI and therefore is a potent modulator of end-organ dysfunction. Interleukin-1 (A), tumor necrosis factor-alpha (B), basic fibroblastic growth factor (D), and keratinocyte growth factor (E) do not mediate dermal fibrosis.

Answer 154-3: D

Discussion 154-3

Dietary factors (D) have not been shown to be associated with varicosity. Although implicated as a possible cause, there is no direct evidence that dietary factors play a role in varicose vein development, other than their leading to morbid obesity. All of the remaining factors (A, B, C, and E) have been reported to play a role in varicose vein development.

■ ANSWERS AND DISCUSSION FOR CHAPTER 155

Answer 155-1: C

Discussion 155-1

CEAP clinical class 3 is edema attributed to a venous cause. Lipedema (E) is not mentioned in the classification and is a term used to describe limbs enlarged from localized adiposity; thus, patients with lipedema do not belong to CEAP clinical class 3.

Lipodermatosclerosis (A) is included in clinical class 4, and the term refers to indurated tissue resulting from chronic inflammation, which is frequently localized to the "gaiter" area of the ankle. A healed leg ulcer (B) with typical distribution at or above the ankle is most likely to be of venous origin; however, as noted in the text, support for this assumption is the role of the Etiology, Anatomy, and Pathophysiology (E, A, P) components of the classification.

The clinical classification includes the designation of C-0 to accommodate those individuals in whom no objective E, A, or P evidence of venous reflux or obstruction is found and who have (D) no clinical findings of venous disease. Telangiectases or reticular veins (E) constitute clinical class 1 and are distinguished from class 2, varicose veins, by size criterion. Patients with veins of less than 3 mm in diameter belong to class 1; those with larger veins belong to class 2 (varicose veins). The CEAP classification of chronic venous disease was originally published in 1995 and revised in 2004.

Answer 155-2: D

Discussion 155-2

Several longitudinal studies have confirmed that proper treatment of a healed leg ulcer is efficacious in preventing recurrence. Both surgical intervention and compliant use of compression stockings or devices have a role in reducing ulcer recurrence; between 20% and 30% of patients will still have recurrences in this treated population; however, if untreated, the likelihood of recurrence approaches 100%. When appropriate therapy is administered, ulcers that have healed are likely to remain healed (D). Ulcer recurrence is much more frequent in patients with postthrombotic syndrome than in those with primary valvular incompetence (E). According to a 25-year, population-based study in Olmstead County, Minnesota, 6% of limbs with clinical signs of chronic venous stasis will go on to develop ulceration within 5 years (A). The likelihood of a patient developing the most severe symptoms of CVI increases with increasing age and obesity (B, C).

Answer 155-3: D

Discussion 155-3

Items A, B, C, and E are considered essential to the assignment of the complete CEAP classification. A major focus of the CEAP initiative is to facilitate a uniform international assessment of venous diseases. The ease of study, availability, and reliability of duplex scan examination contribute substantial accuracy to the previous standard classification, which only considered clinical findings. Even the new basic

CEAP should be formulated by combining clinical and duplex examinations.

The addition of other minimally invasive diagnostic studies, such as CT angiography or magnetic resonance angiography, is recommended for more specific evaluations and longitudinal clinical research. Air plethysmography (D) contributes to the clinical estimation of disease severity and physiologic dysfunction, but it is *not* considered an essential part of the routine clinical assessment. More extensive investigations such as MRV or computed tomography (CT) have a greater role in the assessment of the suprainguinal venous system and may be combined with venography for endovascular correction of some abnormalities.

Answer 155-4: C

Discussion 155-4

The Venous Clinical Severity Score (C) has been validated against the CEAP classification and found to have reasonable correlation in separate studies. The original 18-point clinical severity score (A) was probably useful, but never subjected to clinical validation. The Venous Segmental Disease Score (D) has failed to correlate consistently in studies performed to date. The Nottingham Health Profile (B) and Short Form-36 (E) are both generic instruments for assessment of Health Related—QOL; although both are extensively validated for this purpose, neither has correlated well with venous disease severity.

■ ANSWERS AND DISCUSSION FOR CHAPTER 156

Answer 156-1: B

Discussion 156-1

A. Hospital admission with local wound care was the standard of care many years ago when admission to the hospital was basically unrestricted. It worked, not because of the local wound care, but because the rest and elevation eliminated the underlying cause, venous hypertension. However, prolonged bed rest would *not* be good for the described patient.

B. Unna boot dressing changed weekly by a health care professional is the best solution for this patient. A number of different health professionals can be trained in the proper application of an Unna boot, and applications at weekly intervals (longer as the ulcer cleans up and approaches healing) have proven effective in the ambulatory treatment of venous ulcers.

C. The main benefit from oral antibiotics and bed rest *with elevation* is in the latter. But prolonged bed rest would *not* be good for the described patient.

D. There are aids to make elastic support stockings easier, but even if this patient is not too weak for this, he has an *open* ulcer.

E. Stanozolol is an androgenic steroid with fibrinolytic activity. Studies with it in treating venous ulcer brought mixed results and were not impressive. It has been (or should have been) abandoned for this use.

Answer 156-2: D

Discussion 156-2

A. Although some physicians have used diuretics, particularly hydrochlorothiazide, in the past, as an adjunct in this setting, it does not address the underlying pathophysiology.

B. Unna boot applications are primarily for the outpatient treatment of venous ulcers, which this patient does not have.

C. Pentoxifylline has no role here.

D. New compression stockings are required approximately every 3 months to maintain an effective pressure gradient. This is the most appropriate next step; she was doing well on conservative therapy until recently, and her stockings have been worn for 9 months!

E. Reconstructive valve surgery should be considered in active patients but only after a good conservative therapy program has failed and, where present, superficial and perforator incompetence and any proximal occlusion have first been corrected.

Answer 156-3: B

Discussion 156-3

This patient could have a venous ulcer, for this is a typical location, but there is associated arterial occlusive disease, and the ABI suggests that ischemia is the reason for it not healing with Unna boot application, and likely the severe pain, because the ABI is in the ischemic rest pain range. Patients who have responded to conservative therapy for CVI in the past and then fail to respond should always be considered for associated peripheral arterial disease and obtain an ABI.

A. Continuing with a failing regimen is inappropriate.

B. Complete lower extremity arteriogram with run-off visualization, with a view to correcting the underlying arterial occlusive disease, is needed with an ABI of 0.3.

C. Oral antibiotics would not help heal this ulcer.

D. Venous ulcer healing can be accelerated by skin coverage, for example, by an Apligraf skin substitute, but the underlying problem in nonhealing is arterial insufficiency.

E. Stripping or SEPS should not be performed in limbs with severe arterial ischemia.

■ ANSWERS AND DISCUSSION FOR CHAPTER 157

Answer 157-1: D

Discussion 157-1

Duplex ultrasonography (D) performed on a patient in the standing position is the best technique to study venous valvular incompetence of the deep, superficial, and perforating veins. Magnetic resonance examinations (E) are performed with the patient supine where reflux evaluation is unreliable. The supine position is not useful in evaluating venous incompetence. Venous plethysmography can evaluate venous reflux by estimating venous return time and its correction by tourniquet application to obstruct different levels of the superficial venous system, but little else (C). Segmental reflux is assessed with difficulty with the handheld Doppler (B) but is clearly mapped out by duplex. Air plethysmography studies (A) are used to estimate venous physiology of the whole limb, not segmental function.

Answer 157-2: E

Discussion 157-2:

There is level I evidence that proximal great saphenous vein ligation with ligation and division of all proximal tributaries, and saphenous stripping has the lowest rate of recurrence of varicose veins in the long term (E). All other modalities listed (A, B, C, D) have higher recurrence for the following reasons: missed collaterals at the groin, neovascularization, thigh perforators, or persistent patency and incompetence of the main or accessory saphenous vein. Ligation alone (A) even when all tributaries are ligated (B), leaves behind variable lengths of refluxing saphenous vein. This becomes a major source of recurrent varicose veins. Sclerotherapy (C, D) has been compared with stripping with inferior results.

Answer 157-3: E

Discussion 157-3

Class 1 applies to telangiectasias, a condition that usually requires no anatomic or physiologic testing (E). Any evidence of saphenous incompetence, such as skin changes, varicose veins, veins greater than 3 mm in size, or a history of deep vein thrombosis, however, warrants evaluation with DS (C). Ankle venous pressures are rarely used today and even then only selectively before reconstructions for deep vein occlusion (B). Air plethysmography (A) is used to assess leg venous function, usually for CEAP class 3 to 6. Descending venography (D) is used selectively before interventions to correct valve incompetence.

■ ANSWERS AND DISCUSSION FOR CHAPTER 158

Answer 158-1: C

Discussion 158-1

The presence of ICPVs is of clinical significance, and they are present more frequently in patients with advanced CVI and venous ulcers. Incompetent perforators occur in at least two thirds of patients with venous ulceration and are found together with superficial or deep venous incompetence in most patients. The diagnosis of ICPV is based on the finding of flow from the deep to the superficial system after release of compression distal to the site under study (not in the opposite direction, which is normal, as in A). The best test to confirm that is DS, which is superior, not inferior, to phlebography (B). Ascending phlebography, as a diagnostic method in the evaluation of ICPVs, has a low incidence of false-positive findings but a high rate of false-negative findings. (C) Duplex scanning is far superior to physical examination in the diagnosis of the presence *and localization* of the site of ICPVs, the latter (PE) not even being a good screening method (D).

(E) The addition of a handheld Doppler to PE can help but does not achieve an accuracy anywhere close to that of DS.

Answer 158-2: D

Discussion 158-2

(D) is false. In the mid- and distal calf the most important direct medial perforators are the upper and middle posterior tibial perforators, the so-called *Cockett II* and *III* perforators but they do *not* originate directly from the great saphenous vein but from the posterior arch vein (also called posterior calf accessory saphenous vein or Leonardo's vein). Stripping of the greater saphenous vein in the calf, therefore, does not interrupt these important perforators, which are usually located 7 to 9 cm and 10 to 12 cm proximal to the lower border of the medial malleolus (E). Perforating veins connect the superficial to the deep venous system, either directly to the main axial veins (direct perforators) or indirectly to muscular tributaries or soleal venous sinuses (indirect perforators). (A) The term "communicating veins" refers to interconnecting veins within the same system. (B) It has been shown that perforating veins of the foot are valveless and that these veins paradoxically direct flow from the deep to the superficial venous system and not from the superficial to the deep system (C) as do calf perforators.

Answer 158-3: B

Discussion 158-3

First introduced by Hauer in 1985, the SEPS procedure is the best surgical technique to interrupt incompetent perforating veins in the medial calf. There are single-port and double endoscopic-port techniques to perform SEPS (C). The technique frequently involves using CO_2 insufflation (A), with a pressure of 15 to 30 mm Hg (D); the use of a thigh tourniquet is helpful to decrease bleeding and enlarge the working space in the subfascial area (E). Incision of the fascia of the deep compartment close to the tibia (paratibial fasciotomy) *is routinely needed* to explore the deep space and more important to interrupt the Cockett II and III perforators, so B is false and therefore the correct answer.

■ ANSWERS AND DISCUSSION FOR CHAPTER 159

Answer 159-1: D

Discussion 159-1

A. Although descending venography has identified the severity of distal valve reflux and the location of incompetent valves, the latter has not had a one-to-one correlation with surgical observations.

B. Although results of venous valve repair are worse with secondary (postthrombotic) disease, this is not absolute and some valves are amenable to in situ repair. In addition, other reconstructive techniques can be applied.

C. Primary deep venous insufficiency *can* lead to vein wall thickening, similar (but not commonly as severe and widespread) to that seen with the postthrombotic syndrome. However, it certainly can lead to fibrotic changes in the valves and walls of some vein, leading *in the past* to confusion and debate as to whether there had been superimposed thrombosis.

D. The postthrombotic syndrome can lead to vein wall thickening *without* valve cusp involvement leaving a valve suitable for in situ repair. This observation has refuted the long-held position represented by B and undermined the generalization that valves in primary disease are amenable to repair/reconstruction, whereas those with secondary disease are not. It remains valid that results with secondary disease are worse; it is just that case selection has to be individualized after proper evaluation.

E. Following on the above discussions (B, C, D), it is clear that primary and secondary causes of deep venous insufficiency are not mutually exclusive processes, as viewed by the later status of the venous valve and walls.

Answer 159-2: B
Discussion 159-2

In this discussion one has to accept the point made in 159-1A, that descending venography does not have a one-to-one direct correlation with the status of the valve (presence, absence, incompetence) observed during surgery, and answer on the basis of surgical observations.

A. Ligation of the profunda femoris vein would control its reflux, but if thrombosis of the femoral vein repair occurred, the main collateral channel would have been excluded.

B. Transposition of the profunda femoris vein has had initial good but deteriorating late outcomes, reported in an earlier study from Northwestern, but this was when a competent profunda femoris was transposed as a primary procedure with concomitant ligation of an incompetent (superficial) femoral vein. The late deterioration was probably related to the dilation of the now main outflow channel, the profunda femoris, with secondary incompetence of its valves. This situation is different; the (superficial) femoral vein is patent and its valve has been rendered competent by repair. To avoid profunda reflux, its transposition into the femoral vein distal to the competent valve is preferable to its ligation, for reasons given in A.

C. Axillary valve transplantation is not an appropriate procedure to apply to the profunda femoris vein.

D. The same can be said for intimal flap reconstruction of a valve for the profunda femoris vein. In addition, this old concept has not been proven to be a feasible solution in locations other than the saphenofemoral junction, and even this (Japanese) application is not likely to replace saphenous ablation or stripping, with or without high ligation (another debatable subject), let alone in the profunda femoris.

E. A trial of cryopreserved allograft valve transplantation gave initially encouraging results, but later was abandoned. Furthermore, it was applied to the femoral and popliteal veins, not the profunda femoris vein.

Answer 159-3: C
Discussion 159-3

The risk of experiencing clinically significant DVT at the time of femoral vein internal valvuloplasty is in the 5% to 10% range, and the prospect for long-term ulcer healing without recurrence at 5 years is approximately 70% according to most recent reported experience. C is the correct answer. A higher risk of DVT (D, E) or a lower risk of healing (B) would make this procedure much less acceptable. The

result listed in A hopefully can be achieved in the future and would certainly boost its acceptance in patients with recurrent venous ulceration refractory to conservative therapy and not contributed to by uncorrected superficial or perforator incompetence.

■ ANSWERS AND DISCUSSION FOR CHAPTER 160

Answer 160-1: B
Discussion 160-1

Iliac vein obstruction, caused by acute deep vein thrombosis, usually can be treated effectively with iliac vein stenting. Left iliac vein occlusion is frequently caused by the May-Thurner syndrome, in which left iliac vein occlusion or stenosis is caused by the overriding right common femoral artery. The most useful test to plan the procedure is an ascending venography with bilateral femoral vein injections to visualize the occluded segment(s) and assess any IVC involvement (B). It should be noted that there are two techniques for ascending phlebography. The technique using injection of contrast into a foot vein may not visualize the iliac vein well, unless a prolonged infusion is used (Paulson technique). However, by cannulating the femoral vein the iliac morphology is not only seen better but one can recheck the femoral central pressure gradient and then continue with angioplasty and stenting as needed.

Color duplex examination (D) is frequently unreliable to assess the pelvic veins because of bowel gas and obesity. Hemodynamic information is provided by measuring arm/foot venous pressure differential in the supine patient (A). A value of more than 4 mm Hg signifies hemodynamic obstruction at rest. Alternatively, a femoral-central venous pressure gradient that is greater than 5 mm Hg, or if it doubles after exercise (10 forceful foot movements), provides evidence of significant obstruction. However, these give no anatomic information.

Outflow strain-gauge plethysmography will also quantitate the degree of proximal occlusion (E), but it also does not localize or visualize the obstructed segment so is not helpful in planning. Descending venography (C) is used for delineating valve reflux, not obstruction. However, IVUS can be helpful to define details of the obstruction and assist in stent placement.

Answer 160-2: E
Discussion 160-2

A. If history, physical examination, and noninvasive venous tests indicate significant obstructive venous disease, ascending and descending phlebography and foot and femoral venous pressure measurements are all mandatory studies before venous reconstructive surgery. More recently, venous pressure measurements have not routinely been taken into consideration, because the use of IVUS has gained popularity.

B. Large, profuse collaterals around an obstructed venous segment on phlebograms can be *hemodynamically inadequate* because of the presence of stenosis or other high-resistance areas not readily seen with phlebography.

C. A hemodynamically significant iliofemoral venous stenosis/obstruction exists if (1) a vertical gradient of more than 2 mm Hg exists at rest or if the horizontal gradient (compared with the contralateral femoral pressure) is more than 2 mm Hg with the patient supine and at rest, or (2) if an exercise venous pressure (using a pedal ergometer) increases more than 3 mm Hg from the resting level.

D. An arm/foot venous pressure differential at rest of more than 4 mm Hg and a foot venous pressure elevation with reactive hyperemia more than 6 mm Hg are also indicators of a hemodynamically significant venous obstruction.

E. Patients with phlebographic obstruction may have normal hemodynamic function because of extensive collateral formation, whereas patients with venograms showing patent but recanalized main venous channels may demonstrate significant hemodynamic abnormality. Thus, statement E is false.

Answer 160-3: E
Discussion 160-3

A. To prevent excessive tension, it is advisable to interpose a graft longer than the excised vein segment.

B. There is unanimous agreement that the least thrombogenic conduit in the venous system is autogenous vein. However, when autogenous vein is not available or of poor quality, or when large-diameter veins need to be replaced (e.g., thoracic caval or iliocaval), a prosthetic externally supported PTFE conduit can achieve acceptable patency.

C. Adjunctive temporary AVFs improve long-term patency of both autogenous and prosthetic venous bypass conduits.

D. The exact timing of closure of an adjunctive AVF remains unsettled. Most data support closure of adjunctive fistulas before 6 months. They can be closed surgically or nonoperatively by percutaneous deployment of a detachable balloon or coils in the fistula under direct radiographic control.

E. Traumatic injury/occlusion to the proximal femoral vein can be treated with ligation without reconstruction. Collateral circulation usually develops.

■ ANSWERS AND DISCUSSION FOR CHAPTER 161

Answer 161-1: E
Discussion 161-1

A. Some physicians would treat this patient conservatively, but the response to elastic stockings alone by patients who work upright all day has been shown to be disappointing.

B. A Palma procedure is a major undertaking, and even with an adjunctive AVF initially, the long-term patency of PTFE grafts has been disappointing.

C. Stent-mounted venous valves are still in development and are not proven effective, and would be disadvantaged below an iliac obstruction.

D. An axillary vein transfer to the femoral vein would also be disadvantaged below the iliac obstruction, even if it did fit the femoral vein diameter, which it does not (it is a better diameter fit in the popliteal vein).

E. This patient is relatively young, is actively employed in a job in which he works upright, and has symptoms typical of CVI. Studies show he has iliac vein stenoses above a refluxing deep system. At this point an invasive procedure, venogram with pressure gradients, has already been undertaken. Iliac vein percutaneous transluminal angioplasty and stenting have achieved encouraging results in observational studies to date and are the best of the alternatives listed for mitigating CVI symptoms.

Answer 161-2: C
Discussion 161-2

A. The greater saphenous vein is normal in diameter, as is the refilling time. Saphenous reflux may exist but is not the main underlying problem and does not deserve this intervention.

B. Better elastic support hose may help in a compliant patient, but this patient deserves further evaluation.

C. Of the diagnostic options listed this one is the most likely to demonstrate the underlying problem, especially because a DS has not done so. (One might want to repeat an "outside" DS.) The complaint may represent a May-Thurner syndrome.

D. The CT scan would also involve a contrast load but would focus on a long shot. The femoral venogram would also demonstrate extrinsic compression.

E. The varicosities may deserve this treatment, if thorough evaluation shows otherwise negative results. Calf varicosities can develop in the absence of saphenofemoral incompetence.

Answer 161-3: B
Discussion 161-3

A. These are *not* normal findings; they indicate iliac vein obstruction.

B. Iliac obstruction can be missed on a single-plane, anteroposterior view. Multiplane phlebographic views are needed. IVUS would also give definitive information about the lumen of the iliac vein.

C. A femoral vein-central vein pressure gradient, with and without leg exercise, could detect a hemodynamically significant venous obstruction proximally, but this is already evident from the collaterals visualized.

D. Diaphragmatic depression during inhalation can slow venous outflow but will not produce these collaterals, which are a response to a chronic obstruction.

E. Evidence of an iliac obstruction *is visualized.*

■ ANSWERS AND DISCUSSION FOR CHAPTER 162

Answer 162-1: C
Discussion 162-1

A. A combined transfemoral and internal jugular access is a good secondary option to access central veins.

B. The best technique to start venogram is with access through both basilic veins.

C. When there is an SVC occlusion with extension of acute thrombus into both brachiocephalic veins, *each* subclavian vein must be traversed with catheters and wires advanced into the SVC and right atrium, so statement C is false. The risk of PE is very small.

D. Once vascular access has been achieved in both arms and the basilic venipuncture sites are converted to 5F or 6F angiographic side-arm sheaths the best way to proceed is to pass a 5F angiographic catheter with a simple curve (Berenstein glide catheter, Boston Scientific, Watertown, Mass) and a 0.035-inch steerable hydrophilic guidewire (Glidewire, Boston Scientific) through the occluded vein segment.

E. For more organized fibrotic occlusions, extra stiffness may be needed to avoid buckling of the catheter when it encounters resistance. In this situation, one can convert to a coaxial system consisting of a 7F or 8F braided coronary guiding catheter fitted with a Touhy-Borst adapter to allow placement of the 5F catheter and guidewire. The guiding catheter provides a better mechanical advantage and reduces the tendency of the 5F catheter to recoil.

Answer 162-2: B

Discussion 162-2

A. Balloon-expandable stents, *such as Palmaz stents* (not the Wallstent as stated), are susceptible to plastic deformation when external, two-point compression is applied.

B. Using a Wallstent for the treatment of brachiocephalic vein stenosis and a Palmaz stent in the SVC are excellent choices. This is the only true statement.

C. The Gianturco Z-stent is an excellent *self-expanding* (*not balloon expandable*) stent for large vein reconstructions.

D. The Wallstent (not a Palmaz stent) is a longitudinally flexible, self-expanding metal stent.

E. The *disadvantage* of the Wallstent is that it *does* foreshorten when it is deployed in the vein.

Answer 162-3: D

Discussion 162-3

This patient has membranous occlusion of the IVC associated with Budd-Chiari syndrome. The best option at this stage is (D) to attempt to place a Gianturco Z-stent into the IVC to decrease venous outflow obstruction because of the IVC stenosis. The Gianturco Z-stent is a relatively rigid, self-expanding stent. Among its advantages, the Z-stent comes in a wide variety of diameters (8–40 mm), possesses good hoop strength, and does not foreshorten during deployment. In addition, its small surface area, large interstices, and low thrombogenicity allow it to be placed across tributary veins like the renal veins. It is used with very good results for IVC occlusions.

A Wallstent (E) is not a good option in this location; it has a relatively low radial force. (A) Medical management will not relieve the patient's symptoms, and endovascular techniques should be tried before (C) open surgery. Thrombolysis of the hepatic veins (B) is not indicated at this stage.

■ ANSWERS AND DISCUSSION FOR CHAPTER 163

Answer 163-1: D

Discussion 163-1

Vascular leiomyosarcomas are rare and involve veins more often than arteries. Primary venous leiomyosarcoma occurs most often in the IVC compared with other central or peripheral veins (A). The tumors are usually polypoid or nodular in appearance, and the most common growth pattern is intraluminal (B), although the tumor can invade adjacent structures. Primary venous leiomyosarcoma is more prevalent in women than in men (C), and the tumors have been reported in patients over a wide age range (E). Most patients with primary caval tumors present with symptoms or signs of metastatic disease or obstruction of the vena cava. Early detection is rare and occurs in only 2% to 3% of patients with this problem. Thus D is the false statement.

Answer 163-2: B

Discussion 163-2

Renal cell cancer with intraluminal tumor thrombus (B) is the most common type of malignancy that involves the vena cava. The tumors are more often on the right than the left side. The presence of cardiac arrhythmias and syncope suggests extension of the thrombus into the right side of the heart. Cardiac arrhythmias and syncope would be unusual symptoms for a patient with (D) renal cell cancer with tumor thrombus only involving a short segment of the suprarenal IVC. Although the tumor type *could be* an adrenal cortical carcinoma (A) or pheochromocytoma (C), these tumors are much rarer than renal cell cancer. A retroperitoneal sarcoma (E) would usually involve tissues beyond Gerota's fascia, and the CT scan showed a free tissue plane. This description of the relationship between the tumor and the IVC makes it unlikely that there is invasion of the vena cava.

Answer 163-3: C

Discussion 163-3

This patient has a retroperitoneal tumor that has obstructed the vena cava. There is no evidence of metastatic disease, and the scans suggest the tumor is locally resectable. The most common tumor types to involve the infrarenal segment of the IVC are retroperitoneal sarcomas.

A. Preoperatively, chemotherapy and radiation are rarely warranted in these cases.

B. The location of the tumor, the absence of para-aortic or pericaval adenopathy, and no metastatic lesions in the liver make the likelihood of adenocarcinoma or germ-cell tumors to be low. Therefore, preoperative needle biopsy of the mass would not significantly alter treatment.

C. The vena cava is chronically occluded based on the lack of recent lower extremity edema and the dilated veins in the pelvis and left perivertebral region. Therefore, the IVC can be resected en bloc with the tumor and not replaced under these conditions. Thus, C is the correct answer.

D. Collateral venous drainage was noted by the dilated veins in the pelvis and left paravertebral region. *If* large collateral veins required ligation and division during the tumor resection, then the vena cava could be replaced, *but* this is usually done with an externally supported ePTFE graft rather than autogenous vein. Autogenous vein for replacement of the abdominal IVC is reserved for patients in whom there has been violation of the bowel or other contamination during the tumor resection.

E. There is nothing in the case presentation or description of the location of the tumor that makes it unresectable. Untreated, the patient's mean survival would be less than 1 year for most tumors in this location. Because the patient is young, is physically fit, has no major medical comorbidities, and has no evidence of metastatic disease, tumor resection remains the best chance for cure or local control of the tumor.

■ ANSWERS AND DISCUSSION FOR CHAPTER 164

Answer 164-1: B

Discussion 164-1

This young patient has mediastinal fibrosis, which is the most frequent benign cause of SVC syndrome. Today, lung cancer (squamous, small cell, and adenocarcinoma) with mediastinal lymphadenopathy and primary mediastinal malignancy are the most frequent causes of SVC syndrome, accounting for 60% to 85% of cases. Benign disease, as in this patient, is less common, accounting for only 15% to 22% of cases. Mediastinal fibrosis and granulomatous fungal disease, such as histoplasmosis, have been the most frequent benign causes of SVC and innominate vein obstruction. However, the exponential increase in the use of indwelling central venous catheters and cardiac pacemakers over the last 2 decades has resulted in postthrombotic SVC obstructions with scarring secondary to irritation and inflammation around the indwelling catheters and wires, and a greater proportion of patients presenting with SVC obstruction of benign cause.

(A) It is necessary to perform a good-quality bilateral upper extremity venography to plan treatment, and it may be justified to try once more to cross the obstruction with a guidewire with the hope of performing angioplasty and stenting. If unsuccessful, SVC occlusion can be bypassed successfully with PTFE, spiral vein graft, or femoral vein graft (C, D, E). Although the internal jugular vein is a good vein graft for IVC, iliac, or femoral vein repairs, it should not be harvested in patients with symptomatic SVC syndrome (B).

Answer 164-2: B

Discussion 164-2

Currently, lung cancer with mediastinal lymphadenopathy is the most common malignant cause of SVC syndrome. Primary mediastinal malignant tumors may also cause SVC syndrome; these tumors include mediastinal lymphoma, medullary, or follicular carcinoma of the thyroid, malignant thymoma, teratoma, angiosarcoma, and synovial cell carcinoma. (A) CT scan and treatment of the malignant disease take priority, and radiation treatment may produce a rapid and striking diminution of the signs and symptoms of SVC syndrome. (B) Not true, and this is the correct answer. Although SVC syndrome can cause blindness and cerebral hemorrhage, these complications are rare in this setting, so there is almost always time for cancer treatment.

Options C, D, and E are all true and would come into play *after* the cancer treatment, when its effect on the SVC syndrome is assessed and the prognosis is more apparent.

Answer 164-3: C

Discussion 164-3

Doty et al. first reported excellent results with spiral saphenous vein grafts for the SVC syndrome. The Mayo Clinic group reported on the long-term results in 29 patients who underwent 31 SVC reconstructions for nonmalignant SVC obstruction. Five-year primary and secondary patency rates for all grafts used were 53% and 80%, respectively.

A. Spiral vein grafts performed the best of the different graft types, with 90% secondary patency at 5 years.
B. Externally supported ePTFE is the best prosthetic material for use in the venous system. A review of results from multiple series from the literature reveals a 2-year patency of ePTFE grafts of approximately 70%. Thrombosis occurred more frequently when the distal anastomosis was performed to the internal jugular or subclavian veins, and the results were much better in patients with innominate anastomosis or SVC interposition grafts.
C. Increasing success with "superficial" femoral vein as an arterial conduit has caused a resurgence in the use of this autologous graft for large vein reconstructions as well. It *can* be used for SVC reconstruction, although concerns about distal thrombosis at the harvest site and chronic venous insufficiency have been voiced. Nonetheless, it is a good conduit in patients with unavailable or inadequate saphenous vein for spiral graft. So this is the only false statement (correct answer).
D. Saphenous vein is usually too small for central vein reconstruction.
E. Bovine pericardial patch has been used successfully as a patch material in the venous system.

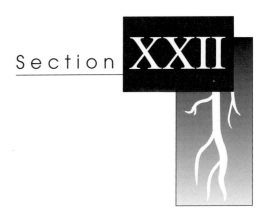

Section **XXII**

THE MANAGEMENT OF LYMPHATIC DISORDERS

STUDY QUESTIONS

■ QUESTIONS FOR CHAPTER 165

Question 165-1

The discovery of the lymphatic system is attributed to:

A. William Harvey.
B. Gasparo Asellius.
C. Jean Pecquet.
D. William Hunter.
E. E. Starling.

Question 165-2

The most frequent local or regional cause of chronic swelling of the extremity in North America is:

A. Primary lymphedema.
B. Secondary lymphedema.
C. Chronic venous insufficiency.
D. Congenital vascular malformation.
E. Acquired arteriovenous fistula.

Question 165-3

The term "Milroy's disease" should be reserved for patients with:

A. Primary lymphedema.
B. Primary congenital hereditary lymphedema.
C. All patients with lymphedema praecox.
D. Lymphangiectasia.
E. Lymphangiosarcoma in a limb with chronic lymphedema.

■ QUESTIONS FOR CHAPTER 166

Question 166-1

The primary mechanism by which lymph is propelled forward is:

A. Contractions of surrounding muscles, like the venous pump.
B. Negative pressure phases of the respiratory cycle.
C. Intrinsic lymphatic contraction.
D. Fascial constriction (compartmental pressure changes).
E. A forward thrust from arterial pulsations (vis a tergo).

Question 166-2

The pathophysiology of *secondary* lymphedema (chronic lymph stasis) is characterized by:

A. Progressive loss of truncal contractility and proximal occlusion with distal intraluminal valve incompetence, leading to eventual progressive deposition of fluid, fat, and collagen in the skin and subcutaneous tissues.
B. Rapid onset of limb swelling, accumulation of protein-poor edema fluid, and progressive insufficiency of the superficial and deep lymphatics followed by dermal hyperpigmentation and paramalleolar skin ulceration.
C. Acute, unremitting extremity swelling, prompt response to diuretic drugs, and gradual remission of edema over many years.
D. Low-protein edema fluid, progressive improvement with diuretic drugs, and dietary salt restriction, often in conjunction with limb-threatening ischemic foot ulcers.
E. Progressive limb swelling, hyperpigmentation, subcutaneous fibrosis, and development of ulceration.

Question 166-3

Which of the following statements is *most* accurate?

A. Veins and lymphatics are both thin-walled conduits that propel liquid back to the heart under *high* intraluminal pressure and *high* vascular resistance.
B. Veins and lymphatics are both thin-walled conduits that propel liquid back to the heart under *low* intraluminal pressure and *low* vascular resistance.
C. Veins and lymphatics are thin-walled conduits that propel liquid back to the heart, but whereas venous blood flows at *low* intraluminal pressure and *high* vascular resistance, lymph flows at *low* intraluminal pressure and *low* vascular resistance.
D. Veins and lymphatics are thin-walled conduits that propel liquid back to the heart, but whereas venous blood flows at *low* intraluminal pressure and *low* vascular resistance, lymph flows at *low* intraluminal pressure and *high* vascular resistance.
E. Veins and lymphatics are thin-walled conduits that propel liquid back to the heart, but whereas venous blood flows at *high* intraluminal pressure and *low* vascular resistance, lymph flows at *low* intraluminal pressure and *low* vascular resistance.

203

■ QUESTIONS FOR CHAPTER 167

Question 167-1

The test of choice to diagnose lymphedema is:

A. Direct-contrast lymphangiography.
B. Indirect-contrast lymphangiography.
C. Computed tomography (CT).
D. Magnetic resonance imaging (MRI).
E. Isotope lymphoscintigraphy.

Question 167-2

Which of the following is *not* one of the characteristic signs and symptoms associated with chronic *primary* lymphedema?

A. Nonpitting edema of the ankle and foot.
B. Squaring of the toes (Stemmer's sign).
C. Hyperkeratosis.
D. Yellow fingernails.
E. Moderate to severe aching pain.

Question 167-3

Which of the following statement about lymphedema is *true*?

A. Lymphangiosarcoma develops in approximately 10% of all patients with lymphedema of more than 15 years' duration.
B. Emotional problems are common in patients with lymphedema and should be addressed when identified.
C. Severe lymphedema, although unsightly, rarely causes significant physical or emotional disability/limitation.
D. Nonoperative measures to control lymphedema are generally inferior to surgical treatment.
E. Skin ulcers are common in severe lymphedema.

■ QUESTIONS FOR CHAPTER 168

Question 168-1

The most common cause of *secondary* lymphedema worldwide is:

A. Cancer surgery.
B. Radiation therapy.
C. Infection.
D. Tumor obstruction.
E. Obesity.

Question 168-2

Which of the following treatment interventions is *least* useful in *lymphedema reduction*?

A. Sequential pneumatic compression device.
B. Compression wrapping.
C. Combined complex decongestive therapy program.
D. Graduated compression garment.
E. An exercise program.

Question 168-3

Which of the following treatment interventions is *least* well documented by scientific studies in terms of its effectiveness in the prevention of lymphedema?

A. Meticulous skin care of limb at risk.
B. Antifilarial drug prophylaxis.
C. Sentinel node biopsy.
D. Weight management.
E. Control of nutritional factors.

■ QUESTIONS FOR CHAPTER 169

Question 169-1

Which of the following statements is *true* regarding the surgical treatment of lymphedema?

A. Approximately 30% of patients with lymphedema require surgery to treat it.
B. Functional impairment is the best indication for surgery.
C. The best excisional surgical procedure is the Charles operation (circumferential excision of the skin and subcutaneous tissue with skin grafting of the extremity).
D. Both the Thompson and modified Homans procedures are intended to be both excisional and physiologic in approach.
E. The function of microsurgical lymphatic grafts in humans has *not* been documented by lymphoscintigraphy.

Question 169-2

Which of the following statements concerning patients with lymphangiectasia and reflux of chyle is *not* true?

A. Symptomatic patients should be evaluated with lymphoscintigraphy and selectively with direct-contrast lymphangiography.
B. These patients are at risk for chylous effusions, such as chylous ascites or chylothorax.
C. These patients most frequently have bilateral lower extremity lymphedema.
D. These patients can have associated protein-losing enteropathy.
E. These patients can be treated successfully with retroperitoneal ligation or sclerotherapy of the dilated incompetent lymph vessels.

Question 169-3

Which of the following statements regarding surgical lymphovenous anastomosis for the treatment of chronic lymphedema is *true*?

A. This operation is now an established surgical procedure.
B. Lymphovenous anastomoses are particularly good for patients with primary lymphedema praecox.
C. This operation can be applied to patients with secondary lymphedema, if conservative measures fail.
D. This operation has documented long-term patency in humans.
E. This operation is best reserved for the late stage of lymphedema.

ANSWERS AND DISCUSSION

■ ANSWERS AND DISCUSSION FOR CHAPTER 165

Answer 165-1: B

Discussion 165-1

A. William Harvey described the arterial and venous circulation but did not recognize the importance of the lymphatic system.

B. The discovery of the lymphatic system is attributed to Gasparo Asellius (or Aselli), a professor of anatomy and surgery at Pavia, Italy. On July 23,1622, he observed the mesenteric lymphatics during vivisection of a well-fed dog. Asellius named the lymphatics *vasa lactea* and recognized their function of absorbing chyle from the intestines.

C. Jean Pecquet, whose name is attached to the receptaculum chyli, first described the exact route of the mesenteric lymphatic drainage to the thoracic duct.

D. William Hunter was one of the first to emphasize that the lymphatic vessels are the absorbing vessels that are similar to the lacteals, and that with the thoracic duct they constitute one system for absorption dispersed through the entire body.

E. The *modern* investigation of lymph formation began with E. Starling, who at the turn of the twentieth century confirmed the relationship between the hydrostatic pressure in the blood capillaries and the oncotic pressure of the plasma proteins (Starling's Law). He suggested that lymph was formed by filtration of the blood through the wall of the capillaries.

Answer 165-2: C

Discussion 165-2

The most frequent local or regional cause of chronic leg swelling in North America is chronic venous insufficiency (C), caused by either primary venous valvular incompetence or previous deep venous thrombosis. In third-world countries, and worldwide, however, secondary lymphedema (B), caused by filariasis, is the most frequent cause. Filariasis, which was eradicated in Europe and North America with public health measures and wide control of mosquito breeding, is caused by the developing and adult forms of three parasites: *Wuchereria bancrofti, Brugia malayi,* and *B. timori*. Of the estimated 90.2 million people in the world who are infected, more than 90% have bancroftian filariasis. The disease is most frequent in subtropical and tropical countries, such as China, India, and Indonesia. In developed countries, however, the most important secondary lymphedema is postmastectomy lymphedema. (A) Primary lymphedema is less common than secondary lymphedema; it occurs in young patients more frequently than secondary lymphedema. (D, E) Of the conditions listed, congenital vascular malformation and acquired arteriovenous fistula are the least frequent causes of leg swelling.

Answer 165-3: B

Discussion 165-3

The report by Milroy in 1892 described lower limb lymphedema in 22 members of the same family over six genera-

tions. In all but two of these patients the edema was present at birth. (B) The term "Milroy's disease," therefore, should be reserved for patients who have primary hereditary lymphedema that was present at birth or noticed soon thereafter. (A) In a collected series of 291 patients with primary lymphedema, 14% had a family history of lymphedema, but only 5% had true Milroy's disease with congenital hereditary lymphedema. (C) Lymphedema praecox includes patients who develop lymphedema between the ages of 1 and 35 years, and the cause of the swelling is congenital hypoplasia, obstruction of the lymphatic system, or acquired obstruction of the lymph-conducting elements of the lymph vessels and lymph nodes. The term "Meige's disease" is reserved for the hereditary form of lymphedema praecox. (D) Patients with lymphangiectasia usually have congenital valvular incompetence and dilated mesenteric and retroperitoneal lymphatics; they frequently have chylous effusion and chylorrhea from vesicles of the skin. (E) The term "Stewart-Traves syndrome" is used for patients who have lymphangiosarcoma in a limb with chronic lymphedema.

■ ANSWERS AND DISCUSSION FOR CHAPTER 166

Answer 166-1: C

Discussion 166-1

Extensive research in both humans and experimental animals has firmly established that contraction of the lymph vessels is the main mechanism by which the lymphatic system propels lymph back to the bloodstream (C). Lymph propulsion originates predominantly from spontaneous intrinsic segmental contractions of larger and probably smaller lymph trunks, and to a much lesser extent from "haphazard" extrinsic forces such as breathing, sighing, yawning, surrounding muscular contractions, and transmitted arterial pulsations (A, B, D, E). Contractions of lymphatic segments between intraluminal valves (i.e., the lymphangions) are highly responsive to lymph volume. Thus, an increase in lymph formation is accompanied by more frequent and powerful lymphangion contractions. Lymphatic truncal contraction, like venous and arterial vasomotion, is mediated by sympathomimetic agents (both alpha- and beta-adrenergic agonists), by-products of arachidonic acid metabolism (thromboxanes and prostaglandins), and even neurogenic pacemaker stimuli. These characteristics of the lymphatics give researchers hope for developing more effective drug therapy for lymphedema in the future.

Answer 166-2: A

Discussion 166-2

The pathophysiology of secondary lymphedema is described in A. In secondary lymphedema, caused by tumor invasion, radiation, excision of lymph nodes, or infection, extensive impairment of lymph drainage is the cause of chronic protein-rich lymphedema. Proximal lymphatic occlusion results in dilation, valvular incompetence, and progressive loss of truncal contractility of the distal lymph vessels. There is usually a long interval between the disruption of the lymph trunks and the development of refractory edema, which helps to explain the unpredictability of limb swelling after radical operations for treatment of cancer and other disorders of defective lymphatic drainage.

Venous occlusive disease (B), or venous valvular incompetence (E), are associated with valve destruction, venous stasis, and eventually overt edema (postthrombotic syndrome) with characteristic tropic skin changes (hyperpigmentation and ulceration). In a similar progression, the absence or obliteration of the lymphatics is associated with lymphatic valve incompetence, lymph stasis, and eventually intractable edema (postlymphangitic syndrome) with its characteristically different trophic skin changes (thickened toe skin folds or Stemmer's sign, warty overgrowth, and brawny induration).

Acute edema caused by cardiac failure responds well to diuretics (C). Patients with critical limb ischemia and rest pain (D) may develop low protein chronic edema from dangling the feet, which improves arterial inflow but impairs venous (and some lymphatic) return (see also Chapter 1 for differential diagnosis of the swollen limb).

Answer 166-3: D

Discussion 166-3

Although both veins and lymphatics transport liquid back to the bloodstream, the flow-pressure dynamics of the two systems are distinctly different. In contrast with venous flow, which receives its circulatory boost from the thrust of the heart and external compression (e.g., calf muscular contraction), lymph flow is regulated by lymphatic truncal contraction and responds to an interstitial fluid challenge with an increase in both contractile frequency and amplitude. The pumping capacity of these lymphatics overcomes high vascular resistance by generating intermittent pressures in excess of 30 mm Hg. In general, however, pressure in the lymphatics is low. Of the options given, D describes their differences most accurately. Temperature, alpha-adrenergic agonists, neurogenic stimuli, hormones, and cytokines, in turn, modify vascular resistance and thereby affect lymphatic flow.

■ ANSWERS AND DISCUSSION FOR CHAPTER 167

Answer 167-1: E

Discussion 167-1

A. Direct-contrast lymphangiography should be used very selectively in patients to diagnose the type and exact site of the lymphatic obstruction. This test, which is invasive and uncomfortable to the patient, has a small but definite rate of complications that include worsening of lymphedema. It is restricted now to the perioperative evaluation of patients with lymphangiectasia or used selectively for some patients who undergo lymphatic reconstructions.

B. Indirect-contrast lymphangiography includes the subepidermal infusion of a water-soluble contrast material (dye). Usually only dermal lymphatics and some distal lymph collectors can be visualized with this technique.

C and D. CT (C) and MRI (D) may be useful to demonstrate underlying lymphangiectasia, chylous effusions, or iliocaval venous obstruction. They are also used frequently to exclude any underlying mass, tumor, or retroperitoneal fibrosis. MRI is excellent to evaluate congenital vascular malformation but *not* very useful to confirm the diagnosis of lymphedema.

E. Radionuclide lymphoscintigraphy, using ^{99m}Technetium-labeled antimony trisulfide colloid or ^{99m}Technetium-labeled human serum albumin, is the test of choice to confirm that edema is lymphatic in origin (E). Semiquantitative evaluation of lymphoscintigraphic images has an excellent sensitivity (92%) and specificity (100%) for the diagnosis of lymphedema.

Answer 167-2: E

Discussion 167-2

A. Lymphedema is nonpitting or only very slightly pitting and involves the ankle and, in most patients, the foot.

B. The edema of the dorsum of the forefoot resembles the "buffalo hump," and it is characteristic of patients with lymphedema. Squaring of the toes (Stemmer's sign) is also a characteristic feature and is caused by the high protein content of the excess tissue fluid.

C. Chronic eczematous dermatitis and excoriation of the skin occur in longstanding lymphedema, as does hyperkeratosis (C) and lichenification *(peau d' orange)*. Frank ulcerations are rare.

D. Yellow nails may occur in patients with primary lymphedema. Yellow nails, clubbing, transverse ridging, friability of the nails, and decreased rate of nail growth are the characteristic features of the yellow nail syndrome.

E. Patients with chronic primary lymphedema characteristically present with *painless swelling* of the limb. Painful lymphedema is almost always associated with *secondary* lymphedema and may reflect associated end-stage malignancy or combined, massive venous, and lymphatic obstruction. Superimposed lymphangitis can be painful.

Answer 167-3: B

Discussion 167-3

A. Cancer such as lymphangiosarcoma occurs, albeit rarely, in patients with long-standing lymphedema. Nevertheless, careful and periodic surveillance of the edematous limb should be performed. Nonhealing "bruises," the development of multiple rounded, purple-red nodules with persistent ulcerations, should alert the physician to the possibility of malignancy. Lymphangiosarcoma after longstanding secondary lymphedema, originally described by Stewart and Treves, frequently results in loss of a limb or even the life of the patient. More commonly, the complications of lymphedema are related to the disfigurement and limitations caused by the disease.

B. Psychologic problems are common in those with lymphedema, especially younger patients, and the physician should address these.

C. In patients with severe lymphedema the physical limitations caused by limb enlargement may significantly interfere with activities of daily living, job performance, and so forth.

D. In general, conservative nonoperative measures are *more effective* and universally applicable than surgical measures.

E. Whereas ulceration frequently occurs in chronic venous insufficiency, it is very unusual in patients with lymphedema.

ANSWERS AND DISCUSSION FOR CHAPTER 168

Answer 168-1: C

Discussion 168-1

Infection (C) is the most common cause of secondary lymphedema because of the high incidence of tropical lymphedema associated with filariasis, caused by *Wuchereria bancrofti* and *B. malayi* in the populated tropical climates. Surgery for cancer resection (A) with subsequent radiation (B) has been reported as a common risk factor for secondary lymphedema in North America. Obesity (E) has recently been reported to be a risk factor in the literature for the development of secondary lymphedema. This is important because of the increasing epidemiologic health issue with markedly increasing rates of obesity in the United States.

Answer 168-2: D

Discussion 168-3

The graduated compression garment (D) is typically not considered part of an *active* edema *reduction* program. A well-fitted garment is the most significant component of the edema *maintenance* program. Compression wrapping by itself (B) or as part of a complex decongestive therapy program (C) are both documented in the literature to be useful in *reducing* lymphedema. There are a variety of programs of edema management and some advocate exercise as primary therapy for edema reduction. However, lymph is produced peripherally in direct proportion to blood flow, so exercise alone might be debated. Nevertheless, a part of a prescribed exercise program is a helpful adjunct. Although the program of complex decongestive therapy has assumed the preferred treatment role in most edema management programs, it should also be recognized that success in edema reduction by use of pneumatic compression devices (A) has been repeatedly substantiated in the literature and that new innovative devices continue to be developed.

Answer 168-3: E

Discussion 168-3

Nutritional factors (E) including dietary restrictions (e.g., low salt, no alcohol consumption, no dairy products) and advocacy for the use of a variety of nutritional supplements have received little documentation in the scientific literature. Scientific, controlled studies are needed. Meticulous skin care (A) and antifilarial drug prophylaxis (B) can assist in reducing secondary infection through the skin, a leading cause of development of secondary lymphedema worldwide and capable of aggravating primary lymphedema. Obesity is now a known risk factor, with rates of secondary lymphedema reported to be less with better weight management (D).

Sentinel node biopsy (C), by avoiding more extensive lymph node dissection, is reported convincingly to be associated with a decreased incidence of *secondary* lymphedema.

ANSWERS AND DISCUSSION FOR CHAPTER 169

Answer 169-1: B

Discussion 169-1

A. Nonoperative management has become the mainstay of treatment of lymphedema and physical therapy, using different forms of a complete decongestive therapy program, and has largely replaced surgical management of these patients. For the *less than 10%* of patients with lymphedema who ultimately require some form of surgical treatment, the likelihood of benefit and satisfaction depends in large part on the indication for surgery.

B. The patient with restricted movement from massive extremity enlargement is most likely to benefit from surgical intervention. *Functional impairment* is the best indication for surgery. Less important are cosmetic results. The aim of surgery is to improve limb function and appearance by improving lymphatic drainage or excising the lymphedematous skin and subcutaneous tissue.

C. Operations for lymphedema can be divided into two major groups: physiologic procedures and excisional procedures. Excisional procedures recognize that lymphedema is limited to the skin and subcutaneous tissue. These operations involve removal of varying amounts of this compartment. The Charles operation is radical, and it should be reserved for those few patients who have extreme lymphedema with severe skin changes. Because of the poor cosmetic results this operation is seldom performed today, although occasional successful cases have been reported. The best results from an excisional operation have been reported by Miller, who popularized the staged subcutaneous excision beneath flaps.

D. Whereas the Thompson procedure is intended to be both excisional and physiologic, the Homans procedure is purely excisional.

E. Baumeister reported several patients with functioning lymphatic grafts many *months* after lymphatic grafting, documented with lymphoscintigraphy. However, documenting *late* patency of lymphovenous anastomoses in humans has been problematic, because only invasive contrast lymphangiography irrefutably proves late patency. The literature therefore lacks evidence of *late* function after microsurgical lymphovenous anastomoses.

Answer 169-2: C

Discussion 169-2

Congenital lymphangiectasia may result in reflux of the chyle, causing lymphedema and chylorrhea (draining chyle through small vesicles of the skin of the lower extremity or perineum).

A. Evaluation should be performed in symptomatic patients with lymphoscintigraphy and, selectively, direct-contrast lymphangiography.

B. Patients with this disorder have dilated, incompetent lymphatics, may have rupture of mesenteric lymphatics, and may present with chylous ascites or (if the thoracic duct or thoracic lymphatics rupture) chylothorax.

C. It is interesting that the lower-extremity lymphedema associated with this syndrome is most frequently *unilateral,* not *bilateral.*

D. The lymphatics in the wall of the bowel may also rupture toward the lumen, and patients may present with protein-losing enteropathy and diarrhea.

E. The so-called antireflux operation involves staged ligation of the dilated retroperitoneal lymphatics; it effectively decreases reflux of lymph. In most cases, even though the lower-extremity lymphatics are ligated, lymphedema of the lower extremity improves because reflux is prevented. The operation is also effective in reducing chylorrhea from skin vesicles. Bilateral retroperitoneal ligation may be required for optimal clinical results. If the lymphatics are large enough, percutaneous CT-guided sclerotherapy of these lymphatics is also possible. Otherwise, intraoperative ligation can be combined with injection of a sclerosing solution (tetracycline) into the lymphatics.

Answer 169-3: C

Discussion 169-3

A. Microsurgical lymphovenous anastomoses have been performed for four decades. The procedure, however, is still not a well-established treatment for lymphedema.

B. Secondary lymphedema, and not primary lymphedema (as in lymphedema praecox), responds to this operation.

C. The operation can be attempted in patients with secondary lymphedema if conservative treatment fails.

D. Although 50% to 80% patency of the anastomoses were documented several months after the operation in animal experiments performed with normal lymph vessels, no objective documentation of long-term patency of these anastomoses exists in humans. Recently, Campisi from Italy reported on the treatment of 665 patients with obstructive lymphedema using microsurgical lymphovenous anastomoses, with *subjective* improvement in 87% of their patients. A total of 446 patients were available for long-term follow-up; the authors observed volume reduction in 69%, and conservative measures were discontinued in 85%. This is a remarkable result but has not been duplicated elsewhere. However, lymph node vein anastomoses *in patients with filariasis* do show clinical benefit.

E. Microsurgical lymphovenous anastomoses should be performed *early* in the course of lymphedema when it can be more effective, because intrinsic contractility of the lymphatics is still maintained and chances of normalization of the lymph circulation are better before significant chronic inflammatory changes in the subcutaneous tissue develop.

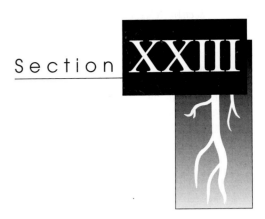
EXTREMITY AMPUTATION FOR VASCULAR DISEASE

STUDY QUESTIONS

■ QUESTIONS FOR CHAPTER 170

Question 170-1

The ratio of below-knee amputation (BKA) to above-knee amputation (AKA) performed worldwide is:

A. 4 to 1 because preserving the knee joint is essential for ambulation.

B. 2 to 1 because a BKA will heal in most patients with peripheral vascular disease.

C. 1 to 1 for primarily systemic and functional reasons.

D. 1 to 4 because most patients with vascular disease are near the end of life and gain no real benefit from preserving the knee joint.

E. 1 to 1 for primarily wound healing reasons.

Question 170-2

Which of the following is *true* regarding the natural history of a dysvascular amputee?

A. The majority of amputees will ambulate after rehabilitation.

B. A high rate of incisional healing makes amputation good palliative therapy for many patients with critical limb ischemia (CLI).

C. Life expectancy is similar regardless of amputation level.

D. There is poor survival (AKA<BKA), with 15% undergoing a contralateral amputation at 2 years.

E. More than 80% of patients who have undergone BKAs and 50% of patients who have undergone AKAs will walk with prosthesis.

Question 170-3

Postoperative pain in amputees:

A. Has both central and peripheral components.

B. Is infrequent once incisions have healed.

C. Is constant in nature.

D. Is quite debilitating for most patients.

E. Is usually manageable with analgesics.

■ QUESTIONS FOR CHAPTER 171

Question 171-1

A 76-year-old man with a history of diabetes mellitus, congestive heart failure (CHF), and end-stage renal disease (ESRD) presents with a 1-month history of gangrene of the left heel that is not painful. On physical examination the patient has a 10-cm eschar over the left heel with minimal surrounding erythema. The patient has a palpable left femoral and popliteal pulse but no left pedal pulses. Doppler signals are weak at the dorsalis pedis and posterior tibial positions, and the ankle-brachial index is falsely elevated because of noncompressible arteries. Transcutaneous oxygen measurements are 8 mm Hg in the forefoot, 10 mm Hg in the hindfoot, and 29 mm Hg below the knee. Foot x-ray film reveals osteomyelitis of the calcaneus. At this point, which of the following is the most appropriate next management step?

A. Left AKA.

B. Left BKA.

C. Foot debridement and long-term intravenous antibiotics.

D. Arteriography and femoral-distal bypass.

E. Further observation under *strict* non–weight-bearing restrictions.

Question 171-2

Which of the following patients with limb-threatening ischemia would have had the most to gain, in terms of limb salvage, from *earlier* referral for evaluation by a vascular surgeon?

A. A 70-year-old woman with toe gangrene and an arteriogram that visualizes no distal arterial bypass targets.

B. A 70-year-old man with a 4-month history of digital gangrene progressing to involve the entire forefoot.

C. A 65-year-old nonambulatory nursing home resident with a deep nonhealing foot ulcer.

D. A 75-year-old man with recurrent rest pain and a history of two leg bypasses.

E. An 80-year-old man with ESRD, difficult-to-manage CHF, and heel gangrene.

Question 171-3

Which of the following is *true* regarding transcutaneous oxygen measurements?

A. A reading of 0 mm Hg indicates no nutrient tissue blood flow.

B. They are very accurate even in the setting of edema and cellulitis.

C. A value of 40 mm Hg at the below-knee level predicts successful healing of a BKA.

D. Successful revascularization produces little change in tcPO$_2$ readings in the first month postoperatively.

E. The degree of intraobserver and interobserver variability makes them unreliable.

■ QUESTIONS FOR CHAPTER 172

Question 172-1

A 69-year-old insulin-dependent diabetic woman presents with gangrene of the right first and second toes, extending onto the medial plantar surface above the base of the affected digits. There is also a deeply necrotic "decubitus" ulcer of the right heel measuring 3 cm in diameter. The right leg is edematous to the knee, and cellulitis extends from the gangrenous digits to the level of the medial malleolus. The patient previously underwent a left femoropopliteal vein bypass that remains patent. Cultures from the heel ulcer grew *Staphylococcus aureus* and mixed coliforms, with antibiotic sensitivities not yet reported.

Which is the *most appropriate definitive* surgical management of this patient?

A. Right BKA under flucloxacillin and gentamicin coverage.

B. Partial right foot amputation with delayed closure of the wound, under penicillin, gentamicin, and flucloxacillin coverage.

C. Guillotine supramalleolar amputation under metronidazole, gentamicin, flucloxacillin coverage.

D. Angiography and subsequent right limb revascularization procedure with concomitant amputation of the gangrenous toes and adjacent necrotic tissue.

E. Right BKA under antibiotic cover with flucloxacillin, metronidazole, and gentamicin.

Question 172-2

A 75-year-old man with a previous right BKA presents with established moist gangrene extending to the bases of the second, third, and fourth digits of the left foot. He has a 3-month history of rest pain. Before that he was mobile, using his right lower limb prosthesis. He lives alone and is self-caring, although he no longer drives. Digital subtraction angiography shows the presence of a left common iliac stenosis and patent left common femoral and profunda femoris arteries. The left superficial femoral artery is occluded beginning at its origin. Visualized distally are a tibioperoneal trunk with a diseased peroneal artery and a good-quality posterior tibial artery that crosses into the foot. The Doppler-derived ankle-brachial pressure index is 0.2 at the left ankle.

What is/are the *most appropriate* surgical procedure(s) for this patient?

A. Left BKA.

B. Left femorodistal bypass graft and amputation of second, third, and fourth digits.

C. Left common iliac angioplasty, femorodistal bypass graft, and amputation of second, third, and fourth digits.

D. Left common iliac angioplasty and left BKA.

E. Left common iliac angioplasty, femorodistal bypass graft, and transmetatarsal amputation.

Question 172-3

A 65-year-old woman who is a smoker presents with dry gangrene affecting the left forefoot to the level of the metatarsal bases. This followed occlusion of the left limb of an aortobifemoral bypass placed 10 years previously for occlusive disease. Angiography confirms that both limbs of the graft are occluded, and that the native common iliac vessels are not visible, but diseased external and internal iliac arteries are seen. Diseased right common and profunda femoral arteries are visualized as being in continuity with the right external iliac artery, but no recognizable arteries are seen below this level. In the left groin only collateral arteries are identified, and no named vessels are visualized throughout the left lower extremity. The patient has a history of multiple myocardial infarctions and CHF, and has a cardiac ejection fraction of 20. There is dry gangrene of the left foot and fixed flexion deformities of 60 degrees at the right knee and 20 degrees at the right hip.

With respect to this patient's *left* leg, the *most appropriate* management is:

A. Axillobifemoral grafting and left BKA.

B. Left hindquarter amputation.

C. Left AKA.

D. Axillobifemoral grafting and left through-knee amputation.

E. Redo aortic bifurcation grafting and left BKA.

■ QUESTIONS FOR CHAPTER 173

Question 173-1

Which of the following subgroups has/have an increased operative mortality after major lower extremity amputation?

A. Those with ESRD.

B. Those with acute limb ischemia.

C. Those with sepsis.

D. Those with multiple bypass failures.

E. All of the above.

Question 173-2

Deep venous thrombosis (DVT) in amputees:

A. Is rarely observed because of the common associated use of anticoagulants.

B. Is seldom suspected because of the lack of edema resulting from the reduced arterial inflow to the stump.

C. Has an incidence of 50%, with one in five leading to pulmonary embolism.

D. Its incidence justifies routine prophylaxis and/or close surveillance.

E. Is uncommon enough that prophylactic high ligation of the superficial femoral vein has been abandoned.

Question 173-3

Depression in amputees:

A. Leads to a major depressive disorder in more than one third of amputees.
B. Is situational, but temporary, and usually resolves with stump healing and prosthesis fitting.
C. Leads to overeating and obesity.
D. Affects the patient, not the amputation outcome per se.
E. Is not life threatening.

■ QUESTIONS FOR CHAPTER 174

Question 174-1

In general, healing in surviving patients after major amputation is *best* described by which of the following statements?

A. Most BKAs heal primarily and are ready for prosthetic use in 6 weeks.
B. All AKAs heal primarily in 6 weeks, and 50% of BKAs heal primarily.
C. Sixty to seventy percent of BKAs heal primarily; half of the remainder will heal with wound care, and the other half will require conversion to AKA level.
D. With correct preoperative testing, all BKAs should heal.
E. One third of BKAs heal primarily, one third heal secondarily, and one third fail and require AKA.

Question 174-2

Which of the following *best* describes long-term survival after BKA and AKA?

A. They are similar, because both groups have CLI and the amputation level predicts function but not survival.
B. Survival is much worse for patients undergoing AKA because this population has more significant comorbidity.
C. It is worse for patients who have undergone BKA, because many of them require conversion to AKA over time, with additional mortality.
D. Long-term survival in amputees is worse in patients who undergo BKA but do not use a fitted prosthesis.
E. Because amputation eliminates the life-threatening limb necrosis, survival is no different in patients who have undergone AKA or BKA.

Question 174-3

Ambulation after BKA performed for vascular indications is *best* described by which of the following?

A. Up to 90% within 1 year.
B. Approximately 80% within 1 year, with decline after that.
C. Approximately 60% are referred for prosthesis, and most ambulate to some extent at 1 year.
D. Approximately 40% ambulation at 1 year because of wound problems and delayed fitting of prosthesis.
E. Approximately 40% ambulation at 1 year because of phantom and residual stump pain and contralateral amputations.

■ QUESTIONS FOR CHAPTER 175

Question 175-1

A 47-year-old electrician has pain and stiffness of the amputation stump 1 year after sustaining a crush amputation of the dominant left index finger at the level of the proximal interphalangeal joint. At the time of the injury, primary closure was performed in the emergency department.

Which of the following is the *most appropriate* management now?

A. Injection of formaldehyde into the amputation stump.
B. Desensitization of the stump with iontophoresis.
C. Repair/excision of digital nerve neuromas.
D. Revision amputation to the level of the metacarpophalangeal (MCP) joint.
E. Ray amputation of the injured digit.

Question 175-2

A 32-year-old student sustains a sharp amputation of the volar pad of the nondominant index finger. Which of the following is the *most appropriate* management of the defect?

A. Dressing changes.
B. Cross-finger flap.
C. Moberg advancement flap.
D. Neurovascular island flap.
E. Thenar flap.

Question 175-3

A 29-year-old laborer sustains an *incomplete* amputation of the dominant index finger at the level of the distal third of the proximal phalanx while working with a band saw. Examination shows minimal damage to the soft tissues. There are no other injuries. The patient desires maximum strength and function in the hand and wants to return to work as soon as possible. Surgical exploration shows division of all structures, including the neurovascular bundles. A skin bridge on the ulnar side of the finger is intact.

Which of the following is the *most appropriate* initial management?

A. Amputation of the digit at the level of the injury and primary closure.
B. Amputation of the digit at the level of the injury and toe-to-hand transfer.
C. Ray amputation.
D. Disarticulation of the digit at the MCP joint.
E. Replantation of the digit.

■ QUESTIONS FOR CHAPTER 176

Question 176-1

A failed infrainguinal bypass can adversely affect the outcome of a subsequent amputation by which one of the following?

A. Increasing the incidence of an AKA.
B. Increasing the wound complications and amputation healing time.
C. Increasing the perioperative mortality risk for the subsequent amputation.

D. Reducing the muscle mass in the amputated limb.
E. Increasing the risk of infection of the thrombosed bypass graft in the amputated limb, with increased morbidity but without significant increased mortality.

Question 176-2

Infrainguinal bypass for CLI in patients with ESRD is characterized by which of the following?

A. Similar perioperative mortality rates compared with all patients with CLI.
B. Similar long-term survival compared with all patients with CLI.
C. Reduced bypass incision and pedal wound healing.

D. Reduced autogenous conduit available for bypass.
E. The policy to perform infrainguinal bypass in patients with ESRD, despite increased risks, is supported by acceptable limb salvage rates in most reported series.

Question 176-3

Which of the following risk factors for poor outcome in patients with CLI undergoing revascularization has the best chance of significant modification in the future?

A. ESRD.
B. Lack of autogenous conduit.
C. Premature atherosclerosis.
D. Extent of pedal necrosis before operation.
E. Advanced age.

ANSWERS AND DISCUSSION

■ ANSWERS AND DISCUSSION FOR CHAPTER 170

Answer 170-1: C

Discussion 170-1

The ratio of AKA to BKA worldwide is 1 to 1 and has not changed in the last decade. The reasons are more often (C) systemic and functional than related to healing potential (E). Primary healing rates with AKA are far superior to BKA (contrary to answer B) in most series. However, prosthetic limb ambulation is only achieved by a limited portion of patients with CLI because of balance problems and the cardiovascular load of ambulating with a prosthesis. Patients are often at the end of life and gain little benefit from preserving the knee joint, but the ratio is not 1:4, but 1:1. (D) The knee joint is *not essential* for ambulation, but it certainly helps; nevertheless, the ratio is not 4:1, but 1:1 (A).

Answer 170-2: D

Discussion 170-2

A. Available data indicate that a decided minority of dysfunctional ever ambulate. The number of patients who have undergone BKAs and are ambulating is reported to be as low as 50% and as high as 80% and AKAs do much worse. Therefore, even optimistic reports indicate that less than half of vascular amputees ever ambulate.

B. Incisional healing after amputation is slow over time, with up to 15% of patients after BKA requiring reoperation and/or revision to AKA.

C. Survival after amputation is dismal and much worse for patients after AKA. However, this is because of the poor medical status of many patients having AKA, rather than a result of the operation.

D. In addition to poor survival, worse for AKA than BKA, because of the systemic nature of atherosclerotic arterial occlusive disease, 15% will undergo a near-term contralateral amputation. Thus, D is the only correct answer.

E. Few patients with AKAs ever ambulate with a prosthesis. The number of patients who have undergone a BKA and are ambulating is reported to be as low as 50% and as high as 80%, so the estimate in E is far too optimistic.

Answer 170-3: A

Discussion 170-3

A. Postamputation pain (phantom and residual limb pain) has both central and peripheral pain mechanisms. These include ectopic activity originating from afferent fibers in a neuroma and cortical reorganization/spinal cord sensitization. This answer is correct.

B. In surveys of amputees, more than 70% report some level of postoperative pain, and it typically does *not* subside with incision healing.

C. For the majority, it is episodic, not constant.

D. The pain is often mildly troublesome, but in one of four (not most) it is severe.

E. Current medical therapies and modern analgesics are commonly ineffective.

■ ANSWERS AND DISCUSSION FOR CHAPTER 171

Answer 171-1: B

Discussion 171-1

A and B. Both patient and surgeon alike want to preserve as much of the limb as possible when amputation is necessary. The presence of a palpable popliteal pulse and a TCO_2 level greater than 20 mm Hg below the knee indicate that this patient has adequate circulation to heal a BKA.

C. Foot debridement and long-term antibiotic administration might be indicated if the patient had good circulation, but they would not help here.

D. Patients with ESRD and large foot lesions with tissue necrosis rarely get significant benefit from heroic attempts at limb salvage by revascularization procedures. Far more morbidity, and even mortality, results from futile attempts at limb salvage and multiple failed procedures in this particular subgroup (diabetes with ESRD) than from primary amputation.

E. Non–weight-bearing restrictions are important in healing foot lesions in diabetic patients with neuropathy, but this heel necrosis is also associated with both osteomyelitis and chronic critical ischemia, based on transcutaneous oxygen levels.

Answer 171-2: B

Discussion 171-2

In CLI the risk factor that has the greatest potential for future modification to improve limb salvage is *delay in referral*. Available data indicate that patients with CLI and nonhealing foot lesions usually have had symptoms for weeks and months before referral to a vascular specialist. The majority of this time has been under the care of a health care provider, and improved education of these providers presumably would lead to earlier referral before pedal necrosis progresses to the point of an unsalvageable limb regardless of revascularization.

Having said this, certain subgroups are least likely to benefit from prompt referral leading to attempts at arterial reconstruction and may well benefit from primary amputation. These include (A) patients with unreconstructable arterial anatomy (although this must be based on good vascular imaging), (C) nonambulatory patients, especially those with other problems that mandate nursing home care, (D) patients with repeated bypass failures, and (E) patients with ESRD, especially those manifesting other comorbidities, such as intractable CHF. On the other hand, the patient in B, with none of the preceding problems, might have had limb salvage surgery if referred to a vascular surgeon earlier, when the ischemic lesions were limited to the toes. By definition, limb salvage, more aptly foot salvage, requires preservation of sufficient foot anatomy to allow independent ambulation. High forefoot or Syme's amputations do not qualify for this standard definition.

Answer 171-3: C
Discussion 171-3

Transcutaneous oxygen levels have been shown to have an accuracy of 87% to 100% in predicting wound healing. The sensors can be placed anywhere on the body, and readings are given in millimeters of mercury. Absolute readings may be recorded, or readings in areas may be indexed to a reference site (often the chest). The probes are small and atraumatic, and multiple simultaneous sites can be tested depending on the equipment used. The readings in the supine position are more predictive than measurements in the dependent position or during supplemental oxygen breathing.

A. In general, transcutaneous partial pressure of oxygen (tcPO$_2$) readings of greater than 40 mm Hg are associated with healing and those less than 20 mm Hg are associated with failure. The lack of a consistent minimum level is most likely because some nutrient blood flow may be present even in the setting of tcPO$_2$ readings of 0 mm Hg.
B. The tcPO$_2$ may be artificially low in the setting of infection, inflammation, or edema, and repeat measurements are advised once such processes have resolved.
C. The tcPO$_2$ has shown not only to accurately predict wound healing but also to accurately predict amputation level healing. A BKA should heal if the tcPO2 is 40 mm Hg at that level.
D. In predicting outcome after revascularization, increases in tcPO$_2$ of greater than 30 mm Hg are predictive of a successful outcome, and this can be detected shortly (within days) after the procedure.
E. The values recorded are reliable and show an acceptable day-to-day variability in repeat measurements. The degree of intraobserver and interobserver variability is reasonable, and thus variability does *not* make it an unreliable test.

■ ANSWERS AND DISCUSSION FOR CHAPTER 172

Answer 172-1: E
Discussion 172-1

The extent of this patient's tissue loss on the plantar aspect of the foot, coupled with evidence of spreading sepsis extending to the level of the ankle joint, and a large infected, necrotic ulcer of the heel, preclude successful limb (foot) salvage.

A. BKA is appropriate, but this is not the right antibiotic coverage (see E).
B. Open amputation of the toes with delayed closure might suffice if there was no heel decubitus and no sepsis progressing proximally. It would be inadequate here, even with proper antibiotic coverage.
C. Guillotine amputation at the level of the ankle joint would be an acceptable temporizing (*not definitive*) measure, allowing the edema and inflammation to subside before the definitive BKA, which would then be carried out distant from any actively infected tissue.
D. In a diabetic patient such as this, it is mandatory to remove all necrotic and actively infected tissue to prevent life-threatening sepsis. This would leave a foot with little

functional value and little prospect of successful salvage with a vascular reconstruction, if it were deemed otherwise appropriate. However, the bypass is patent, and the tissue loss in this diabetic patient is likely independent of underlying ischemia.
E. BKA can be successfully undertaken as the *definitive* procedure here. The use of loose skin-apposing sutures and a rigid stump dressing should minimize the effects of the tissue edema on stump healing. In this answer, as opposed to A, the perioperative antibiotics chosen do appropriately cover the *Staphylococcus aureus* species and coliforms already cultured, as well as the anaerobic clostridial species commonly associated with necrotic tissue, particularly in diabetic patients.

Answer 172-2: E
Discussion 172-2

Because the patient is a self-caring unilateral amputee, independence and aggressive treatment aimed at preserving this patient's remaining limb are appropriate. The extent of tissue loss does not preclude this, and successful revascularization combined with an appropriate amputation offers a reasonable prospect of functional limb salvage.

A. Therefore, left BKA is not appropriate.
B and C. Although a femorodistal bypass graft and toe amputations may suffice, correction of more proximal occlusive disease offers improved long-term patency, and any proximal disease should be treated before, or at the same time as, the femorodistal bypass. However, the level of amputation in these two answers is not appropriate (see E).
D. Iliac angioplasty without femoral distal bypass and BKA give up the opportunity of limb salvage and will rob this patient of his self-care independence.
E. Amputation of the necrotic digits should be undertaken at the same time because of the presence of wet gangrene, and because the loss of the second, third, and fourth toes will leave isolated toes at the medial and lateral aspects of the foot, a transmetatarsal amputation is preferred, providing a more functional foot and offering the likelihood of primary wound closure. The presence of a good-quality distal vessel crossing in continuity with the pedal vessels optimizes the prospect of such an amputation healing successfully. Thus, proximal and distal revascularizations, and this amputation level, constitute the best combination of procedures.

Answer 172-3: C
Discussion 172-3

In the absence of any recognizable arteries in the left groin, successful revascularization is unlikely, and the prospect of healing a BKA is remote. There is, however, the possibility of any open surgical procedures (even axillofemoral bypass under local anaesthetic, answers A and D) to improve arterial inflow into the right leg, which may ensure survival of this limb. However, the severe and fixed flexion deformities of the *contralateral* limb ensure that this patient will almost certainly remain wheelchair-bound after any major limb amputation.

Therefore, in the presence of such poor inflow, the most appropriate option is to amputate at a level that is most likely to heal and that remains compatible with the patient's predicted postoperative functional capacity. Healing at the above-knee level (C) can be expected on the basis of the angiogram findings and would be preferable to (B) a primary hindquarter amputation. The patient's cardiac status makes (E) redo aortic surgery unrealistic, and the low ejection fraction is likely to compromise the long-term patency of an extra-anatomical reconstruction (A and D). Thus, C is the correct answer.

■ ANSWERS AND DISCUSSION FOR CHAPTER 173

Answer 173-1: E

Discussion 173-1

Overall perioperative mortality for major lower extremity amputation is 5% to 10% for BKA and 10% to 15% for AKA. However, perioperative mortality for amputation in patients with (A) ESRD, (B) acute limb ischemia, and/or (C) sepsis is often double that, being higher for AKA. Physiologic amputation (tourniquet isolation and freezing the leg in dry ice) and two-stage amputation (lower guillotine followed by proximal formal amputation) have been used by many to reduce the high perioperative mortality rate in septic patients. Those with (D) multiple bypass failures have not only a much lower success with additional bypass attempts but also a higher associated mortality with amputation. The underlying reasons are multifactorial, but the patients' associated comorbidities and the physiologic insult that accompany the amputation play major roles. Most often, amputations under these conditions are carried out at the AKA level. All of the above are true, so E is the correct answer.

Answer 173-2: D

Discussion 173-2

A. The incidence of perioperative DVT in amputees is 12% to 15%, and anticoagulants are *not* routinely used.
B. Inflow must be adequate to allow stump healing. Postoperative DVT is a well documented complication, and can cause severe swelling.
C. The incidence of DVT is well less than 50% (see A), and the incidence of fatal pulmonary embolus in amputees ranges from 1% to 3%. Therefore, C is a gross exaggeration and wrong.
D. Nevertheless, routine DVT prophylaxis and/or careful perioperative screening for DVT with duplex scanning in amputees is prudent and justified on the basis of the associate rates of DVT and PE. This answer is correct.
E. In the days when high ligation of the superficial femoral vein was practiced as prophylaxis against PE, its use in AKA was almost routine. Tying off that slow-flowing column of blood is *still* practiced.

Answer 173-3: A

Discussion 173-3

A. Depression is a common problem in amputees, with one series demonstrating 35% of patients harboring a major depressive disorder, so A is correct.

B. Associated depression may seem a natural response to limb loss, but assuming that the patient will get over it is a mistake. Even positive outcomes, such as successful healing and prosthesis fitting, do not guarantee spontaneous resolution.
C. To the contrary, amputees with depression do not overeat and gain weight, but most often are malnourished, with weight loss, poor albumin, and lack of interest in their environment as predominate signs.
D. Depressed amputees will often have decubitus ulcers and contractures from apathy and inactivity. These affect ambulation with prostheses.
E. In addition to depression complicating care and increasing morbidity, suicide attempts have been reported.

■ ANSWERS AND DISCUSSION FOR CHAPTER 174

Answer 174-1: C

Discussion 174-1

Despite a tremendous amount of research to determine whether an amputation will heal at the below-knee level, a percentage of BKAs will fail primary healing and require either additional wound care to achieve healing or conversion to the AKA level. The actual percentage of BKAs that heal primarily varies from series to series, but answer C best expresses the outcome, "Sixty to seventy percent of BKAs heal primarily; half of the remainder ($\frac{1}{6}$) will heal with wound care, and the other half ($\frac{1}{6}$) will require conversion to AKA level." The cause of failure to heal is multifactorial, including circulation issues, postoperative trauma from falls, and so forth. Unfortunately, this leads to a tremendous amount of morbidity and waste of health care resources. (A) Although the majority of BKAs heal primarily, the majority are not ready for prosthetic fitting by 6 weeks. (B) *Not all* AKAs heal primarily in 6 weeks, and *more than* 50% of BKAs heal primarily. (D) Although correct preoperative testing will increase the healing rate of BKAs, it will not reach 100%. (E) One-third rules are nice to remember, but this one is wrong!

Answer 174-2: B

Discussion 174-2

Worldwide, the ratio of BKA/AKAs performed is approximately one, with many patients undergoing AKA because it is considered the best palliative procedure in a population so functionally impaired because of severe comorbidity that they are not considered prosthetic candidates. Therefore, (B) is correct. Perioperative mortality and long-term survival in large series of major amputees *are* worse for patients who have undergone AKAs compared with patients who have undergone BKAs, who are considered to benefit functionally from salvage of the knee joint. Patient survivals in the Veterans Affairs amputation series for BKA and AKA were 57% and 39% at 3 years, respectively. Survivals in A and E were said to be similar, but for different reasons, and both are wrong. Survival in patients who have undergone BKAs is not worse because of (C) conversion to AKA, nor has it been shown to be worse in patients with BKAs just because (D) they do not use their prosthesis (although theoretically it could be worse if death or worsening of associated comorbidities prevented them from using their prosthesis).

Answer 174-3: C

Discussion 174-3

The energy expenditure for ambulation with a below-knee prosthesis is substantial, and many vascular amputees are unable to manage the increase in oxygen consumption because of cardiovascular issues. This problem is even great in those with AKAs. In addition, balance and proprioception are important factors in bipedal ambulation with a prosthesis, and many diabetic patients with vascular disease lack this. A number of adverse clinical events (contralateral ischemia and cardiovascular events) work to reduce the number of ambulating amputees during follow-up. Finally, in the United States, readily available wheelchair access (Americans with Disabilities Act) acts as a disincentive to many older patients who struggle with the physical demands of rehabilitation to bipedal gait with a prosthesis. Answer C best describes the current ambulation outlook for BKAs. Answers A and B conceivably might be achievable in the future but are too optimistic, and D and E are too pessimistic. Although most amputees have some phantom and residual stump pain, for most of them the pain is not debilitating and does not prevent ambulation with a prosthesis.

■ ANSWERS AND DISCUSSION FOR CHAPTER 175

Answer 175-1: E

Discussion 175-1

In this patient, who has functional impairment of the dominant left index finger after trauma, the most appropriate management is (E) a Ray amputation. Amputation is often the procedure of choice in patients who have functional impairment or disability of one digit after trauma. This patient has stiffness and pain in the index finger remnant after sustaining a crush amputation at the level of the proximal interphalangeal joint. In addition, the stump is not functional and actually interferes with hand usage. Ray amputation will relieve this patient's symptoms and remove the amputation stump, thus resulting in unhindered hand function; the middle finger will perform the functions of the index finger during hand use. The other options, (A) injection of formaldehyde into the amputation stump, (B) desensitization of the stump with iontophoresis, (C) attempted repair/excision of digital nerve neuromas, and (D) revision/amputation at the MCP joint, would not appropriately address this patient's problem.

Answer 175-2: A

Discussion 175-2

A. This patient has a small ($<10 \times 10$ mm) defect of the volar tip of the nondominant index finger, without exposed bone, tendon, or nerve. Dressing changes are effective in the management of this type of injury and will prevent the need for additional surgery and a secondary donor site. This is the most appropriate treatment.
B. A cross-finger flap is appropriate for amputations of the finger with exposed bone, tendon, or nerve, but *not* here.

This flap can be lifted from the dorsal aspect of a healthy finger and transferred to cover the palmar aspect of the affected finger.
C. In patients who have palmar oblique amputations of the thumb, the Moberg advancement flap can be used to preserve as much length as possible. However, the flap cannot be advanced more than 2 cm. Contractures of the interphalangeal joint may occur.
D. A neurovascular island flap is typically transferred from the *ulnar side of the ring or long finger* to cover amputations involving the thumb. Complications with venous congestion are not uncommonly associated.
E. Thenar flaps are used for amputations involving the tip of the index or long finger to provide adequate soft-tissue padding over exposed bone and to preserve as much length as possible. Neither of the latter two are problems here. Stiffness of the proximal interphalangeal joint and painful donor site scarring are frequent postoperative problems with this approach.

Answer 175-3: A

Discussion 175-3

This patient has a single digit injury in Zone II; two tendons are located within the flexor tendon sheath. (A) The most appropriate initial management in this patient is amputation at the level of injury and primary closure. Although (E) replantation is feasible in a patient with minimal soft-tissue damage, it will result in greater loss of function than an amputation. Recent studies have compared replantation of a single digit with amputation and found significant differences between the two procedures. Replantation was associated with increased treatment and therapy and a longer period of inactivity. In patients who had single-digit amputations, approximately 90% rated their hand function as good or excellent; only 44% of the replantations were similarly rated. Amputation at the level of injury will salvage as much viable tissue as possible. The index finger stump should be preserved because it may be needed for key pinch. Flexion of the remaining digit will be accomplished through the intrinsic muscles. (B) A toe-to-hand transfer is rarely performed at the time of initial injury. (C) Ray amputation should be performed as a delayed procedure and should only be considered in a patient with severe functional impairment that renders the digit useless. This procedure has been shown to result in diminished power grip, key pinch, and supination strength. (E) Disarticulation of the digit at the level of the MCP joint will result in a shortened digit that interferes with key pinch and thumb opposability.

■ ANSWERS AND DISCUSSION FOR CHAPTER 176

Answer 176-1: B

Discussion 176-1

A. A number of published reports have demonstrated that a failed infrainguinal bypass does *not* adversely affect the level of subsequent amputation (BKA vs. AKA).
B. However, a failed infrainguinal bypass increases the healing time for the subsequent BKA, increases the num-

ber of secondary procedures required to achieve healing, and by default increases the global perioperative mortality rate in the compromised population with CLI.

C. However, the perioperative mortality of a subsequent amputation is *not* increased.

D. The failed bypass does *not* reduce the muscle mass in the subsequently amputated limb.

E. Because of the problematic nature of amputation incisional healing after failed infrainguinal bypass, the potential for prosthetic graft infection is increased. This results in a significant increase in morbidity *and mortality*.

Answer 176-2: C

Discussion 176-2

Infrainguinal bypass for CLI in the population with ESRD has received mixed reviews in the vascular surgery literature in the past, but these answers reflect current views.

A. Perioperative mortality rates are greater, 5% to 10%, compared with 2% to 3% in patients with non-ESRD CLI undergoing infrainguinal bypass in modern series.

B. Long-term survival is 50% or less at 2 to 3 years, compared with 50% at 5 years for populations with non-ESRD CLI.

C. Postoperatively, wound healing is definitely poorer, and this applies to the bypass incisions and areas of tissue loss and ulceration, particularly on the foot. Factors in addition to bypass success are also at play.

D. The problem is *not* inadequate autogenous graft availability, even though use of arm veins can be expected to be compromised because of hemodialysis access. In

fact, a higher rate of use of autologous vein is driven by the condition of distal target arteries.

E. On the basis of reported series, with significant length of follow-up, the majority of vascular surgeons now consider these greater risks to be prohibitive and only perform infrainguinal bypass *very selectively* on the best-risk patients with ESRD. Those who consider the risk acceptable and remain uniformly aggressive regarding limb salvage attempts in these compromised patients are not practicing evidence-based medicine.

Answer 176-3: D

Discussion 176-3

Of the risk factors listed, (D) the extent of pedal necrosis on presentation to vascular surgery offers the best chance for modification through improved education of other health care providers, especially primary care physicians and podiatrists. Available data indicate that most patients with CLI and pedal necrosis have had symptoms for weeks and months, and are rarely under the care of a vascular specialist. Therefore, the portion of severe pedal lesions that complicate or preclude limb salvage could be reduced and converted to potential salvageable pedal lesions, with better education leading to a timelier referral.

Age (E) and (A) the prevalence of ESRD are not likely to decrease, nor is (B) the availability of autogenous conduits likely to increase. Atherosclerosis is likely to be better controlled in the future, but reducing the *incidence* of premature atherosclerosis will require massive screening programs and very early institution of, and compliance with, lipid abnormality, and other risk factor-controlling measures.